S0-DUW-397

# The Behavioral Effects of Drugs

DOUGLAS W. MATHESON
*University of the Pacific*
*Stockton, California*

MEREDITH A. DAVISON
*Medical Center*
*The University of Oklahoma*
*Oklahoma City*

HOLT, RINEHART AND WINSTON, INC.
*New York Chicago San Francisco Atlanta*
*Dallas Montreal Toronto London Sydney*

Library of Congress Catalog Card Number: 70-186960
**ISBN: 0-03-085307-9**
Printed in the United States of America
4 5 090 9 8 7 6 5 4 3 2

# Preface

Drug abuse is only one problem currently facing the people of the world, and it is not a new one. Presently, the drug problem has hit the "straight" generation hard. There is an abundance of misinformation proliferating among both young and old, a problem that the present book is intended to reduce. Although we do not cover all the drugs being misused, we do include discussion of most of the popular categories, with special emphasis on the drugs most used by young people.

The purpose of this text is to familiarize the reader with the behavioral effects of drugs and the behavior of drug users. We have attempted in the present collection to blend material written for the layman with some cold hard facts in the form of data for the professional. The book was prepared with the student in mind and can be used as a textbook or a reference book for students of psychology, sociology, medicine, nursing, law, and any other area where people are interested in behavior. In addition, many of the articles included are appropriate for high school students, for example, the first article, "About Drugs," and the second article by Farber, entitled "Ours Is the Addicted Society." Parents can also profit from reading this textbook.

Each chapter is preceded by a very brief introduction of the articles that it includes. Chapter 1 consists of a general introduction to drugs. The articles blend both theoretical and philosophical notions about drug use and, in some cases, drug abuse. Chapter 2 follows with several articles on popular social drugs such as alcohol and marihuana and clarifies some of the misconceptions about the use of both. Chapter 3 covers the psychotropic drugs, the uppers and downers. Here, drugs such as amphetamines and barbiturates are discussed, and a comparison is drawn between the behavioral effects of amphetamines and LSD. Chapter 4 is concerned with the hallucinogens, such as LSD and mescaline. Finally, Chapter 5 gives a brief introduction to the problem of heroin addiction and its treatment. Specifically, methadone therapy is discussed. Also included are two articles on the use of behavior modification with heroin addicts.

We wish to thank all of the contributing authors and publishers for allowing their articles to be reprinted here. In addition, we wish to thank Debby Doty, Psychology Editor, and Barbara Gibbons, both of Holt, Rinehart and Winston, Crystal Henderson, and Gwenda Nylen for their help in preparing the manuscript. Finally, we would like to thank the students at the University of the Pacific who classroom-tested most of the readings in this book.

*Stockton, California*
*Oklahoma City, Oklahoma*
*January 1972*

Douglas W. Matheson
Meredith A. Davison

# Contents

# 1
# Introduction

The first section is a general introduction to the most commonly used drugs and their general effects. To be sure, drugs have had an enormous effect on the lives of most people in the United States. The discovery and development of many drugs have helped us to live longer, healthier, and fuller lives. No one can deny that antibiotics have helped most of us at one time or another, or that the Salk and Sabin discoveries have saved thousands of lives and prevented many hardships. It is also true that drug therapy (primarily tranquilizers) has been invaluable in the treatment of behavior problems such as schizophrenia. On the other hand, the abuse of drugs has rendered many in our midst helpless, hapless, and, in many cases, addicted either psychologically or physically, and their addiction in turn forces these people into situations at odds with the rules of our society. As you read the articles in this book, ponder the following question: Are drugs a problem in themselves, or are they a symptom of other problems?

The first article, "About Drugs," was prepared by a group at the University of Michigan to acquaint the reader with the most commonly abused drugs. The paper was written for students and presents information about drugs in a very lucid fashion. It provides an excellent introduction to the collection.

The second article, "Ours is the Addicted Society," is both philosophical in its orientation and frightening in its implications. The article portrays our society as being "hooked" as a result of advertising. The author may not be too far from the truth.

The third article, "Drugs and the Law," briefly describes some of the legal aspects of drug use. The final article by Kuehn provides an interesting psychoanalytic approach to counseling the college student drug user. Parents as well as students should profit from Kuehn's article.

# 1

# *About Drugs*

OFFICE OF ORIENTATION,
UNIVERSITY OF MARYLAND

Thousands of drugs and chemicals are capable of altering an individual's perceptions and behavior. Often, students are fascinated by the described experiences and second-hand recountings of others involving the use of many of these drugs. This abstract of factual information about drugs and their effects should make it possible to be informed on the subject and to discuss it without appealing to the common misconceptions, incorrect information, and emotional attitudes that usually pervade discussions of this interesting topic.

## BACKGROUND INFORMATION

### Variables Influencing Drug Effects

Generalizations about the effects of any drug on human beings are not easy to make. Many different variables increase the complexity and difficulty that is encountered in attempting to make generalized statements.

A few of these variables can be described as follows:

1. Any drug, whether aspirin or opium, has a "no effect" dose and a lethal dose with a multitude of effects in between for any individual.
2. A single dose may have different effects than those produced by chronic repetitive administration of a drug.
3. Very few people are similar to the "average" person. People vary a great deal physically as well as psychologically.
4. Society is not the same for all Americans but is composed of many hundreds of subcultures with differences in ethical, religious, and social characteristics. These subcultures or reference groups influence the behavior of any individual to the degree he accepts their values and attitudes as being "correct" for him. These values and attitudes tend to become his standard for making decisions about correct behavior.

### Dependence

Several terms, such as drug addiction or drug habituation, have been used to describe the extreme results of repeated use of many drugs. To eliminate the confusion and overlap between these terms, the World Health Organization suggests the more general term "drug dependence." Drug dependence may result from repeated administration of any drug on a periodic or continual basis. This dependence may be psychological, physical, or both psychological and physical depending on the drug.

Individuals may become dependent upon a wide variety of chemical substances that produce central nervous system effects ranging from stimulation to depression. All of these drugs have one effect in common, that is, creating a particular state of mind that is termed "psychological dependence." In this situation, the individual learns to interpret his reactions to the drug as pleasurable and satisfying. Thus the individual requires periodic or continuous use of the drug to regain or maintain this feeling of pleasure and satisfaction. To some, the drug offers a means of escape from physical and emotional stress. These drug-induced mental states are the most powerful of all the factors involved in the chronic use of many drugs. Even in cases of intense craving and compulsive use, psychological dependence may be the only factor involved with certain types of drugs.

Some drugs also induce physical dependence. This is a state of adjustment by the individual's body to the drug. This change becomes apparent when repetitive administrations of the drug are suspended and the individual manifests a series of physical disturbances. The disturbances (withdrawal or abstinence syndrome) are composed of specific patterns of psychological and physical symptoms that are characteristic of each drug type. The withdrawal syndrome is relieved by re-administering the same drug or another drug of similar pharmacological action. A casual observer can not usually determine if an individual is physically dependent as long as adequate doses are maintained. Physical dependence is a powerful factor in continuing the use of a drug and reinforces the influence of psychological dependence.

Psychological dependence can and does develop without any evidence of physical dependence. This means that withdrawal of the drug can take place without physical symptoms developing. Also, physical dependence can be induced without notable psychological dependence. Indeed, physical dependence is an inevitable result of the pharmacological action of some drugs taken in sufficient amounts and with short time periods between administrations (e.g., morphine for pain of widespread cancer).

Many of the drugs that induce dependence, especially those that create physical dependence, also induce tolerance. Tolerance is a state of physical adjustment characterized by diminished responses to the same amount of drug or by the requirement of a larger dose to reproduce the same degree of either physical or psychological effects.

## Abuse

An individual abuses the use of any drug when he becomes either psychologically or physically dependent on the drug resulting in harm either to himself or to society.

A look at the abuses of psychoactive drugs in the United States reveals the following picture: from any point of view, alcohol constitutes the major drug problem today. Approximately 4 percent of the estimated 125–150 million users of alcohol abuse the drug to become individual or social problems. These five or six million alcoholics constitute about 3 percent of the total population.

Also there is an unknown number of emotionally disturbed people who become dependent upon a wide variety of other drugs such as heroin, barbiturates, pep pills, marijuana, etc. Assuming that the abuse of these psychoactive drugs involves 2 percent of the population, the total number of people dependent on drugs as a means of solving personality difficulties or just reliving an intensely pleasurable experience may be as high as four million people. Thus when considering both alcohol and these other drugs, nine or ten million people may be dependent on either one or several drugs. This is about 5 percent of the total population.

Most harm to the individual arises from preoccupation with drug-taking. Personal neglect (i.e., lethargy, malnutrition, and infection) is frequently a consequence. Some drugs, such as the barbiturates, result in impairment of mental functioning, with confusion, poor judgment, loss of emotional control, and occasionally coma and death. Sometimes drugs produce feelings of increased capability which do not stand up to reality testing.

Harm to society is chiefly related to the preoccupation of the individual in obtaining and taking the drugs. He may become an unproductive member of society. His interpersonal relationships can be disrupted and he may attempt to withdraw from the world around him. Often there is economic loss due to the individual's inabilities to maintain a job. Further there can result a proneness to accidents.

The Joint American Medical Association and American Bar Association Narcotic Committee deplores the hysteria which sometimes dominates the approach of persons in positions of public trust to problems of drug abuse. In terms of numbers affected, and in negative effects on others in the community, drug abuse is a problem of far less magnitude than alcoholism. Crimes of violence are rarely, and sexual crimes are almost never, committed by users of certain drugs. In most instances, the abuser's sins are a result of being an ineffective person whose great desire is to withdraw from the world and its everyday frustrations. Of course, where large sums of money are needed to support a habit, the drug-dependent person may turn to illegal activities to obtain money or drugs.

If it were practical by legal or other means to limit the individual intake of any drug so that physical or psychological dependence did not occur, no drug would be abused. This is difficult, if not impossible, to do, even for one individual. There exists a range of reactions to any drug, from no effect at all to the development of psychological and/or physical dependence. It is a rare possibility that an individual will be psychologically dependent on the first administration of a drug. Many individuals will not be adversely affected by their initial drug experience but may become dependent on the drug on subsequent administrations. Anyone who is actively seeking to experiment with a drug is going to find it and try it. He should be aware of the difficulty in predicting his reaction to the drug and that there exists no way for him to determine if he is becoming psychologically dependent on it until he is in fact dependent.

## DRUG GROUPS SUBJECT TO ABUSE

### I. Narcotics (Narcotic Analgesics)

Narcotics are drugs which cause depression of the central nervous system. They generally produce sleep and relief of pain, but in excessive doses may produce stupor, coma, or even death. Included in this group of drugs are opium and its derivatives (e.g., morphine, heroin, codeine, paregoric, dilaudid, metopon, patopon, and laudanum) and synthetic morphine substitutes (e.g., meperidine and methadone). Because they can induce marked degrees of dependence, both psychological and physical, and thus have a high potential for abuse, the manufacture, distribution, and use of narcotic drugs is stringently regulated by Federal and state laws. (Although marijuana and cocaine have been classified as narcotics under narcotic laws, they will not be discussed in this section on narcotic drugs but will be examined separately in later sections.)

### *Medical Uses*

Narcotic drugs are very effective in relieving almost any type of pain. They are especially valuable in treating short-term, severe pain caused by trauma, burns, and certain diseases. These drugs are also used to relieve pain in patients suffering from long-term diseases such as cancer, although repeated use leads to tolerance which makes the drugs progressively less effective. They alter the psychological reaction associated with the perception of pain and induce lethargy or sleep. The physician who prescribes narcotic drugs for a patient for a long period of time must balance the beneficial, pain-killing effects of the drug against the possibility of establishing physical dependence.

Some narcotic drugs in small dosages are also used for the suppression of cough (codeine) and for the control of diarrhea (paregoric).

### *Psychological and Physiological Effects*

The appeal of narcotic drugs to the user lies in their ability to reduce sensitivity to both psychological and physical stimuli. The user feels better because he does not experience physical pain or psychological pain such as fear, tension, anxiety, or guilt feelings. While under the influence of narcotic drugs, the user may experience a sense of exhilaration or well-being. The rapid intravenous injection of narcotics, especially heroin, produces an intensely pleasurable sensation localized primarily in the abdomen (pseudo-orgasm). The sensation is short-lived, but experienced users seek to repeat it as often as possible. The frequency is limited only by the supply of drugs and by the accumulation of its depressant effects.

Continued use of narcotic drugs leads to tolerance, the need for ever-increasing doses to produce the desired effect, and psychological and physical dependence. In the early stages of drug administration, the addict's breathing and body temperature are decreased. His eyes become reddened, his pupils pinpointed, and his eyelids droop. He may suddenly become very active physically and then become drowsy and inactive and may drift back to sleep, suddenly awaken, and then drift back to sleep and to dreaming. His aggressive impulses and sexual interests are usually decreased by the drug.

As the user becomes more dependent, his pupils remain constricted and he becomes constipated. Although he becomes tolerant to the drug's effects, he can always take a dose large enough to produce respiratory depression, coma, and death.

### *Withdrawal*

With morphine, the abstinence syndrome appears within a few hours of the last dose, reaches peak intensity in 24 to 48 hours, and subsides spontaneously. The most severe symptoms usually disappear within a few days. The time of onset, peak intensity, and duration of abstinence phenomena vary with the degree of dependence on the drug and with the characteristics of the specific agent involved. Administration of a specific antagonist, such as nalorphine or levallorphan, during continuing administration of morphine-like drugs promptly precipitates the immediate onset of an intense abstinence syndrome.

The unique feature of the morphine abstinence syndrome is that it represents changes in all major areas of nervous activity, including alteration in behavior and excitation of both divisions of the autonomic nervous system. Symptoms and signs include anxiety, restlessness, generalized body aches, insomnia, yawning, lacrimation (tearing), rhinorrhea (runny nose), perspiration, mydriasis (dilated pupils), piloerection (goose flesh), hot flushes, nausea, vomiting, diarrhea, elevation of body temperature or respiratory rate, and of systolic blood pressure, abdominal and other muscle cramps, dehydration, anorexia, and loss of body weight (Isbell and White, 1953). Withdrawal from narcotics is seldom life-threatening unless the person has other diseases which are aggravated by the stress of withdrawal, e.g., heart trouble. It is now possible for the physician skilled in the use of drugs to minimize the discomfort associated with withdrawal from narcotic drugs.

### *Special Note about Heroin*

Heroin is a semisynthetic substance made from morphine found in the opium poppy. It is no more effective from the medical point of view than any other analgesic; therefore it is not used for medical purposes, not legitimately manufactured, and not legitimately available in this country. Heroin is illegally imported raw, then diluted by the wholesaler, usually by adding milk sugar and quinine. It may be diluted again by the dealer, so the final strength, composition, and purity of "street heroin" is unknown.

Its properties are the same as for the entire group of drugs discussed in this section. Heroin has always been used by the despairing, oppressed, and miserable, many of whom live in urban ghettos, not so much to obtain a "high" as to numb their abject misery. More recently, the use of heroin has spread to all parts of society as a part of the general increase in the use of illicit drugs. There now is an increasing demand and enlarging potential market for the drug. A proportion of those who try heroin will try again, and will become dependent—thus establishing an even greater demand for a highly profitable drug.

Unlike some drugs, heroin is a big business of organized crime; profits are enormous, with $35 worth of crude opium eventually being marketed for $40,000 on the street in a many-times-diluted form.

## II. Barbiturates

Like the narcotic analgesics, barbiturates are drugs which exert a calming or depressing action upon the central nervous system. All of the barbiturates are synthetics derived from barbituric acid and are available in solution, capsule, or tablet form. Legally, they can be obtained only with a doctor's prescription.

There are three general classifications of barbiturate drugs: the long-acting, slow starters such as phenobarbital; the intermediates such as amobarbital (amytal) and butabarbital (butisol); and the short-acting fast starters such as secobarbital (seconal) and pentobarbital (nembutal).

### *Medical Uses*

Because of their depressant action on the central nervous system, barbiturates have numerous medical uses. The most important of these is to produce sleep. Due to the large number of barbiturate drugs available, the physician can choose from short-acting, intermediate-acting, and long-acting barbiturates, depending on the patient's symptoms.

Barbiturates, in small doses, are also used frequently for their sedative or calming effect. This effect is particularly valuable in treating nervous tension and high blood pressure.

Certain barbiturates are used to prevent or minimize convulsive episodes in epileptic patients. They are also used in combination with other drugs (e.g., to increase the soporific effects of pain-killing drugs, to decrease the stimulant effects of amphetamines).

When properly prescribed and taken as directed, barbiturates have no lasting adverse effect upon the patient.

### *Psychological and Physiological Effects*

If barbiturates are carelessly used, they may lead to psychological and physical dependence. A large, single overdose may lead to death because barbiturates are capable of depressing the brain's respiratory center to the point where breathing ceases. Because persons under the influence of barbiturates are befuddled, lose their sense of time, and are incapable of logical thought, accidental overdoses are common. Unlike alcohol, which has a sort of built-in safety mechanism that requires a person to remain sober enough to continue to drink, barbiturates may be taken in large doses all at once. That is, many capsules may be swallowed before the full effect is experienced. This is a result of the slow absorption of the drug from stomach and intestine and is often the underlying cause of many inaccurately labeled suicides.

Use of barbiturate drugs in excessive amounts produces confusion, slurring of speech, staggering and falling due to interference with balance mechanisms, difficulty in thinking, defective judgment, quick temper, and a quarrelsome disposition. The superficial signs of excessive barbiturate use are quite similar to the classic stages of alcohol intoxication: first relaxation and increased sociability, then gloominess and irritability, followed by staggering, incoherence, and a lapse into deep sleep and then coma and marked respiratory depression.

One would expect that the mechanism of physical dependence involving barbiturates would be set in motion by the first dose, but there is no evidence that this is the case. There is, indeed, no evidence that physical dependence develops to a detectable degree with continuation of the therapeutic doses for the production of sedation or hypnosis. The daily dose must be increased appreciably above the usual therapeutic level and intoxication must be maintained continuously before abstinence signs will appear on abrupt withdrawal. Some degree of psychological dependence facilitating continued administration may occur with therapeutic doses, but low doses of the depressants can usually be discontinued without serious psychological disturbance. Factors that may lead to increasing consumption and eventual overt physical dependence include, in addition to tolerance, gaining a pleasurable feeling, incomplete relief of emotional problems and tension, and impairment of judgment, so that larger doses are taken without regard to need. The degree of tolerance that can develop to depressants is much less than that seen with narcotic analgesics (e.g., heroin). Thus, it is relatively easy for the person to take a lethal overdose of the depressants.

### *Withdrawal*

The abstinence syndrome is the most characteristic and distinguishing feature of drug dependence on barbiturates. It begins to appear within the first 24 hours after the last dose, reaches peak intensity in two or three days, and subsides slowly. At present there is no agent which is known to precipitate the barbiturate abstinence syndrome during continuation of drug administration. The complex of symptoms constituting the abstinence syndrome, in approximate order of appearance, includes: anxiety, involuntary twitching of muscles, tremor of hands and fingers, progressive weakness, dizziness, distortion in visual perception, nausea, vomiting, insomnia, with weight loss due to dehydration, a precipitous drop in blood pressure on standing, convulsions, and delirium. Generally, a patient may have one or two convulsions during the first 48 hours of withdrawal, and then may become psychotic during the succeeding 24 to 48 hours. With respect to the psychotic episodes, paranoid reactions, reactions resembling schizophrenia with delusions and hallucinations, withdrawn semistuporous state, and disorganized panic have been seen.

Unlike the situation with narcotics, withdrawal of depressant drugs from a person physically dependent on them is always a serious, life-threatening ordeal. It requires a skillful, experienced physician to minimize the risks of convulsions and death.

## III. Other Sedatives

There are numerous drugs of a chemical structure different from that of the barbiturates but able to produce very similar effects to those of the barbiturates (e.g., librium, equanil or miltown, chloral hydrate). Also the similarity extends to the medical uses, psychological and physiological effects, and withdrawal symptoms of barbiturates.

A distinction should be made between the above noted barbiturate-like sedatives and the specific group of drugs referred to as tranquilizers (e.g., thorazine, compazine, reserpine). Although tranquilizers produce calmness, sedation, etc., as do the barbiturates, they also produce numerous undesirable side effects, especially as the dosage is increased. These side effects are almost never interpreted by the user as pleasurable so that psychological dependence seldom results. It is generally agreed that the tranquilizers do not cause physical dependence and have little potential for abuse.

## IV. Stimulants

Drugs in this group stimulate the central nervous system causing wakefulness, excitation, alertness, some increased physical activity, a temporary rise in blood pressure and respiration and, in moderate doses, euphoria. The amphetamines, benzedrine and dexedrine for example, are the best-known and most widely used of the stimulant drugs. However, phenmetrazine, benzphetamine, diethylpropion, mephentermine, pipradrol, ephedrine, and methylphenidate are also included in this group as is the strong stimulant, cocaine.

### *Medical Uses*

The only legitimate medical use of cocaine is to produce local anesthesia, and even for this purpose there are many synthetic drugs which are equally as effective and which do not possess the dependence-inducing potential of cocaine. Amphetamines and other stimulant drugs have few legitimate medical uses although they are widely used and misused in current medical practice. Because they often improve mood disturbances, these drugs have been used for many years by physicians in treating mild forms of mental depression. They are used effectively in treating certain relatively rare diseases of the nervous system such as narcolepsy, a disease characterized by an almost overwhelming compulsion for sleep. These drugs are used to counteract the excessive depressant effects of large doses of antiepileptic and other types of depressant drugs. Although it appears to be paradoxical, the amphetamines, which are stimulants, have been used effectively in calming the exaggerated behavior of hyperkinetic children.

Physicians frequently prescribe stimulant drugs, especially the amphetamines, for patients who are overweight. These drugs appear to facilitate dieting by exerting an effect on the appetite center in the brain, and also, by improving the patient's mood, lessen his psychological dependence on food. However, even with continued daily administration, the appetite-suppressing effects disappear within a few weeks. Some physicians and patients have been unaware of this tolerance to the anorexic effects of amphetamines and have continued to use the drug for prolonged periods. Not infrequently, marked psychological dependence on these drugs has been a consequence of such medical misuse.

### *Psychological and Physiological Effects*

Because of their very nature, stimulant drugs tend to produce a feeling of alertness in tired people and an elevation of mood in depressed people. Unfortunately, this ability to make tired people feel alert and depressed people feel "alive" seems to have a special appeal to some people and is the major factor underlying the abuse of these drugs.

Dependence on stimulant drugs can occur without the awareness of the user. Someone might use one of the drugs to increase his capacity for work. As he develops a dependence on and tolerance to the drug, he may increase the dosage. The individual who is using one of these drugs under a physician's supervision may pay no attention to his doctor's direction and use larger amounts than prescribed. He, too, is likely to develop a psychological dependence on the drug.

Still other cases of stimulant drug abuse arise among college students looking for "pleasurable experiences" or those who use the drugs for increased performance for athletic events, to stay awake while studying for exams or the like. Here again, continued use results in dependence on the drug for a "normal" feeling and a need to use increasing amounts to produce the desired effect.

Amphetamines and other stimulant drugs may increase alertness and efficiency for a short time, but this effect is often followed by headache, dizziness, agitation, irritability, decreased ability to concentrate, and marked fatigue. The most important fact in considering the use of stimulant drugs is that excessive, unsupervised use interferes with the body's normal protective symptoms of drowsiness and fatigue. The feeling of exhaustion is short-circuited, causing a person to use up reserves of body energy until a sudden and total collapse may occur.

The stimulant drug user, taking large doses, is usually active and excited and the pupils of his eyes are dilated. He may have bad breath and have gone for long periods of time without sleep and with little food. Daily use in excessive amounts can cause tremor, insomnia, mental confusion, assaultiveness, panic, and convulsions. Hallucinations, both visual and auditory, and other signs and symptoms of psychoses can occur. Especially frequent are the appearance of paranoid delusions and panic states. These symptoms usually disappear upon dosage reduction or upon withdrawal of the drug.

Like the narcotic "mainliner," the stimulant abuser derives a unique, intensely pleasurable sensation (pseudo-orgasm) from rapid injection of the drug intravenously. It is with repeated intravenous use of large doses that the more serious side effects (hallucinations, psychoses, convulsions) are most frequently experienced. Indeed, the intravenous route is employed by some for the express purpose of obtaining bizarre mental effects, often associated with sexual functions, even to the point of orgasm.

More generally, the symptoms of stimulant drug abuse are milder than those mentioned above. They include excitability, talkativeness, restlessness, irritability, tremor of hands, enlarged pupils, sleeplessness, and profuse perspiration.

A unique feature of the amphetamines is their capacity to induce tolerance, a quality possessed by few central nervous system stimulants. (Repeated use of cocaine does not produce tolerance to its effects.) Although tolerance develops slowly, a progressive increase in dosage permits the eventual ingestion of amounts that are several hundred fold greater than the original therapeutic dose. Apparently, all parts of the central nervous system do not become tolerant at the same rate, so that the user will continue to experience increased nervousness and insomnia as the dose is increased. Although an individual may survive the oral administration of very large quantities, such ingestion may produce profound behavioral changes that are often psychological in nature, such as hallucinations, delusions, etc. As noted above, the latter effects are much more likely to occur after intravenous injections than after ingestion.

### *Withdrawal*

Although the amphetamines do not induce physical dependence, as measured by the criterion of a characteristic and reproducible abstinence syndrome, the withdrawal of the stimulant drug leaves the individual in a state of chronic fatigue and the need for sleep. Thus, the withdrawal period is characteristically a state of depression, both psychological and physical, which probably reinforces the drive to resume the drug. Although stimulant withdrawal does not compare in the magnitude of its physical effects with that seen during withdrawal from morphine, barbiturates, alcohol, and other drugs that create physical dependence, withdrawal of drugs of the amphetamine type can nevertheless be serious. The withdrawal of stimulants may lead to profound psychological depression even to the point of suicidal intent. Obviously such persons require proper psychological therapy.

## V. Hallucinogens

Hallucinogens are drugs which have the ability to produce hallucinations. They may also be known by other names such as psychedelics (mind-manifesters) and consciousness expanders. Included in this group of drugs are lysergic acid diethylamide (LSD-25), mescaline, peyote, psilocybin, and various forms of the *cannabis* plant, discussed in Section VI. In large doses, the hallucinogens produce a temporary psychological state which is similar in many respects to schizophrenia or psychoses—a separation from reality. Hence, these drugs are also called psychotomimetics.

### *Medical Uses*

Some of these drugs (e.g., LSD) may be useful in treating certain types of mental disorders and in treating alcoholism, but there is not yet enough evidence to substantiate this. Legally, the hallucinogens are available only for bona fide experimental purposes and not for routine medical practice or for personal use.

### *Psychological and Physiological Effects*

The drugs are taken for thrills, to partake in an intensely pleasurable feeling, to change and clarify perception, and to obtain "psychological insight" into the personality problems of the user. Generally, the drugs are taken orally and in the company of other users. Ingestion of a single dose or of several doses over a period of two or three days is the customary pattern; prolonged or continuous use is unusual. Periodic, rather than continuous, use is favored by difficulty in obtaining the drugs, rapid development and disappearance of tolerance, and a lack of physical dependence on these drugs.

Drugs of the LSD type induce a state of excitation of the central nervous system and central autonomic hyperactivity manifested by changes in mood (usually euphoric, sometimes depressive), anxiety, distortion in sensory perception (chiefly visual), visual hallucinations, delusions, depersonalization, dilation of the pupils, and increases in body temperature and blood pressure. There may be nausea, chills, as well as flushes, irregular breathing, sweating of the hands, and trembling of the extremities. Sleep is virtually impossible until the drug experience is over. The major physical dangers related to the hallucinogenic experience are physical and emotional trauma resulting from impulsive acts (e.g., leaping from a window) and from panic reactions.

A high degree of tolerance to LSD (Isbell, et al., 1956) and to psilocybin (Wolbach, Isbell, and Miner, 1962) develops rapidly and disappears rapidly. Tolerance to mescaline develops more slowly. People who are tolerant to any of these three drugs are cross tolerant to the other two (Wolbach, Isbell, and Miner, 1962).

There is increasing concern about the mental and physical side effects of the hallucinogens, especially with regard to their long-term effects. Mental side effects include the acute panic reaction during the drug experience, a prolonged continuing psychotic state, and the periodic recurrences ("flashbacks") of the drug experience without taking the drug. It is still not certain that these drugs induce brain damage, although a number of users and physicians report apparently permanent changes in the behavior of persons who have used one or more of these drugs repeatedly. The occurrence of mental side effects is unpredictable; they have been observed with the first dose as well as with the next dose following many previous pleasurable drug experiences. Serious mental side effects are most frequently encountered by emotionally disturbed persons.

Much less is known about the long-term physical effects of the hallucinogens. To date there is no concrete evidence that use of these drugs leads to the production of defective offspring in humans. But concern is raised by observations of the occurrence of abnormal chromosomes in the blood cells of humans taking LSD (or a variety of other drugs) and by studies in animals of the incidence of fetal resorption and birth defects following the administration of LSD. As is often true in the early phases of experimentation, the relevance of studies of animals to the human situation remains to be evaluated. However, society is generally advised to take a cautious or conservative approach in such situations, especially when the benefits of drug usage remain uncertain.

### *Withdrawal*

No evidence of physical dependence can be detected when the drugs are withdrawn abruptly.

## VI. Marijuana

Marijuana comes from the dried flowering tops of the hemp plant *cannabis sativa*. This plant grows as a weed throughout most of the world and can be grown in all parts of the United States. The most potent plants are grown in a hot, moist climate such as is found in India. The most potent forms of *cannabis* contain the greatest quantities of tetrahydrocannabinol, one of the pharmacologically active substances in the *cannabis* plant. Although marijuana is classified as a narcotic under federal laws, it is different from the narcotic drugs in that it does not create physical dependence and it is not a potent analgesic.

### *Medical Uses*

The drug is not used currently in medical practice, and the growth, distribution, or sale of it in the United States is illegal.

### *Psychological and Physiological Effects*

Among the more prominent of marijuana-induced psychological effects for which it is taken occasionally, periodically, or chronically, are: hilarity, often without apparent motivation; carelessness; feelings of happiness and satisfaction with increased sociability as a result; distortion of sensation and perception, especially of space and time. The intensity of the effects produced by marijuana are dependent on the dosage taken, and large doses can cause impairment of judgment and memory; distortion of emotional responsiveness; irritability; and confusion. Other effects which appear especially after repeated administration and as more experience is acquired by the user include: lowering of the sensory threshold, especially for optical and acoustical stimuli, thereby resulting in an intensified appreciation of works of art, paintings, and music; hallucinations, illusions, and delusions often of a paranoid type which may predispose to aggressive and antisocial behavior; anxiety as a result of the various intellectual and sensory derangements; and sleep disturbances.

Whereas marijuana often attracts the mentally unstable and may precipitate temporary psychoses and lead to changes in behavior patterns in predisposed individuals, no unequivocal evidence is available that lasting mental changes are produced.

In the psychomotor sphere, increased motor activity occurs without obvious impairment of coordination. The effects of marijuana intoxication on driving skills remains to be determined, but distortions of time and space sense suggest that it may be unsafe to operate complex machinery under the influence of marijuana. Among somatic effects are injection of conjunctival vessels (red eyes), oropharyngitis (sore throat), and bronchitis. These conditions are symptoms of intoxication and exposure to irritants in marijuana smoke. Not infrequently, there is an increase in appetite and sleepiness following the use of marijuana. No long-term physical effects have been demonstrated to result from the use of the drug.

### *Withdrawal*

Typically, the abuse of marijuana is periodic, but, even during long and continuous administration, no evidence of the development of physical dependence can be detected. That is, no characteristic abstinence syndrome appears when use of the drug is discontinued.

Whether administration of the drug is periodic or continuous, tolerance to its psychological and psychomotor effects has not been demonstrated in humans.

Frequently repeated use of the drug in this country and in others (e.g., Africa, India), has demonstrated that psychological dependence can occur to marijuana as well as to the stronger forms of the *cannabis* plant.

## VII. Alcohol

Abuse of alcohol may be said to occur when the consumption of alcohol by an individual exceeds the limits that are accepted by his culture, when he consumes alcohol at times that are deemed inappropriate within that culture, or when his intake of alcohol becomes so great as to injure his health or impair his social relationships. Since the use of alcoholic beverages is a normal, or almost normal, part of the cultures of many countries, dependence on alcohol is usually apparent as an exaggeration of culturally accepted drinking patterns, and the manifestations of dependence vary according to the cultural mode of alcohol use. Thus, in the United States, alcohol is frequently taken in concentrated forms for brief periods as an aid to social intercourse. Dependence on alcohol in the United States is usually characterized by heavy consumption of strong spirits, by a tendency to drink regularly or continuously throughout the day, and by overt drunkenness. In some countries, on the other hand, alcohol is customarily consumed as wine, usually with meals. In these countries, dependence on alcohol is characterized by the drinking of wine throughout the day often with relatively little overt drunkenness. A similar pattern applies where beer is the common beverage.

### *Medical Uses*

Alcohol is used as an antiseptic and is sometimes prescribed as a sedative or appetite stimulant. If nothing else is available, alcohol may be used as an analgesic.

### *Psychological and Physiological Effects*

Psychological dependence on alcohol occurs in all degrees. In the mildest grade, alcohol is missed or desired if not available at meals or at social functions. A moderate degree of psychic dependence exists when the individual feels compelled to drink in order to work or to participate socially and takes steps to ensure a supply of alcohol for these purposes. Strong dependence is present if the individual uses alcohol in amounts far exceeding the cultural norm, drinks in situations that culturally do not call for drinking, or is obsessed with maintaining a supply of alcohol even to the extent of drinking unusual or poisonous mixtures.

As with other drugs, psychic dependence on alcohol results from an interplay between the pharmacodynamic effects of the drug and the personality problems of the user. The consciously verbalized reasons for the use of alcohol cover a wide gamut and may include a need to stimulate the appetite, to alleviate anxiety or fatigue, to remove boredom, or to induce sleep. For some people, alcohol provides a temporary escape from a hostile, threatening world, or it releases them from their mental and moral inhibitions and allows them to express their aggressive impulses toward that world.

Tolerance to alcohol does develop. During continuous drinking there is a slight but definite increase in the amount of ingested alcohol required to maintain a given blood level. In addition, physiological and psychological adaptation occurs so that the alcoholic appears less intoxicated and is less impaired in performance tests at a given alcohol concentration in the blood than is a nonalcoholic. But, as is true for other depressant drugs, the person tolerant to alcohol can still ingest a lethal dose.

There is no question that long-term, continuous use of alcohol is associated with detrimental physical and mental changes, some of which are permanent. Some of the changes may be related to the poor nutritional and health practices followed by the alcoholic. The detrimental effects include low resistance to infectious disease, cirrhosis of the liver, and a variety of neurological and mental syndromes. There is a very definite association of alcohol intoxication with serious detrimental effects on society, such as accidental injury and death, property damage, absence from work and school, and disruption of family life.

### *Withdrawal*

Physical dependence on alcohol definitely occurs and the abstinence syndrome resulting when the intake of alcohol is reduced below a critical level is manifested by tremors, sweating, nausea, tachycardia, rise in temperature, hyperreflexia, postural hypotension, and, in severe grades, convulsions and delirium. The last mentioned condition is characterized by confusion, disorientation, delusions, and vivid visual hallucinations. The symptoms of alcohol withdrawal are very similar to those seen after barbiturate withdrawal. The intensity of alcohol abstinence syndrome probably varies with the duration and amount of alcohol intake, but as yet little quantitative information on this point is available. The mortality rate, when the alcohol abstinence syndrome is severe, averages at least 8 percent.

## GLOSSARY OF DRUG SLANG[1]

This glossary is incomplete and probably out of date. The use of slang or jargon is to enable the "in-group" to communicate without the "uninitiated" being able to understand what is meant. When a street term or slang word becomes clear to the uninitiated and falls into common usage, another term will take its place. For a more complete listing and a more extensive discussion of terms, see the book *Drugs from A to Z: A Dictionary*, by R. R. Lingeman, McGraw-Hill, 1969.

acid—chemical hallucinogen drug (e.g., LSD)

bad trip—undesirable physical and psychological reactions to drug use
beans—amphetamine pills, benzedrine
benny, bennies—amphetamine, benzedrine
blue cheer—hallucinogen drug (e.g., LSD)
bluebirds—amobarbital (Amytal), a barbiturate
boo—marijuana
boot—drawing blood out of, then putting it back into a vein to get the last bit of drug from syringe
booze—alcoholic beverage
bummer—undesirable drug experience; a bad trip
busted—arrested

cap—capsule or dose of LSD
chipping—injection, but not intravenous.
coke—cocaine
copping—obtaining drugs
crank—homemade methamphetamine
crashing—undesirable after-effects of stimulant drug (e.g., headache, dizziness, marked fatigue, decreased ability to concentrate); withdrawal symptoms; profound psychological depression
crystal—a type of methamphetamine

dex—dexedrine
downer—a barbiturate
drop—oral intake of drugs, usually a chemical hallucinogen

feno—phenobarbital
flash, flashback—recurrence of drug influence without having taken the drug
freak—one who uses drugs
freaked-out—undesirable drug experience; a bad trip

girl—cocaine
goofballs—amphetamine tablets
grass—marijuana

"H"—heroin
hard stuff—a narcotic analgesic (e.g., opium and derivatives)
hash—hashish; loosely, marijuana
head—one who uses drugs
high—under the influence of a drug; intoxicated
holding—having drugs in your possession
horse—heroin

"J"—marijuana cigarette; a joint
joint—marijuana

[1] From *Drugs from A to Z: A Dictionary* by R. R. Lingeman. Copyright 1969 McGraw-Hill Book Company. Used with permission of McGraw-Hill Book Company.

jones—heroin
junk—a narcotic analgesic (e.g., opium and derivatives)
junk works—homemade equipment for injecting drugs
key, kilo—kilogram, or 2.2 pounds, usually in reference to heroin or marijuana
lid—a little less than an ounce of marijuana
lucy—LSD
mainliner—one who uses intravenous injections
mainlining—intravenous injection, usually rapid
mary jane—marijuana
mesk—mescaline
munchies—increased appetite, as during marijuana intoxication
nark—narcotics agent; policeman
O.D.—overdose of drugs; death from overdose
oding—showing symptoms of an overdose of drugs
ope—opium
pacifier—homemade equipment for injecting drugs
pheno—phenobarbital
pot—marijuana
pot-head—marijuana user
purple owsley—chemical hallucinogen (LSD)
purple-white dome—type of chemical hallucinogen
rainbows—mixture of amobarbital and secobarbital (tuinal); both are barbiturates
red devils, reds—secobarbital (Seconal), a barbiturate
reefer—marijuana cigarette
roach—butt of a marijuana cigarette
rushing—quick sensation, high or low
scag—heroin
scag boy—cocaine
shooting up—injecting drugs with a syringe
shotgun—equipment for injections
skinpopping—injection, but not intravenous
slider—barbiturate
smack—heroin
speed—a stimulant drug (e.g., amphetamine)
speedball—mixture of cocaine and heroin
spike—needle for syringe
spoon—about 1/16th of an ounce of heroin
spoonful—a narcotic analgesic (e.g., heroin)
stash—drugs on hand
stoned—intoxicated, as on alcohol, marijuana, or other drugs
strawberry flats—chemical hallucinogen (LSD)
street heroin—heroin cut with quinine and milk sugar, usually 3 to 11 per cent heroin content
stuff—marijuana
strung out—symptoms of stimulant drugs (e.g., excitability, talkativeness, irritability, enlarged pupils, sleeplessness)
sunshine—chemical hallucinogen (LSD)
supercharging—particular method of smoking marijuana
tea—marijuana
toke—puff of a marijuana cigarette
tracks—skin marks left by injections
trip—drug experience; under the influence of a drug; intoxicated
uppers—stimulant drugs (e.g., amphetamines)
tips—stimulant drugs (e.g., amphetamines)
weed—marijuana
white orange—type of chemical hallucinogen
white owsley—type of chemical hallucinogen
wired—daily use of stimulant drugs
works—equipment for injecting drugs
yellow flats—type of chemical hallucinogen
yellow jackets—pentobarbital (Nembutal), a barbiturate
yellow wedges—type of chemical hallucinogen

## REFERENCES

BELLEVILLE, R. E., and FRASER, H. F., "Tolerance to Some Effects of Barbiturates," *Journal of Pharmacology and Experimental Therapeutics*, 1957, Vol. 120, p. 469

COHEN, S., "Lysergic Acid Diethylamide: Side Effects and Complications," *Journal of Nervous and Mental Disease*, 1960, Vol. 30, pp. 30–40.

DEPARTMENT OF JUSTICE, COMMONWEALTH OF PENNSYLVANIA, OFFICE OF THE ATTORNEY GENERAL, "A Guide for High School and College Officials in Dealing with the Use and Abuse of Drugs by Students," 1966.

DEPARTMENT OF MENTAL HEALTH OF THE AMERICAN MEDICAL ASSOCIATION, "Narcotics Addiction," 1963.

EDDY, N. B., HALBACH, H., ISBELL, H., and SEEVERS, M. H., "Drug Dependence: Its Significance and Characteristics," *Bulletin of World Health Organization*, 1965, Vol. 32, pp. 721–733.

FOOD AND DRUG ADMINISTRATION, UNITED STATES DEPARTMENT OF HEALTH, EDUCATION, AND WELFARE, "Fact Sheets 1–7," 1967.

ISBELL, H., and WHITE, W. M., "Clinical Characteristics of Addictions," *American Journal of Medicine*, 1953, Vol. 14, p. 558.

ISBELL, H., ATTSCHUL, S., KORNETSKY, C. H., EISENMAN, A. J., FLANASY, H. G., and FRASER, H. F., "Chronic Barbiturate Intoxication," *Archives of Neurology and Psychiatry*, 1950, Vol. 64, No. 1.

ISBELL, H., BELLEVILLE, R. E., FRASER, H. F., WILKER, A., and LOGAN, C. R., "Studies on Lysergic Acid Diethylamide (LSD-25)," *Archives of Neurology and Psychiatry*, 1956.

SEEVERS, M. H., "Marijuana in Perspective," *Michigan Quarterly Review*, 1966, Vol. 5, No. 4.

WOLBACH, A. B., Jr., ISBELL, H., and MINER, E. J., "Cross Tolerance between Mescaline and LSD-25 with a Comparison of the Mescaline and LSD Reactions," *Psychopharmacologia*, 1962, Vol. 3, No. 1.

WHO EXPERT COMMITTEE ON ADDICTION-PRODUCING DRUGS, "Thirteenth Report," *World Health Organization Technical Report Series*, 1964, Vol. 273, No. 9.

# 2

## *Ours Is the Addicted Society*

LESLIE H. FARBER

This has been called the "Age of Anxiety." Considering the attention given the subject by psychology, theology, literature, and the pharmaceutical industry, not to

From *The New York Times Magazine*, December 11, 1966. 

mention the testimony from our own lives, we could fairly well conclude that there is more anxiety today, and, moreover, that there is definitely more anxiety about anxiety now than there has been in previous epochs of history. Nevertheless, I would hesitate to characterize this as an "Age of Anxiety," just as I would be loath to call this an "Age of Affluence," "Coronary Disease," "Mental Health," "Dieting," "Conformity," or "Sexual Freedom," my reason being that none of these labels, whatever fact or truth they may involve, goes to the heart of the matter.

Much as I dislike this game of labels, my preference would be to call this the "Age of the Disordered Will." It takes only a glance to see a few of the myriad varieties of willing what cannot be willed that enslave us: We will to sleep, will to read fast, will to have simultaneous orgasm, will to be creative and spontaneous, will to enjoy our old age, and, most urgently, will to will.

If anxiety is more prominent in our time, such anxiety is the product of our particular modern disability of will. To this disability, rather than to anxiety, I would attribute the ever-increasing dependence on drugs affecting all levels of our society. While drugs do offer relief from anxiety, their more important task is to offer the illusion of healing the split between the will and its refractory object. The resulting feeling of wholeness may not be a responsible one, but at least within that wholeness—no matter how perverse the drugged state may appear to an outsider—there seems to be, briefly and subjectively, a responsible and vigorous will. This is the reason, I believe, that the addictive possibilities of our age are so enormous.

Let me be more specific about the addictive consequence of this disability of will which, in varying degree, affects us all. Increasingly, I believe we are addicted to addiction. This is to say that, with few exceptions, we subscribe to the premise—whether implicit or explicit—that this life cannot be lived without drugs. And those who would repudiate this unpleasant premise by living without drugs are still more or less captive to it, in that so much of their consciousness must be given over to withstanding the chemical temptations that beset them. Withstanding is a lesser evil than yielding, but it is no escape from the issue of addiction, so that I would have to characterize the predicament as one of being addicted to not being addicted. I do not mean to suggest that we choose one course or the other, but rather that both the premise and its negative variation exist in all of us. Even the most debilitated heroin addict retains his pride in the few items to which he has not become addicted.

Not many years ago, we had best remind ourselves, the problem of addiction seemed confined to a few chemicals—narcotics, alcohol and, perhaps, barbiturates—and it was then possible to make fairly clear distinctions between addiction and habituation, based mainly on the presence or absence of physiological withdrawal symptoms. However, today, even the well-publicized and allegedly extreme agonies of heroin withdrawal have been disputed by the Lazaruses who came back. Recently, a member of Synanon expressed to a reporter his disagreement with the fictional clichés which have acquired the status of scientific fact, remarking: "Kicking the habit is easy. It's not like that Frank Sinatra movie, crawling all over the walls. Sure, it's tough for a couple of days, but it's more like getting over a bad cold."

Fearing this view might be as extravagant in one direction as Nelson Algren's violent imaginings were in another, I checked with a friend who had been a staff member at Lexington. He thought the "bad-cold" analogy an accurate one, and added: "We had far more trouble with withdrawal symptoms in barbiturate users."

Our appropriation of the drug-user's vocabulary for our own purposes shows the extent to which the problem of addiction has invaded our daily existence. When our absorption with not only a chemical but a person, an activity, a distraction, an ideology seems to have more weight than is warranted, we say we are "hooked," meaning either that we wish we could be cured of our vice or else that we value the passion contained in our infatuation.

If someone or something excites us pleasurably, we say he or it "turns us on," but if our response is indifference or boredom, we are "turned off." Our extension of these terms for our own purposes is, to some degree, a fashionable reaction to the notoriety drugs have earned in the mass media. However, my own belief is that we resort to the junkie vocabulary because it expresses a metaphysical or addictive shift in our existence that the older vocabulary did not quite account for—at least in ordinary usage.

Even if we try to restrict ourselves to drug-taking, statistics about the extent and degree of addiction are hard to come by. Certainly we are no longer surprised to learn of the growing proportion of college students who resort to such drugs as marijuana, amphetamines, barbiturates, LSD, tranquilizers. One expert is quoted in *The New York Times* to the effect that about 40 percent of the students at the University of California use drugs from time to time. This figure falls somewhat short of Timothy Leary's immoderate proclamation: "Today, in the molecular age, the issue is not what books you read or which symbols you use, but which chemicals are part of your life and your growth."

Numerical estimates notwithstanding, on the theory that convicts tend to riot for those privileges society deems essential, such as humane treatment, recreation, adequate food, civil rights, I am more persuaded by this news release:

> WALPOLE, Mass., Aug. 13 (AP)—Inmates rioted outside a medication dispensary at the Massachusetts State Prison in an attempt to steal drugs late last night, injuring nine guards . . . Two guards were stabbed and five others beaten as the inmates pushed their way into the "pill" room, yelling, thrashing and literally gobbling down as many pills as they could at one time . . . State Police Cpl. James Dunne, who led the squad equipped with 12-gauge shotguns, gas masks and crash helmets, said about 18 of the inmates were reeling "on Cloud Nine" when he arrived . . .

And from industry, where access to drugs is sufficiently relaxed not to require riots, I offer this item:

> LOS ANGELES, Oct. 9 (Los Angeles Times)—Use of illegal drugs in industry, especially among production-line workers, is so common that to arrest everybody who sold or used them would mean some plants would have to hire whole new shifts of employes, according to a police narcotics specialist. The drugs most commonly used are amphetamine sulfate compounds and barbiturate derivatives, which keep workers awake, or put them to sleep . . .

Since it is forbidden to peddle or "push" most drugs, including whisky, on television, Madison Avenue has responded to the double dilemma of addiction by advertising aspirin as though it were *the* drug for every tribulation we must undergo. On television we are shown scenes in which mothers snap at their children, employers lose their tempers with employes. With only an awkward swipe at the questionable ethics of permitting this poor old headache remedy to carry such a heavy burden, advertisers show these embattled and suffering creatures putting one hand to their heads while a kindly neighbor advises them that this new aspirin combination is the perfect cure for "tension." The happy scenes following their use of the drug are deliberate efforts to imitate the style in which the pharmaceutical companies persuade physicians of the virtues of their products.

Most touching are aspirin commercials in which an aging movie star, long past his prime and no longer regularly employed, sits thoughtfully in his well-appointed study, telling the television audience that movie-making is a hectic and demanding affair. To avoid tension and headache, intrinsic to such activity, he has always resorted to this particular remedy.

Although probably unintentional, such a commercial goes to the heart of addiction, for we must contemplate the pathos of this formerly glamorous creature whose powers have so dwindled that he is reduced to doing headache commercials in which, fooling no one, he pretends nothing has changed. As he holds his bottle of pills to the audience, he seems to say life is really impossible without these pills. But we know, and he knows, that aspirin is not enough; for the vast restitution he demands of life, more powerful drugs are needed.

Should he seek them, he will not have to resort to any illicit drug traffic. He will have no trouble finding a physician who will prescribe amphetamines or psychic energizers to brighten his mood as he waits for calls from his agent. And if the phone refuses to ring, one or several of the many tranquilizers can be prescribed so that he can endure the waiting. Whatever insomnia may have originally been his lot will now be painfully exacerbated by his drug-taking so that other sedatives, fortified often by alcohol, will insure his sleeping. As he moves from one drug to another, mixing and testing the chemicals he believes his state requires and countering their disagreeable effects with still other chemicals, from time to time the sheer immodest scope of his undertaking will strike him; he has become a deranged chemist, his only laboratory his own poor body.

No matter how haggard that body becomes, he must unfortunately depend on it for fresh chemical inspiration. And, if everything else fails, there is LSD for instant revelation, if not wisdom, about the pretentious games that have brought him to this impasse, allowing him the death and rebirth that are now accepted pieties of the LSD mystique.

While it is true that the medical profession and the pharmaceutical industry together are the largest and most powerful group of pushers for the new drugs, I see no conspiracy on their part to make addicts of us all. It has long been common knowledge that physicians are the most devoted users of the drugs they prescribe, unlike the more disreputable pushers whose livelihood depends on abstaining from the drugs they peddle. The men who devise and merchandise these pills and the physicians who dispense them are, by and large, decent human beings who share the same disability of will that afflicts everyone.

Believing, as we do, that we should be able to will ourselves to be calm, cheerful, thin, industrious, creative—and, moreover, to have a good night's sleep—they simply provide the products to collaborate in such willing. If the satisfactions turn out to be short-lived and spurious and if their cost in terms of emotion, intellect and physical health is disagreeable, these scientists are ready to concoct new drugs to counter this discomfort. In other words, they offer us always new chances—virtually to the point of extinction—to will away the unhappiness that comes from willing ourselves to be happy.

Recently, Dr. Carroll L. Witten, president-elect of the American Academy of General Practice, was quoted in the press as being in agreement with a report issued this year by the United Nations Commission on Narcotics which expressed concern over "the alarming rise in the sale of barbiturates, tranquilizers and amphetamines."

The report suggested further that the "explosive expansion of the use of drugs . . . was most likely a result of their being used less as medication than as agents for producing sleep, a sense of happiness and relaxation." Dr. Witten declared:

> I believe these drugs are not only used wrongly, to excess and without adequate indication, but that in many cases their indiscriminate use has led to dependency, habituation and addiction, with all of the consequent results thereof.

Dr. Witten said he was referring specifically to the nonnarcotic drugs used as "psychic energizers, stimulators, activators, deactivators, depressants, alleviators, levelers, elevators or in whatever imaginative category one might place them. One must note with a great deal of alarm," he declared, "that the vast majority of cases first obtained their drugs through the prescription of a physician."

If willing what cannot be willed has led us to being addicted to addiction, it would seem that our addictive appetite will always be more than a match for the ever-mounting number of chemicals that are fashioned to gratify that appetite. And even if we eliminate actual drugs from our consideration, the addictive possibilities are endless: cigarettes, chocolate, detective and spy stories, football on television, psychoanalysis—to mention only a few of my own excesses, which I would unhesitatingly characterize as addictive. Everyone, I am convinced, has his own list, as well as another more prideful list of those objects and activities whose addictive claims he has successfully withstood.

If the term is not to be altogether meaningless, some distinction must now be made between one addiction and another. Concretely, when it comes to putting myself to sleep, how shall I distinguish between detective stories and sleeping pills? Or between watching football on TV and enduring my Sunday with tranquilizers? Or completing a tedious chore on amphetamines and procrastinating as usual?

The first generalization I would make about these sets of alternatives is that in an immediate sense drugs are clearly more effective. Detective stories, for me at least, are not entirely reliable as sedatives. If the story is so poor as to outrage or challenge my diminished sensibilities, I am in trouble, whereas I can always take another sleeping pill.

Watching even an exciting, well-played football game on TV, I cannot entirely obliterate from my awareness the perception that there are other ways in which I could more profitably spend my time. And if the game is inept and boring and still I do not turn the set off, my view of my condition is grim indeed. On the other hand, with tranquilizers, I could achieve a state of not unpleasant relaxation, unruffled by the sort of nagging self-concern which interrupts my absorption with even a good football game.

It is the last set of alternatives that will prove the most troublesome. If I have a group of evaluations of psychoanalytic candidates to write, I am inclined to put it off. The reasons and/or rationalizations for my procrastination will be various: I don't feel well; such reports are too tedious to be endured; I resent the bureaucratic rule requiring these reports; I am reluctant to set myself up as a judge of the performance of these young men; I am convinced I am not equal to the imaginative discriminations that would do these human beings justice.

With a dose of amphetamine, however, my self-concern, with its associated fatigue and hesitations and doubts, will vanish, so that in a single-minded way I shall vigorously engage my task. Within a few hours all the evaluations will be completed. Like a schoolboy who has at the last minute finished his term paper, I shall feel relieved and virtuous to have at long last done what my organization demands of me.

Reading over my reports after I have recovered from the drug, I may be chagrined to note a breathless, assertive and yet self-indulgent quality to my writing that did not trouble me at the time. But I can counter my dissatisfaction by assuring myself these deficiencies matter very little, since I have done all that was asked of me. It was my own sin of pride that initially led me to regard my task as such an intricate and demanding responsibility. Besides, I will tell myself, wasn't it a choice between doing nothing and doing something, however imperfectly?

Thus will my mood of accomplishment prevail, helping me to disown my self-criticism and perhaps persuading me, since I won't have to read these reports again, that I had indeed been discriminating in preparing them. And my earlier doubts as to whether these evaluations should have been written at all can be postponed for another time.

The sensation of being a going, if unquestioning, member of society should not be slighted, because it is hard to come by these days. Nevertheless, we must concede that while the drugs in these sets of alternatives may be more effective, their effectiveness is largely dependent on the chemical deadening of important imaginative and critical capacities, whose privileges are admittedly problematic. Practically every drug invented, from opium to LSD, has had its champions in both science and the arts who insisted that their particular brew was not only not reductive but was actually heightening of human potentiality.

The objective evidence for their claims, however, has always been depressing, and of the same order as my own reports, whether it be the music played under marijuana or heroin, the pictures painted and the poetry composed under LSD, the deadlines met by means of amphetamines, or even—perhaps especially—the perceptions and insights granted by drugs.

At this point, the question must be raised: aren't other addictions—nondrug addictions—also reductive? The answer has to be a qualified affirmative. The friend watching me glued for hours to the television set, isolated from all intelligible life, impervious to the claims of my children who have waited all week to have a few moments with me, has to find my human condition bizarre, to say the least.

Far more seriously incapacitating, of course, are those nondrug addictions that involve ideas and habits of thought. Those who over the years develop an addiction to shopworn ideologies—religious, scientific, political, esthetic, psychological—in a sense forfeit, in willful dedication, the very capacities of spirit and intellect that might set them free.

Nevertheless, there is a difference between drugs and no drugs. While disdain and denial of these capacities will cause them to shrivel and grow ever more paralyzed as years go by, there remains the possibility of a response, however minimal at first, to some human claim. Chemical deadening, on the other hand, if pursued, will, by its very nature, render such capacities eventually heedless to any call.

But to return to my evaluations of those psychoanalytic candidates—my will, with the help of amphetamine, has had its undiscriminating way in my reports, without the reflective give-and-take between me and my writing that could be called dialogic, causing this enterprise to resemble other headstrong monologic sprees in which the speaker is deaf and blind to those about him at the same time that he is convinced of a singular openness and freedom and mutuality to the exchange.

The nonuser has a dispiriting effect on groups enthusiastically consolidated by such convictions, so that they would prefer him to find his own sober companions. And his response to them will be marked by his discouraged observation that, despite the cries of mutual congratulation, all he can hear are colliding monologues, breathlessly composed so that each participant gives in to his own worst headstrong and literal-minded inclinations.

The person who ordinarily must guard against his habit of vast abstraction now becomes even more abstract in his theoretical pronouncements. The person top-heavy with esthetic sensibility becomes even more indulgent to that side of himself, abdicating his ability to temper such estheticism with moral and psychological discriminations.

The most blatant examples of the literal-minded aspect of the drugged state come from the public writings on LSD, but it is by no means restricted to this particular drug. Under LSD, it would seem one is at the mercy of any fancy that strikes him, much like the hypnotic subject responding to the commands of the hypnotist. Should he note that his hand is ugly, that hand becomes literally swollen and grotesque. Should the thought strike him that he is alone in the world, he will quickly and literally find himself as one small mortal in the midst of an endless desolate landscape. In each instance, what properly should be no more than a beginning metaphor has been exalted, at the behest of the will, into physical reality. Similarly, the death undergone with LSD can be regarded as more deathly than death itself. In a section, jarringly titled "Running Smack Into Your Essence," of "LSD: The Acid Test," published in *Ramparts*, one evangelist, Donavan Bess, wrote:

> The psychedelic death is especially lonely—lonelier, perhaps, than for the soldier who physically dies in a Vietnamese field hospital. He at least has the comfort of cuddling up in the image of his mother. Under LSD you have no

such bourgeois comfort; you have no familial figure at all. You die grown up. If you can hang onto that, afterward, you can offer society some adult values. You came to this point in a rite of passage as explicit, as terrible and as meaningful as those rites used in aboriginal Australia.

In considering the addictive state which may result from drugs, narcotic and non-narcotic, I must of course neglect the specific effects each drug has or purports to have on the central nervous system. An unfortunate consequence of such neglect will be to give the false impression that my own addiction to nonaddiction has led me to advocate an impossibly ascetic life, requiring abstention from all chemical assistance, come what may. Let me quickly insist that all the drugs I have mentioned may be taken in nonaddictive ways for reasons that are appropriate to the effects of the particular drug. This is to say, there are times when prolonged sleeplessness can and should be interrupted by sedatives, just as there are painful occasions when morphine is the only answer. Even amphetamines may allow the completion of a low-level chore.

The difficulty, however, here, as indicated earlier, is that the mood of accomplishment may persuade us to disregard the quality, or lack of quality, of our performance, not to mention the disagreeable drug side-effects, so that we turn to the drug in situations that require more of our wits and equanimity than amphetamines will allow. Perhaps a greater danger, as the use of amphetamines becomes more widespread, is that the deadlines asked of us are increasingly determined by the amphetamine intoxications of those who ask. (Another illustration of the manner in which the drugged state influences social values is suggested by the aspirin commercials referred to in this article. The writers of these advertisements seem to be selling not only aspirin but also their conviction—possibly arrived at through their own experience with tranquilizers—that our ordinary difficulties, since they are only subjective and therefore not worth contending with, are best erased with drugs. Thus, an advertisement for meprobamate, addressed to physicians, shows a picture of an overwrought mother with a child, the caption reading: "Her kind of pressures last all day . . . shouldn't her tranquilizer?")

For the sake of completeness, alcohol and marijuana are two drugs whose object is explicitly pleasure, and which may be used nonaddictively. However, too much has been made recently by the younger generation of the nonaddictive properties of marijuana simply because its physical effects are less dramatic than those of alcohol and other drugs. More dramatic is its effect upon relation: the pleasures of monologue experienced as dialogue under the drug, persist as a habit of tolerance for such illusion—which in a sense is the very issue of addiction.

Let us consider briefly the addictive course—from initial pleasure to ultimate disaster—that will result from prolonged and excessive use of any of the drugs I have mentioned, singly or in combination.

The first subjective experience of wholeness and the pleasure accompanying it will acquire its intensity partly through contrast with the discomfort which preceded the use of the drug and partly through the manner a particular drug answers a particular person's need at a particular time. Thus, users are labeled according to their preferences as "Up-Heads" or "Speed-Heads," "Down-Heads," "Acid-Heads," "Pot-Heads," "Lushes," "Junkies."

With further sophistication and availability, and the cooperation of the medical profession, drug-users already are specializing less and availing themselves more of other products and mixtures of products. But the initial feeling of well-being is difficult to duplicate precisely, regardless of the ingenuity of the user. As the drug and the state associated with it begin to wear off, the user returns to a world which has lost none of its oppressiveness and with which, in the midst of the drug hangover, he feels less able to cope.

The distance between himself and the wholeness he sought has grown somewhat, so that he is now vulnerable to the beginning belief that the relief the drug afforded is an extraordinary sort of transcendence which his usual life with others cannot provide, except in the occasional unpredictable and surprising manner in which such moments arise. In other words, he has been burned by the demonic and addictive notion that he need not wait on life for the transcendence he seeks, that he may invoke it whenever he so decrees or wills by returning to the drug or drugs which first allowed him this remarkable feeling.

With this seeming triumph of his will, he will be more impatient of the often frustrating give-and-take of life without drugs, willfully demanding his well-being of those about him and thereby suffering even more the penalties of such willing. In a sense he insists futilely that life now be his drug.

Needless to say, his mounting impatience will be inimical to the exercise or development of such qualities as imagination, judgment, humor, tact. And should he glimpse, however dimly, his impoverishment, he may wish to believe these qualities at least can return with drugs, disowning the evidence accumulating to the contrary. However, without these qualities he is more and more confined to the exigencies of the moment, for he can no longer really remember his drug experience in the past nor can he imagine what may follow. As his intolerance for life without drugs increases, his competence for such life diminishes, so that with every return to the drug he is, in the spirit of Heraclitus, a different and lesser person who attempts to cross the same stream twice.

What seemed the feeling of transcendence at the beginning has long since been abandoned as his drug goal in favor merely of getting from one moment to the next, in favor of mindlessly and minimally staying alive. What began with his will to decree well-being for himself without having to wait on life now culminates in almost a paralysis of will for every trivial action, even getting dressed or feeding himself. It is as though all the taken-for-granted stream of activity had disintegrated into a swarm of tiny yet insurmountable enterprises for his will, every one seeming to require further drugs for its accomplishment.

As the result of the bombardment of his body by such large dosages of drugs, his physical debilitation grows extreme. Yet even this bodily exhaustion and derangement offers a last resort to the will which is now unequal to practically every small movement in his world. Unlike other depleting illnesses that mysteriously overtake us, this one has been induced by himself and seems to be within his control. That is, he may try to assuage his agonies with more chemicals or he can withdraw the noxious agent so that his body can slowly recover its strength.

All other dramas in which his will has been involved have given way now to the one small immediate drama of whether he shall live or die to this world. It is a far cry from the transcendence he sought originally, but every addict knows the drama of his failing body is the last plot his will must confront. Unlike the proponents of LSD, he is beyond metaphysical conceits about the meaning of dying to this world, nor will he glamorize recovery, to whatever degree it may occur, as spiritual rebirth.

Nietzsche, I believe, was not as interested in theological argument about the disappearance of the divine will in our lives as he was in the consequences of its disappearance. Today, the evidence is in. Out of disbelief we have impudently assumed that all of life is now subject to our own will. And the disasters that have come from willing what cannot be willed have not at all brought us to some modesty about our presumptions. Instead, we have turned to chemicals, which seem to enhance our willful strivings. It was only a question of time before man, in his desperation, would locate divinity in drugs and on that artificial rock build his church.

# 3

## *Drugs and the Law*

DAVID W. SCHIESER

Before the turn of the century, opium and its derivatives could be bought legally and inexpensively in any drug store and in many rural general stores. Opium was an ingredient in a host of patent medicines. Mass advertising campaigns promoted these remedies to relieve diverse conditions from arthritis to whooping cough, female problems to male impotence.

The use of patent medicines was intensified by their apparent effectiveness. Promoters seldom admitted that the soothing and pain-relieving effects of a wine-glass-full of their "tonics" were derived from alcohol and opium. As a consequence, many people innocently became dependent upon these products. Repeat sales were assured.

For others the addiction to morphine and its derivatives was more obvious. The invention of the hypodermic needle, the extensive use of morphine during the Civil War, and the introduction of heroin, first thought to be nonaddicting, compounded to incite public alarm.

Finally, a little less than 100 years ago, addiction was recognized as a health problem. Since then, federal, state, and local governing bodies have imposed a variety of "health" laws intended to prevent abuse of drugs. The premises, admit-

From *California Health,* Suppl. 27 (10), 1970, pp. 8–9.

tedly debatable, for these laws are that a substance which is not available cannot be abused, and that the threat of apprehension as a criminal with a stiff penalty will deter most people from possessing or abusing drugs.

Each of the laws was a response to a general alarm or crisis. The various legal restraints may be grouped according to their purposes.

## DISCLOSURE OF CONTENTS

The first federal law to address the problem of drug abuse was the Food and Drug Act of 1906. It required purity and safety for foods and drugs, and listing on the label of names and amounts of alcohol and other habit-forming ingredients. The design was to alert people to the risks of dependence in certain patent remedies.

## LIMITING SALE

In 1901 a special committee of the American Pharmaceutical Association surveyed druggists, and reported that the extent of the public's demand for narcotic drugs was appalling. Studies such as this resulted in the Harrison Narcotic Act of 1914 which required, among other things, that narcotic drugs be dispensed only on the prescription of a physician. As other potent drugs were discovered—barbiturates, sulfanilamide and penicillin are examples—they were added to the list of dangerous drugs with restricted sale. "Dangerous drugs" are those considered unsafe for self-medication for reasons of potential for abuse, other potential harmful effects, or because of difficulty for the layman to diagnose his specific need for a potent drug.

In 1957 the Federal Food, Drug and Cosmetic Act was amended to create two classes of drugs—prescription (Rx) and over-the-counter (OTC). Labels on prescription drugs bear the statement, "Caution, Federal Law Prohibits Dispensing Without a Prescription," and sale of such drugs without a prescription is punishable as a misdemeanor under federal and state laws.

In California there is an additional class of drugs—"restricted dangerous drugs"—which includes hypnotics, stimulants, and certain hallucinogens.

## CONTROL OF IMPORTS AND PRODUCTION

The Narcotic Drugs Import and Export Act of 1922 limits importation of crude opium and coca leaves to amounts deemed necessary for medical and scientific purposes. The Opium Poppy Control Act of 1942 prohibits production of the opium poppy in the United States except under license. The Drug Abuse Control Amendments, 1965, require record-keeping by manufacturers, wholesalers and retailers for all depressant, stimulant, and hallucinogenic drugs. Individual states have adopted laws which closely parallel these federal laws.

## PROHIBITING POSSESSION

Earlier laws implied that possession of narcotics by unauthorized persons was prohibited, but the Boggs Act of 1957 imposed a mandatory sentence for the illegal possession of narcotic drugs. In 1965 California made illegal possession of barbiturates and amphetamines a criminal act, and in 1966, LSD and DMT were added. Federal and state laws also forbid possession of the paraphernalia used by narcotic addicts, such as hypodermic syringes and needles.

## PROHIBITING USE

Federal law does not prohibit the use of a drug, but the California Health and Safety Code, Section 11167 states that "no person shall prescribe, administer, or furnish a narcotic for himself." Thus all narcotic use is illegal unless prescribed by a physician. This prohibition of use does not extend to drugs other than narcotics.

## DRUNK AND DISORDERLY CONDUCT

Local laws prohibiting drunk and disorderly conduct are most frequently applied to those who abuse alcohol, but they are often equally applicable to individuals under the influence of other intoxicants, such as drugs or solvent vapors.

Arrest data indicate that drug abuse is on the rise, but it is difficult to determine how much of this represents a real increase or more concentrated police action. It is generally agreed that present legal controls have failed to prevent abuse of drugs. Laws against possession and use have also been criticized as inhumane to the addict who is, after all, a sick person. Those concerned with the problem emphasize that prevention through public education and treatment for abusers are the real keys to eliminating drug abuse.

# 4

# *Counseling the College Student Drug User*

JOHN L. KUEHN

Excessive drug usage among college students is an overdetermined and exceedingly complex phenomenon. The problems students say drive them to drugs have con-

From the *Bulletin of the Menninger Clinic,* Vol. 34, pp. 205–215, copyright 1970 by The Menninger Foundation. Reprinted by permission.

siderable validity. These include recognition of and identification with widespread use of drugs by adults particularly alcohol, tobacco, and tranquilizers; feelings of altruistic helplessness as a result of genuine flaws in the American political system; and discrepancies between the ideals of "justice," "forgiveness," and "equality" and the actuality of significant deficiencies in legal, criminologic, and social practice depending on race and economic status.

Possibly more important (and something we seem powerless to do much about) is the speedup in the technologic revolution in the last thirty years. It is now a truism that the only constant thing about American life is change. This is particularly true with regard to the important subgrouping of communication developments such as the telephone, the airplane, radio, television and movies. In a concrete sense, these are the technical aspects of our culture we know the most about. But, in terms of ultimate value and long-term effects on human relations, we know very little indeed. It does seem that the speedup and our personal lack of control over such activities, with consequent assaults on the perceptual-motor apparatus could increase feelings of helplessness, reactive hostility and impulsivity.

Similarly, ethologists, geographers, and sociologists make us aware that most men are no longer masters of their own well-defended "territory" as they were in a simpler time when there was more land and fewer people. Much of one's "world" is out of personal control (in the perceptual and phenomenologic sense) for many of us. This gives rise to anxiety in any reasonably intelligent and introspective person from time to time.

Thus, within the context of certain normative developmental problems of youth, rapid and painful change, and profound uncertainty about values in our society, one in three college students has tried illicit drugs such as marijuana and LSD at least once. It is of some reassurance to know that many do not repeat the "experiment." Use of LSD seems to be declining since 1966 when it was estimated that five percent of students tried LSD while in 1969 only about one percent experimented with it (1). On the other hand, use of amphetamines is increasing. In Sweden, this has been of such great concern that the government has recently stopped *all* prescription distribution of the six main types of amphetamines (2).

In our university, 41 out of 433 students (9.5 percent) coming to the Counseling and Mental Health Services for help in the school year 1968–69 had psychedelic drug-related problems. Eight of these students were treated initially for "bad trips" (3 amphetamines, 3 LSD, 2 marijuana). The other 33 students did not complain *primarily* of symptoms they saw arising from drug usage, but were found (from their history) to use drugs repetitively. The incidence of situations involving inappropriate use of drugs would be significantly higher if we could include barbiturate and alcohol-related problems, overdoses of tranquilizers, and data from physicians seeing patients in the medical clinic. At present, however, such data can only be collected in our service of the college hospital and clinics because of staff limitations.

As with the small but important group of students with homicidal impulses reported on previously (3), it is usually necessary to *ask* whether the patient uses "pot," "acid," or "speed." This information is rarely volunteered unless the presenting problem is a "bad trip" or a "flashback." But possibly there is something more in an explicit psychobiologic context that we can say about chronic drug users in the college setting. Such people who have come to our attention in the counseling and mental health center seem to be suffering primarily from neurotic difficulties ("neurosis" is here defined as an arrest of human development) rather than from political and social ennui. The following situation vignettes are more-or-less typical of students coming to us for psychiatric counseling:

### *Vignette No. 1*

A 19 year old male about to enter college was referred to the Center after impulsively taking 100 aspirin tablets while in a period of "meaningless" depression. He was passive, withdrawn, and silent. Articulation of ideas was painfully difficult for him. The only thing he wanted to talk about was his car and his girl. He is called and treated by his parents as "our baby." He has been "given to" and "done for" in order for him to have "every advantage" and "chance for a good life." The mother subtly torpedoes the father's attempts to encourage independence. She is frustrated and bored by her life. In the course of the son's counseling, the mother agreed to enter treatment herself.

Marijuana was used repetitively as an anti-depressant. The youth stated that he takes pot because "I feel happy and can laugh again" (alcohol makes him more depressed) and as a "vacation from the world—outside of my home the world looks too complicated and frightening to me." Parents are characterized as "great people—after all they've done everything they possibly could to help me!"

### *Vignette No. 2*

An attractive but physically immature-appearing ("nice little girl syndrome"), 22-year-old, white, female, college senior, referred to the Counseling Service by one of her professors, complained of long-standing anxiety, confusion, and depression. Her counselor saw it as a sign of strength that she could ask for help from adults. She has used marijuana repetitively which she feels "damps down anxiety and confusion about my value system." However, the last time she smoked marijuana she went into a panic, wondering whether she could "come back to reality" and "felt paranoid."

A psychodiagnostic evaluation revealed a young woman with more than usual intellectual and emotional potential, who bore within herself strong and, at times, overwhelming infantile needs for dependency and affection. As the oldest daughter of nine children, she had functioned earlier as a pseudoadequate "mother's helper." A recent attempt at sexual relations had ended in "disaster" for her. Strong oedipal confusion surfaced during testing, and controls crumbled both there and in external reality. It was predicted she would continue to act out infantile needs in a self-destructive fashion if the process were to continue without clinical intervention. She was advised to go visit her parents in the foreign country where they reside, and was referred for group psychotherapy. She subsequently did both, and has not used marijuana since, to our knowledge.

### *Vignette No. 3*

A single, white, third-semester "freshman" with poor grades came to the Clinic on his own after hearing a talk on student suicides by the university psychiatrist. The student said that he had been depressed and thinking about suicide for one year. Although he wished to be a physician, he was failing math and chemistry. He used LSD, amphetamines, and marijuana repetitively and indiscriminately. Subsequently, he was seen intermittently in the Clinic for two years. One time he came after a girl friend threatened to break off with him after he had exhibited childish pique and anger. He could not understand her "callow" behavior after having sexual intercourse with him. On another occasion he had a "bad trip" and "freaked out" after taking LSD. Again, he came to the Clinic in a panic after receiving a notice to report for a draft physical.

The patient described his father as an alcoholic and his mother as "chronically sick." He was ambivalent about our recommendation for intensive psychiatric treatment. He finally came to trust us, became a "good grouper," and accepted intensive, but brief and time-limited individual counseling with a mature young woman on our junior staff. We heard no more of his drug problems, although many other issues in his life remained seriously unresolved.

## PSYCHOSOCIAL TRAITS OF COLLEGE STUDENTS WHO USE PSYCHEDELIC DRUGS REPETITIVELY

1. A *tendency to live excessively in the present.* These students have an infantile time sense, unable either to imagine or plan for the future, or to accept the significance of their personal past experiences and family history. Initially, they usually spend their time in counseling talking about current friends, dates, and imagined and real "injustices." It is as if their families and culture never existed.

2. *An excessively passive and reactive position in interpersonal relationships.* These students do not "reach out," "act," or assert themselves. Instead, they *re*act excessively. This passive position is accompanied by severe unconscious feelings of helplessness and "placelessness," artfully masked by hostility directed against "the establishment." These young people, who come to us possibly as a "last hope," are severely dependent for their physical survival on others, as well as being about to abandon the necessary search for relevant values and for a personal sense of identity. Analysis of this particular symptom complex exposes drug usage as a regressive and frantic attempt to deal with underlying painful affects by a blatant retreat from coping with the world of "bread-and-potatoes" reality.

3. *Serious cognitive difficulties.* There is a schizophrenoid disturbance of thinking and verbalization. Usually the student is inchoate or "almost catatonic" in his inability to express feelings, motives, fantasies, and ideas in some simple, appropriate cognitive framework. Yet, despite confusion and silence and "cool" behavior, posture and facial features frequently suggest a tremendous wish to communicate accompanied by a severe tension state and damming of affect (the "Billy Budd" phenomenon).

4. *Inexplicable depression.* These students descend into profound melancholia not accompanied by obvious object loss. This is frequently associated with suicidal phenomena of Schneidman's dyadic ("interpersonal message") type (4). Particularly with males, this must be considered an ominous prognostic sign and "cry for help."

5. *Study difficulties, not attributable to reality problems or difficulties in the environment.* Problems in attending to school work and achieving passing grades are often rationalized on the basis of "laziness," "distractibility" or "poor teaching." In Reifler's important study (5) only five percent of students becoming manifestly mentally ill while away at college were "well" when they entered.

6. *Unrewarding sexual behavior.* Although sexual activity may be frequent, relations are ungratifying. According to students seen in psychiatric counseling, sex is used most often as a counterdepressant or tranquilizer, and to make up for mothering perceived by the patients as inadequate or inept. Alliances are frequently dehumanized and transient, with frequent recourse to reciprocal manipulation and "psychological racketeering."[1] Our experience resembled Halleck's with alienated college students (6), of frequent reports of impotence in the male and frigidity in the female. Both men and women complained of severe difficulties in forming any kind of close and trusting relationships with each other, despite the apparent sexual "freedom." It seems the girls came closer to overcoming this than the boys. When the girls were unable to get any human feedback, their depressions increased, accompanied by helpless, tearful rage and guilt.

7. *Regulatory and defensive maneuvers.* The basic regulatory and defensive maneuvers are repression and rationalization. These young patients are, therefore, not in touch with their true feelings when first seen for counseling. Further, they are initially unable to acknowledge the preconscious roots of their problems.

8. *Secondary defenses.* Important secondary defenses are intellectualization and isolation. These students "love" in the abstract but not in the concrete sense of any genuine capacity for appropriate concern for the welfare and feelings of another human being. They are not only out of touch with underlying feelings of hostility but also with inherent and primitive kindness. An estimate of the incidence of these traits in our admittedly small sample is "in excess of 70 percent."

Probably most youthful drug users do not seek psychiatric assistance. However, descriptions given by student patients of their associates convey that a significant number, far from being "healthier" than those who seek psychiatric help, have even more severe difficulties than those who voluntarily come to the Center. In addition to the characteristics which I listed above, some drug users who do not seek psychiatric counseling exhibit traits of externalization and projection. This is manifested as profound suspiciousness and distrust of teachers and counselors, paralyzing fear of dependency, and relatively little anxiety in the sense in which it is a "danger signal" and survival mechanism.

## PSYCHODYNAMICS

The basic problem of the student drug users is an arrest in their psychosocial growth and development. In addition, repetition-compulsion, an important law of neurosis, is operative. They do not seem able to learn by experience and tend

[1] "Psychological racketeering" refers to the buying off of others through variations of the protection racket theme: "If you don't come through for me, I'll punish you."

to repeat the same mistakes over and over. We sometimes ask them in counseling, "Why don't you try a few *new* mistakes for a change?"

Study difficulties often grow out of fear of success because once they succeed they will have to accept additional responsibility. This fear is accompanied by ambivalent worries that they might find out they are *not* as exceptional as they thought they were, as well as the normal resurgence of infantile omnipotence during late adolescence. When sublimated, of course, this may be a source of considerable creativity and achievement; however, it is important to convey to such patients that just because one risks success does not mean you have to win a Nobel Prize. Sometimes the only healthy "way out" of this predicament is for them to fall ill enough to force society to provide residential treatment, wherein they can be protected physically against their self-destructive impulses while they regress to a psychosexual level from whence personal reconstruction of the anaclitic type can begin.

Certainly sociodynamic factors—such as excess leisure time, affluence, and a society in which easy and instant gratification is possible—play a part and must be dealt with in counseling. For many of the young people who seek out help in the college psychiatric counseling center there is an excessive and infantile allegiance to the "fun ethic" which is destructive. These students are rarely campus leaders or effective revolutionaries or campus activists.

Dehumanization, population pressures, inadequate distancing, the college "ghetto" phenomenon in many large university communities, and the "no time alone" problem play their part in the production of much human suffering and discouragement. However, when the repression lifts (after a student has been in counseling and has come to trust us), the story most frequently heard has to do with difficulties explicitly with and within their families. These stories are quite similar to what Halleck described as the "alienated student syndrome." (6) The students are usually from affluent urban or suburban families. They have been routinely exposed to excessive permissiveness, material gratification, and inadequate or inappropriate limit setting earlier in their lives. Parents have histories of severe emotional instability and family conflict. However, this is frequently suppressed behind the facade of the "nice family," which includes presenting a "united front" to the children without regard to the difference between what is *said* by parents and what is *observed* by the youngsters of their parents' behavior. Contradictory communications from parents such as "Don't worry about your grades, just do the best you can," followed by paradoxical anger when grades are poor, are frequent.

Similarly, in regard to sexual behavior, some mothers will convey that, while promiscuity is "bad," the youngster should have more dates, wear adult hair styles, buy (or accept as a present from a parent) seductive clothes, or wear makeup more appropriate to a 35-year-old than a 17-year-old. When the young person takes the parents at their word and tries to operate out of some interests and motives of their own rather than parents' fears and unmet needs, there are explosions that exceed the provocation. The youngsters tell us that their parents' criticism and rage are incomprehensible for, after all, by age eighteen or so, it is their life and their business what their interests are and which direction their career choices will take. Only when they are too sick to work and feed themselves or are suicidal should parents intervene to arrange for hospitalization. They do wish relations with and advice from "people over 30"—but not from their parents!

Parental "love" seems to be more talked about than provided in the form of consistent trust, and support in the development of useful independence. Frequently there seems to be a role reversal of the parents, in which the father is described as the passive, reacting, and compliant ("feminine") figure, while the mother is more active and assertive. The phenomenon in which the youngster is *explicitly* acting out some unconscious needs of the parent has also been observed with several of our young patients (7). The young people feel—but are unable to articulate—that their parents are using them to solve their own difficulties—to live out unmet needs, and to gain satisfaction missing from their own lives. Because these parents repeatedly deny their true feelings, the adolescent experiences further confusion and an increasing sense of helplessness and impotent rage. Of course, the seduction and manipulation of children to satisfy parental needs is one of the less pleasant realities of human nature. Initially, few of the parents we see have the ability and courage to accept such antisocial motives in themselves.

If the adolescent does vent some anger, it is handled hypocritically: anger is "okay" but don't really mean it! Actually the parents of these patients have great difficulty in tolerating angry feelings themselves. They seem unable to "hear out" their child's negative feelings and immediately become defensive, retaliating with even more hostility than the child has expressed. A power struggle and eventual impasse may result.

We have had several incidents on our campus where parents have attempted to violently control their children by literally "kidnapping" them off the street. Hospitalization out of town is indicated when the family conflict becomes this violent. One outcome of family guerrilla warfare is that the young person learns to repress his unacceptable feelings, and to value conformity as a facade. This is facilitated by the emphasis on grades, learning how to take tests, and "how to get into a good college" prevalent in some suburban secondary school systems. One student put it beautifully: "If you're not first rate, there's no place to go."

Then, willy-nilly, they come to college. They have been brainwashed to repress and conform—to "be careful," to follow the family party line, to gratify physical impulses immediately but to live to please family only, and "not to make waves." But most universities worthy of the name operate on completely antithetic principles. The student is encouraged to reexamine previous life experiences and values, to "reach out" and to "risk something." The usual American university tolerates a tremendous flux of ideas, and ambiguities abound—as a built-in "given" of higher education. This new freedom catalyzes students' confusion, anxiety, and depression to intolerable levels. There is a tendency for students to become "as if" individuals who cannot identify what their true feelings are ("full garbage can" cognition) or, at the other end of the scale, who feel hopelessly "empty" of anything they consider their own.

The student has also learned to be a guilty person, specifically when acknowledging and asserting any wishes or feelings of his own. Thus, there is anxiety resulting from conflict between what one *wants* to do and what one thinks he *ought* to do. This guilt also is a reaction to affluence because he has not earned it.

Frequently it is the sophomore year when the mental pain reaches an intolerable level. The young person is now not able to accept the universal adolescent experience of questioning early beliefs and, similarly, cannot cope with the exposure to critical thinking in college because of feelings of helpless dependency and poor tolerance for ambiguity. He is filled with horror and hatred, having found that parents have given him "bum dope." It is common for our patients to tell us after a while that they have fantasies of murdering their parents. These are sometimes quite frightening. The patient not only distrusts his parents, but he repudiates the institutionalized questioning of the university "parents"—the faculty and administration. In the face of this, he opts out. He cannot accept any positive experience learned in his family and rejects an appropriate sense of historical continuity and identity with his family and with western civilization in general. It is then a simple step, in the face of such misery, from "the real world" to the profoundly narcissistic oblivion of the drug experience.

## DEVELOPMENTS IN COUNSELING TACTICS

Halleck (6) makes a number of practical suggestions in structuring and conducting ongoing individual counseling with young people. Elaborations on some of these are:

1. Don't be taken in by the student's intellectualizations about society.
2. Show yourself as a "real person"—at the proper time tell the patient what *you* believe and how *you* solved life's problems when you were his age.
3. Pay close attention to the therapeutic structure because limits will be tested; enforce appointment times and the time limits of the contract explicitly.
4. Wherever possible insist the patient commit himself to psychotherapy and "choose to be a patient" (rather than choosing for him). But because of the basic trust problem, guard his confidences as if they were the crown jewels.
5. If counseling on a fee basis is the way to make your living, charge him if he misses appointments. Outpatient treatment probably shouldn't be attempted unless the student is at least partially self-supporting (so in part he can pay his own fee rather than getting it from his parents).
6. Be alert to our own tendencies to develop impatience and negative countertransference with these young people—particularly where they have long hair, are poorly groomed, are excessively passive and silent, etc.
7. Therapy with this group of patients is not a "brief" matter. In our experience, it goes on from three months to a year. If one sees a student for longer than a year, obtain consultation with a colleague, because of the frequent problem of therapeutic impasse. While family counseling may be the theoretical treatment of choice, considering the dynamics sketched above, the establishment of a contract is often extremely difficult. Frequently schizophrenogenic scapegoating is taking place and, in essence, the family needs the patient sick to maintain their own vital balance as they see it—so they may try subtly to organize against the counselor. Family treatment is also realistically not the cup of tea of many otherwise quite capable counselors.
8. Because of student sensitivity to the betrayal issue, parents should seldom be seen without the patient present, and always with his permission.
9. In many settings, group therapy is practically the most useful primary

modality of counseling. In our experience, it is usually a good adjunct to individual counseling.

Some approaches evolve from the basic community psychiatry concept of "reaching out" to those in need rather than waiting for people to show up at the office. For instance, one member of the junior staff of the Counseling and Mental Health Service lives out in the "pseudo ghetto" ("pseudo" because these "pads" are frequently quite plush, reflecting the affluence and parental dependence problems). Also when students come for help to the Center there are usually a number of others waiting around the fringes to be invited in. One colleague in New Orleans does just this and those students who are invited in join with those who seek help and form a group. The fee is split between those who attend by "passing the hat." (8)

## CONCLUSION

It is important to remind ourselves that despite the incapacity, misery, and hostility of these young people, the willingness to "try drugs" and to "try psychiatry" by voluntarily coming to the clinic suggests that these desperate children in adult clothing have not given up.

Demands for mental health services in colleges by the students continue to grow as enrollments swell, society becomes more complex, and American family life and organization continues its agonizing renewal. The presence of adequately staffed college mental health units, as well as trained and concerned professionals in the private sector, not only for treatment but to provide consultation and education for faculty and administrators, is now no longer a luxury but a necessity if we are to alleviate profound misery and self-destructiveness, and facilitate the development of a large group of our young people.

## REFERENCES


1. Abelson, P. H.: LSD and Marihuana. *Science* 159:1189, March 1968.
2. Citing Abuse, Sweden Bans Amphetamine Distribution. *Psychiatric News* 3(2): 1, 7, Nov. 1968.
3. Kuehn, J. L., and Burton, John: Management of the College Student with Homicidal Impulses—"The Whitman Syndrome." *Amer. J. Psychiat.* 125: 1594–99, May 1969.
4. Shneidman, E. S.: Classifications of Suicidal Phenomena. *Bull. Suicidology,* July 1968, pp. 1–9.
5. Reifler, C. B.: Epidemiologic Aspects of College Mental Health. Unpublished paper presented at the 47th Annual Meeting of The American College Health Association, Oklahoma City, Oklahoma, April 25, 1969.
6. Halleck, S. L.: Psychiatric Treatment of the Alienated College Student. *Amer. J. Psychiat.* 124:642–50, Nov. 1967.
7. Johnson, A. M.: Sanctions for Superego Lacunae of Adolescents. In *Searchlights on Delinquency,* K. R. Eissler, ed. New York: International Universities, 1949, pp. 225–45.
8. Connell, M. L.: Personal communication.

# 2
# Popular Social Drugs

By including both alcohol and marihuana under the title of "Popular Social Drugs," recognition is made of the extensive recreational use of these drugs. Alcohol is a socially accepted part of life, as more than 80 percent of adult Americans are at least occasional drinkers. The number of people who smoke marihuana is hard to estimate, considering the illegality of the drug. However, many have guessed that the number of people who have tried the drug may approach twenty million, with the majority of these belonging to the under-thirty generation. On college campuses, passing a "joint" at a party has become as common as opening a beer can. Despite the laws, many of which are quite harsh, marihuana appears to be gaining acceptance in this country as a harmless way to mild euphoria and relaxation. Alcohol, which has a long history in the Western world, is often held up as an example of a legal drug that is more dangerous than the illegal cannabis. Disagreement over these two drugs and their relative merits and faults continues to persist despite an increase in recent research that has attempted to alleviate some of the misinformation.

The first two articles included in this chapter, by Goodwin et al. (1969) and Ryback (1969), are concerned with state-dependent learning under the effects of alcohol. By state-dependent learning we mean that recall depends on the state of the organism (drunk or sober) during learning and during recall. It may shed some light on the memory-loss aspect often associated with heavy drinking.

The treatment of alcoholism, one of the largest health problems in the United States, has recently taken some new directions. Promise is shown for the treatment of alcoholism in a unique study by Lovibond and Caddy (1970). McBrearty et al. (1968) take a look at the behavioral-oriented treatment programs and offer a comparison of their success with other approaches.

Schwarz (1969) gives an unbiased, general review of the current knowledge of marihuana without moralizing or trying to propagandize. The now-famous study of Weil et al. (1968) on the "Clinical and Psychological Effects of Marihuana in Man" shows that in a controlled situation much of the euphoric effect (the "high") of marihuana may be a learned reaction. His research raises many interesting questions that will lend themselves to further scientific study. Crancer et al. (1969) attempt to clear up some of the disagreement over the relative effects of alcohol and marihuana with their comparison of the effects these drugs have on driving ability. Kalant (1969), in his reply to the article, however, raises several questions that reopen the controversy.

Until the last few years, research on marihuana and alcohol and their behavioral effects has been sparse and often quite poor. The situation has been improving as more competent researchers move into this field and try to find some answers to the puzzling questions that these drugs raise. Because of extent of use and abuse of alcohol and marihuana in our society, these answers, when they come, will be welcome.

# 5

# Alcohol and Recall: State-Dependent Effects in Man

DONALD W. GOODWIN, BARBARA POWELL, DAVID BREMER, HASKEL HOINE, JOHN STERN

Animals trained in a drugged state may "remember" their training better if tested in a comparable drugged state than in a nondrugged state (1). Similarly, learning acquired in a nondrugged state transfers better to the same state than to a drugged state. This "dissociation of learning" has been demonstrated primarily with anesthetic agents (2). Given in sufficient quantities these drugs impair performance, and it could be expected that animals would manifest learned responses better in a nondrugged state than when drugged. The observation, however, that performance may actually improve in a drugged state, provided that original learning was in the same state, cannot be attributed to the drug's depressant effect on acquisition, retention, or performance. Thus, to some extent, learning is apparently state-dependent, that is, it depends for optimum expression on restoration of the original condition in which learning was acquired.

That alcohol produces dissociation has been demonstrated in animals (3) and in man (4). In studying this phenomenon in man we used a higher dosage of alcohol than was previously used and a wider range of learning tasks to determine whether interaction effects are more evident in some tasks than in others.

Forty-eight male medical students, paid to participate in a training session (day 1) and a testing session (day 2) separated by 24 hours, were randomly assigned to four groups of 12 subjects each (Table 1). One group (SS) was sober both days. A second group (AA) was intoxicated both days. A third group (AS) was intoxicated on day 1 and sober on day 2. The fourth group (SA) was sober on day 1 and intoxicated on day 2. Intoxicated subjects, depending on body weight, consumed between 8 and 10 ounces (250 and 300 ml) of 80-proof vodka, diluted in a soft drink, over 1 hour, after which testing began. Concentrations of alcohol in blood, as determined by breath analyses (5), varied from 80 to 140 mg/100 ml, with a mean of 111 mg/100 ml. All subjects drinking this amount showed signs of intoxication. Equivalent amounts of the soft drink were given to nondrinkers. Subjects knew in advance that they might receive alcohol, but had no other knowledge of the experiment.

Tests were administered in the same order to all subjects over a 40-minute period. They included an avoidance task to measure interference and latency of response, a verbal rote-learning task to measure recall, a word-association test to measure recall of "self-generated" learning, and a picture task to measure recogni-

From *Science*, Vol. 163, March 21, 1969, pp. 1358–1360. Copyright 1969 by the American Association for the Advancement of Science. Reprinted by permission of authors and publisher.

tion. A motor task with a pursuit rotor also was used, but proved so easy to master, regardless of state, that the resultant data were unusable.

In the avoidance task, four patterns of lights were randomly presented. Each pattern could be extinguished by a specific switch that could be controlled by hands or feet. An incorrect response or failure to respond resulted in presentation of a noxious tone. Criterion was 20 correct responses, with number of errors to reach criterion taken as the measure of performance. The task was identical on both days, except that on day 2 the pattern-switch relation was altered. Thus, performance on day 2 was assumed to reflect interference; that is, the greater the number of errors on day 2, the greater the degree of interference (6). Latency of response also was recorded.

The rote-learning task involved memorizing four five-word "sentences" of varying meaningfulness (normal sentence, anomalous sentence, anagram, and word list) (7). On day 2 subjects were asked to recall the sentences memorized on day 1, after which a relearning session was conducted. Performance was measured in terms of errors of sequence and omission.

For the word-association test, ten words of low association value (8) were presented. Subjects were instructed to respond to the stimulus words with the first word that came to mind. On day 2 the stimulus words were repeated and subjects were asked to recall their responses on day 1. Performance was measured in terms of errors made in day 2 recall.

In the picture recognition task, subjects were shown 20 pictures on day 1. On day 2 they were asked to select from 40 pictures those seen on day 1. Half of the pictures, showing mail-order catalog models, were designated as "neutral"; half were chosen from nudist magazines and were designated as "emotional."

The means and standard deviations of performance on the four tasks are presented in Table 1. For the avoidance and rote-learning tasks, performance measures were available for both day 1 and day 2, whereas scores for the other two tasks were limited to performance on day 2.

On day 1 performance was significantly better in the sober groups (SS and SA) than in the alcohol groups (AA and AS) for both the avoidance and rote learning ($t = 2.58$, $P < .01$, and $t = 3.78$, $P < .01$, respectively)—the expected depressant effect of alcohol on performance.

Since dissociation or effect of changing state could best be reflected by an interaction effect, the measures of performance on day 2 were subjected to 2 by 2 factorial analyses of variance (Table 2). Preliminary testing with the $F_{max}$ test (9) indicated homogeneity of variance for all data except that obtained from the avoidance task. For the latter, homogeneity was achieved through use of the square-root transformation (10), normalizing distribution of the data.

Table 2 presents the $F$ values obtained from the analyses of variance. The data indicated a significant A by B interaction (state-change effect) for the avoidance, rote-memory, and word-association tasks: Changes in alcohol state from day 1 to day 2 were associated with changes in test performance. Analyses of simple main effects were conducted to assess the source of the interaction effects (Table 1).

In the avoidance task, compared to subjects remaining in the same state those in changed states made significantly fewer errors (were subject to less inter-

TABLE 1. Mean Errors on Memory Tasks for the Four Groups of Either Sober or Intoxicated Subjects

| | Group[a] | | | |
|---|---|---|---|---|
| | *AA* | *SS* | *AS* | *SA* |
| Avoidance[b] (measuring interference) | | | | |
| Day 1 | 8.28 ± 1.15 | 6.91 ± 1.98 | 8.99 ± .67 | 6.02 ± 1.04 |
| Day 2 | 9.12 ± 1.41 | 8.13 ± 1.79 | 7.15 ± 1.34 | 7.20 ± 2.12 |
| Rote-learning | | | | |
| Day 1 | 16.96 ± 5.14 | 12.05 ± 5.90 | 20.56 ± 5.12 | 12.29 ± 5.02 |
| Day 2 | 16.45 ± 6.35 | 13.75 ± 7.09 | 24.55 ± 6.90 | 15.10 ± 7.94 |
| Word Association | 2.50 ± 1.57 | 1.25 ± 1.14 | 4.58 ± 2.13 | 2.25 ± 1.43 |
| Picture recognition | | | | |
| Neutral | 5.08 ± 1.73 | 4.92 ± 2.55 | 5.00 ± 2.09 | 5.08 ± 2.19 |
| Emotional | 3.67 ± 1.88 | 1.67 ± 1.45 | 4.25 ± 2.07 | 2.50 ± 1.51 |

[a]The first letter in group designations refers to condition on day 1; the second letter, condition on day 2; A, alcohol; S, no alcohol. Each group had 12 subjects, with the following exceptions: In the avoidance task, AA and SS had eight, AS had six, and SA had seven subjects. In the rote-learning task, all groups had ten subjects (13). No measure of day 1 errors was possible for the word-association and picture-recognition tasks.
[b]Square root transformations were used to achieve homogeneity of variance (10).

ference from original learning). This difference was primarily due to more errors being committed by the AA group, but the SS group also made more errors than the changed groups, although this difference was not significant.

In both the rote-learning and word-association tasks, the interaction effect was largely due to the fact that the AS group made significantly more recall errors than the AA or SS groups. In neither task did the SA group differ significantly from the same-state groups, although in both tasks the SA group made more errors than the SS group (11).

Latency of response in the avoidance task was not influenced by state change. Nor was there a significant interaction effect in the picture-recognition task, although in the case of "emotional" pictures, a trend toward dissociation was evident.

TABLE 2. *F* Values for Analysis of Variance of Errors on Memory Tasks on Day 2[a]

| *Task* | *A* | *B* | *A* × *B* |
|---|---|---|---|
| Avoidance task | 0.56 | 0.68 | 5.33[b] |
| Rote learning | 7.34[b] | 2.27 | 4.44[b] |
| Word association | 15.05[c] | 1.37 | 11.14[c] |
| Picture recognition | | | |
| Neutral | 0.00 | 0.00 | 0.00 |
| Emotional | 14.09[c] | 0.00 | 2.01 |

[a]*A*, effect on errors on day 2 of being intoxicated on day 1; *B*, effect on errors on day 2 of being intoxicated on day 2; and the *A* by *B* interaction, effect of changed state.
[b]$P < .05$.
[c]$P < .01$.

These results tend to substantiate Storm's finding (4) that learning which the subject acquires while he is intoxicated may be more available to him while he is intoxicated than when he is sober. Conversely, but to a lesser and more variable extent, learning acquired while sober may be more available when sober than when intoxicated. Overton (2) has observed that training often appears to transfer less completely in the direction of drug to nondrug state than in the reverse direction. This asymmetry also was apparent in our findings.

Furthermore certain types of memory appear more sensitive to dissociation than others. The data indicate that simple recall and interference were most clearly influenced by state change, especially where original learning was in the alcohol condition. Picture recognition and latency of response were relatively uninfluenced by state change.

There is evidence that recall of single experiences, where massed practice or "overlearning" is not a factor, may be particularly vulnerable to state change. For example, in Storm's study, subjects were trained to criterion on learning and relearning days. When he used the first relearning trial as a measure of recall, Storm found no tendency for alcohol to enhance recall when original learning was in the alcohol condition. This finding, contrary to ours, may have been due to the overlearning inherent in a training-to-criterion paradigm. Our data suggest that the word-association task, measuring single-trial, "self-generated" learning, may be particularly useful in studying dissociation.

That drinking may facilitate recall of experiences which occurred while previously drinking has support from certain clinical observations. In one study (12), alcoholics frequently reported hiding liquor or money while drinking with no recall of the event until intoxicated again. They also reported difficulty in spontaneously recalling events that happened during a drinking episode and having a return of memory when told about the event. The latter is consistent with our finding that subjects who learned material while intoxicated had difficulty recalling it spontaneously when sober, but, after one relearning trial, performed as well as the other subjects. This suggests that the memory deficit associated with changed state may reflect an impairment of retrieval rather than of registration and retention.

## REFERENCES AND NOTES

1. D. A. Overton, *J. Comp. Physiol. Psychol.* **57**, 3 (1964).
2. D. A. Overton, paper presented at American College of Neuropharmacology Meeting, 12–15 December 1967.
3. L. T. Crow, *Physiol. Behav.* **1**, 89 (1966); D. A. Overton, *Psychopharmacologia* **10**, 6 (1966).
4. T. Storm, W. K. Caird, E. Korbin, in preparation; T. Storm and W. K. Caird, *Psychon. Sci.* **9**, 43 (1967).
5. Breath samples, collected ½ hour after completion of drinking and at the end of each session, were analyzed by the Photoelectric Intoximeter.
6. Interference refers to the detrimental effect on learning a new task of having previously learned a similar task.
7. L. E. Marks and G. A. Miller, *J. Verb. Learn. Verb. Behav.* **3**, 1 (1964).

8. D. S. PALERMO and J. J. JENKINS, *Word Association Norms: Grade School through College* (Univ. of Minnesota Press, Minneapolis, 1964).
9. B. J. WINER, *Statistical Principles in Experimental Design* (McGraw-Hill, New York, 1962). Winer (p. 93) calculates $F_{max}$ by dividing the largest treatment variances by the smallest variances and comparing the results to a table (p. 653).
10. A. L. EDWARDS, *Experimental Design and Psychological Research* (Holt, Rinehart and Winston, New York, 1966), p. 107.
11. The rote-learning task included a relearning session on day 2. After one relearning trial, differences between the groups largely disappeared and, by the third relearning trial, all groups had reached asymptote.
12. D. W. GOODWIN, J. B. CRANE, S. B. GUZE, *Brit. J. Psychol.*, in press.
13. Reduced numbers of observations resulted from mechanical difficulty and subjects becoming too intoxicated to perform the tasks.
14. Supported, in part, by PHS research grants MH-09247 and MH-13002, and training grants MH-07081 and MH-05804.

# 6

## *State-Dependent or "Dissociated" Learning with Alcohol in the Goldfish**

RALPH S. RYBACK

The idea that information learned while under the influence of a drug might not be transferred to the nondrug state was possibly first suggested by Lashley (1) in 1917. He trained rats in a maze after administration of strychnine or caffeine and found that both groups took longer to relearn the maze when tested subsequently without the drug than the undrugged control group. Since then, several investigators (2, 3, 4) have found no transfer of training between the nondrug state and drug states and they named the apparent amnesic effect "dissociation of learning." Response decrements less profound than total loss of the learned response have been reported in several experimental situations (5–8) as a result of the change between the nondrug and drug state. Alcohol has only been used recently in attempts to produce dissociated or state-dependent learning, but the results of different workers have not been the same. Crow (9) demonstrated state-dependent learning with alcohol in avoidance training of rats while Overton (8), using escape from shock in a T-maze, found only partial dissociation of learn-

From the *Quarterly Journal of Studies on Alcohol*, Vol. 30, September 1969, pp. 598–608. Reprinted by permission of the author and publisher.
* From The Alcohol Study Unit, Boston City Hospital and Harvard Medical School. Supported by Grant No. MH-09245-01 from the National Institute of Mental Health.

ing in rats. That the unique attributes of the goldfish might allow resolution of these differences was the hope underlying the present experiment.

Goldfish (*Carassius auratus*) bring several attributes to alcohol research and state-dependent learning with alcohol. As aquatic animals, goldfish can receive alcohol via the water and they actually come into equilibrium with the water-alcohol solution in which they swim within 6 hours. This equilibrium of blood and water alcohol may be expressed as a percentage of the water alcohol concentration. Fish of the size used in maze learning in these experiments reached a mean value of 90.4% at 2.5 hr in 495 mg per 100 ml (w/v) solution; at 6 hr the level had declined to 87% and after 3 days of continuous exposure to water-alcohol solutions of 495 mg per 100 ml, the mean value was 85.8%.[1] Fish of similar size (15 to 20 cm) in a 400 mg per 100 ml solution reached a mean value of 61.7% in 2 hr and 86.3% in 3 hr. At 6 hr the level had declined to 83.6% (10). These findings correspond closely to those of Nicloux (11) who measured the correlation of the alcohol concentration per unit of water in muscles and total bodies of fish with the surrounding water-alcohol solution. He did this in various small freshwater fish after 2 days of immersion in alcohol solutions of 200 to 1000 mg per 100 ml.

Though the goldfish can metabolize alcohol with the alcohol dehydrogenase (ADH) in its liver,[2] it still remains in equilibrium with its environment. The turnover rate of fish-liver ADH is probably very low when compared to that of horse liver or yeast (12). Yet even if the goldfish liver can metabolize ethanol at a rate comparable to man, who can metabolize 10 cc of ethanol per hr (13), it could only metabolize 0.01 cc per hr because the livers from fish of the size used in these experiments weigh only 1.2 to 1.5 g, whereas that of man weighs 1400 to 1500 g (13). Therefore, as soon as the fish removes 0.01 cc of ethanol, it is replaced from the surrounding water-alcohol environment, resulting in a steady-state situation. This is in contradistinction to the rat or mouse, whose very efficient liver removes alcohol from the body much more rapidly than man (14). Consequently, the rise and fall of the blood alcohol curve due to the effect of alcohol absorption and metabolism is avoided and the goldfish can be studied in a steady-state condition. The importance of the latter factor is supported by the findings of Mellanby (15) and Goldberg (16). The latter has suggested that skilled performance may be impaired at a certain level when the blood alcohol curve is rising and not impaired at the same level when the blood-alcohol curve is falling.

The aim of the present study was to demonstrate state-dependent learning with alcohol. The importance of state-dependent learning in alcohol research may be its possible relationship to alcohol amnesia in man and the relative resistance of the alcoholic to the effects of alcohol. The phenomena of state-dependent learning may in the end be explained by the neurophysiologist and neurochemist.

## METHODS

Thirty-two large fish, 15 to 20 cm long, were trained in the winter of 1967–68 in a continuous Y-maze designed by Ingle (17), constructed of three

[1] R. S. Ryback and D. Ingle. Behavioral adaptation to alcohol in goldfish. [Unpublished.]
[2] R. S. Ryback. [Unpublished.]

8-inch arms radiating out from a common junction and ending in a small compartment where the fish can turn around. Fish swim continuously through the arms of the maze and learn to turn in a given direction at the junction in order to avoid bumping into a glass barrier inserted 1.5 inches within the "incorrect" arm. It is assumed that the fish do not avoid the glass barrier through direct visual guidance, since they cannot learn when the glass is randomly interchanged among the arms from trial to trial. The maze problem involved a simple discrimination of direction, e.g., "go right," which was opposite to each subject's spontaneous preference determined the day prior to training by an unimpeded maze run of 30 trials. A criterion of 18 out of 20 correct turns was used. Tables 1 and 3 show the number of trials before the trial which began 18 out of 20 correct trials.

The fish were divided into 4 groups of 8 and trained in the maze daily, up to 50 trials per day, until criterion was obtained. They were then retested the following day for retention in different sequences of alcohol (A) and nonalcohol (N) exposures for a total of 4 possible sequences (AN, NA, AA, NN). All fish trained in alcohol were placed in an alcohol solution of 495 mg per 100 ml for 6 hr and then were trained in a maze filled with a 630 mg per 100 ml solution. Thus the fish first came into equilibrium at the weaker solution and then were trained and tested in the stronger solution, at which time their blood alcohol level was rising slightly. Alcohol solutions of 495 and 630 mg per 100 ml were found to produce minimal sensory loss and motor impairment.

In a second experiment (18), part of which will be reported here, 24 fish of a similar size were divided into 4 groups of 6 and given the different sequences of alcohol and nonalcohol as described above. The conditions differed in that the fish were placed in a 400 mg per 100 ml solution for 2 hr and then trained or tested in the same solution. Testing or training took between 5 and 25 minutes. Therefore, as the blood alcohol is increasing from 61.7% to 86.3% of the surround alcohol solution between 2 and 3 hr after immersion, the fish were trained and tested while their blood alcohol was rising slightly. In addition, the time interval between training and testing or retraining was 3 days rather than 1 day. Finally, 6 additional fish were trained at 400 mg per 100 ml after being in the same solution for 6 hr or when they were in equilibrium with the alcohol solution, and then tested or retrained 3 days later in water (group AAN). Two fish died during the course of the experiment and were discarded.

The alcohol levels of the latter experiments had been determined in a third experiment: 16 medium goldfish, 10 to 15 cm long, divided into 2 groups of 8, were kept in alcohol solutions of 400 and 700 mg per 100 ml and observed for 14 and 7 days, respectively; and 4 fish of similar size were placed in a 1000 mg per 100 ml solution.

## RESULTS

Fish trained and retrained under the same conditions (AA, NN) showed good retention of the maze habit, while fish retrained under a different condition (AN, NA) did not (Table 1). Only two subjects (No. 1 and 13) in groups NA and AN performed better, while all animals in groups NN and AA improved.

TABLE 1. **Trials to Criterion in Y-Maze of 32 Goldfish**

| | *NA* | | | *AN* | | | *NN* | | | *AA* | |
|---|---|---|---|---|---|---|---|---|---|---|---|
| *No.* | *Water* | *Alc.* | *No.* | *Alc.* | *Water* | *No.* | *Water* | *Water* | *No.* | *Alc.* | *Alc.* |
| 1 | 34 | 9 | 9 | 39 | 19 | 17 | 19 | 3 | 25 | 38 | 0 |
| 2 | 21 | 172 | 10 | 72 | 18 | 18 | 25 | 4 | 26 | 46 | 0 |
| 3 | 18 | 100 | 11 | 105 | 28 | 19 | 17 | 6 | 27 | 160 | 10 |
| 4 | 6 | 76 | 12 | 109 | 42 | 20 | 23 | 0 | 28 | 94 | 0 |
| 5 | 13 | 17 | 13 | 62 | 0 | 21 | 9 | 1 | 29 | 106 | 4 |
| 6 | 14 | 110 | 14 | 46 | 31 | 22 | 27 | 3 | 30 | 59 | 3 |
| 7 | 26 | 49 | 15 | 85 | 28 | 23 | 11 | 0 | 31 | 72 | 6 |
| 8 | 8 | 42 | 16 | 49 | 30 | 24 | 15 | 4 | 32 | 43 | 2 |
| *Mean* | *17.5* | *72* | | *70.8* | *24.5* | | *18.3* | *2.6* | | *77* | *3.1* |

Fish were trained in water (N) or alcohol solution (A), then tested the following day in alcohol solution (NA, AA) or water (AN, NN).

An analysis of variance of the basic 2×2 factorial design of the alcohol effects in training and testing appears in Table 2. Difference scores of each animal's total trials to criterion in the two sessions were compared in each of the four groups. The results of the analysis indicate that alcohol (AN, AA) during training sessions significantly impaired learning, but the effects of alcohol during testing sessions were dependent on the presence or absence of alcohol during the training sessions. This latter finding is indicated by the absence of significant main effects of alcohol during testing with significant interaction effects. It should be also noted that, unlike Crow's findings (9), in the first experiment alcohol did not facilitate performance in the testing situation.

In the second experiment (Table 3) subjects showed poor retention of the maze habit when going from alcohol to nonalcohol (AN), but showed good retention of learning in the other three conditions (NA, AA, NN) as Crow (9) found in rats. Differing from Crow's study, however, alcohol was found to facilitate performance only slightly in both the training and testing situation.

An analysis of variance (Table 4) of the same type as in Table 2 obtained significant *F* ratios indicating that the presence of alcohol during either the training ($p < .05$) or testing ($p < .05$) stimulated training and retraining or testing. That the effects of alcohol during the testing sessions were dependent on the presence or absence of alcohol during the training sessions is indicated by the significant interaction effects ($p < .001$). This is seen in the means (Table 3) of group AN with alcohol (10.16) to water (21.8) and group AA with water (17.6) to alcohol (3).

The six fish of group AAN, trained in 400 mg of alcohol per 100 ml after

TABLE 2. **Analysis of Variance of Difference Scores from Training to Testing Situations**

| *Source* | *df* | *MS* | *F* |
|---|---|---|---|
| Alcohol in training | 1 | 51,280 | 43.49[a] |
| Alcohol in testing | 1 | 3507 | 2.97 |
| Interaction | 1 | 19,454 | 16.50[a] |
| Within | 28 | 1184 | |

[a]Significant at the .001 level.

**TABLE 3. Trials to Criterion in Y-Maze of 30 Goldfish**

| *NA* | | | *AN* | | | *NN* | | | *AA* | | | *AAN* | | |
|---|---|---|---|---|---|---|---|---|---|---|---|---|---|---|
| *No.* | *Water* | *Alc.* | *No.* | *Alc.* | *Water* | *No.* | *Water* | *Water* | *No.* | *Alc.* | *Alc.* | *No.* | *Alc.* | *Water* |
| 1 | 27 | 0 | 7 | 27 | 18 | 13 | 25 | 3 | 19 | 14 | 11 | 25 | 3 | 0 |
| 2 | 21 | 11 | 8 | 5 | 23 | 14 | 33 | 6 | 20 | 37 | 4 | 26 | 31 | 10 |
| 3 | 15 | 0 | 9 | 0 | 3 | 15 | 24 | 3 | 21 | 35 | 0 | 27 | 5 | 0 |
| 4 | 28 | 0 | 10 | 5 | 25 | 16 | 27 | 33 | 22 | 10 | 15 | 28 | 10 | 0 |
| 5 | 3 | 3 | 11 | 17 | 35 | 17 | 68 | 9 | 23 | 39 | 0 | 29 | 21 | 0 |
| 6 | 12 | 4 | 12 | 8 | 27 | 18 | 7 | 5 | 24 | 16 | 0 | 30 | 24 | 13 |
| *Mean* | *17.6* | *3* | | *10.16* | *21.8* | | *30.7* | *9.8* | | *25.16* | *5* | | *15.7* | *3.9* |

Fish were trained in water (N) or after 2 hr in alcohol solution (A), then tested 3 days later in alcohol solution (NA, AA) or water (AN, NN). Group AAN was trained in alcohol solution after being in the same solution for 6 hr, then tested 3 days later in water.

6 hr in the same solution when their blood alcohol was in equilibrium with the water-alcohol solution showed good retention of learning when they were retained 3 days later in water (Table 3).

The eight fish kept for 14 days in 400 mg of alcohol per 100 ml showed no obviously abnormal behavior except a temporary failure to eat during most of the first day and a mild temporary excitement lasting 2 to 3 hr.

The eight subjects in 700 mg per 100 ml, however, passed from initial excitement to sluggishness. They swam in an ataxic manner, bumped into the walls and into one another. Furthermore, they showed a delayed avoidance response to a threatening visual stimulus moved suddenly toward one eye. When they did resume attempts to eat food pellets they displayed a consistent habit of spitting food out after each successful attempt to suck it in.

The four subjects in 1000 mg per 100 ml displayed more strongly that which was seen at 700 mg per 100 ml and all died within 48 hr.

## DISCUSSION

Crow (9), using rats in conditioned avoidance response training, found no improvement in performance or transfer of learning when going from alcohol to nonalcohol (AN) sessions and some improvement in performance or transfer of learning going from nonalcohol to alcohol (NA) solutions. He interpreted his results as suggesting that alcohol facilitated performance in the testing sessions. Crow did not find true state-dependent learning in that he found dissociation only in one direction (AN) and not the other (NA). Yet at high levels of alcohol one cannot exclude the debilitating effects of alcohol on performance by in part causing what is found in Group NA (Table 1).

**TABLE 4. Analysis of Variance of Difference Scores from Training to Testing Situations**

| *Source* | *df* | *MS* | *F* |
|---|---|---|---|
| Alcohol in training | 1 | 1093.5 | 3.96[a] |
| Alcohol in testing | 1 | 988.0 | 3.58[a] |
| Interaction | 1 | 2166 | 7.85[b] |
| Within | 20 | 276.6 | |

[a]Significant at the .05 level of confidence (one-tail).
[b]Significant at the .001 level of confidence (one-tail).

In the first study no transfer of learning was found between the alcohol and the nonalcohol sessions (AN) or the reverse (NA), and alcohol did not facilitate performance in either the testing or training session. The difference may be dose dependent (16), but Crow (9) did not report blood alcohol levels. Indeed, facilitation of learning conditioned avoidance responses in the rat has been found at low alcohol doses (19). Accordingly, it is not surprising that in the second experiment, with lower alcohol levels, the results are similar to those of Crow. Nevertheless, the importance of state-dependent learning with alcohol may be its implications for alcoholic amnesia in man and the relative resistance of the alcoholic to the effects of alcohol. Storm and Smart (20), in a commentary, have attempted to explain alcoholismic behavior and alcoholic blackouts in terms of what they called the "dissociation hypothesis" and some evidence supporting the hypothesis has been reported by Storm and Caird (21).

Human alcoholic amnesia has often been interpreted in psychodynamic terms (22) rather than as a neural inhibition as understood by the neurophysiologist (23) or inhibition of protein synthesis as understood by the neurochemist (24, 25). The relationship between alcohol and amnesia has been viewed as (*1*) reduction of tension, alertness or motivation, (*2*) escape from self and (*3*) expression of dissociated impulses (26). However, the data presented here indicate that indeed there may be a neurophysiological or neurochemical basis for alcoholic amnesia, as fish have little "repression" in the psychodynamic sense of the word.

Learning in man is most strongly affected when the blood alcohol curve is rising (15, 16), yet state-dependent learning in fish is readily produced at this time. Indeed, dissociation of learning in group AN at 400 mg per 100 ml was not produced after the fish had come into equilibrium with the alcohol solution. However, one could argue that adaptation had taken place after 6 hr or that the blood alcohol level was not exactly the same as at 2 hr. Yet it is possible that state dependency with alcohol is more closely related to the rate of change of the alcohol level than just to the level of the brain-blood-alcohol alone. Accordingly, it is of interest that alcoholic amnesia in man is generally accepted as occurring after the first three or four drinks. Indeed, state-dependent learning may have some relationship to the early phase of alcoholic amnesia or the "grayout," but not to the total "blackout" per se, as Storm and Smart (20) suggested. I view the major part of the blackout as a retrograde amnesia[3] due to inhibition of memory formation. This disruption of memory formation may be secondary to acutely high alcohol levels, brain amine or catecholamine release, subclinical seizure activity, hypoglycemia, anoxia, etc. That is, there are certain blackouts in which the events occurring in the drunken state could not be recalled even if the same state was again imposed. Furthermore, a simplistic view of memory suggests at least two steps: One, that memory be laid down, and two, that it be made "permanent." High levels of alcohol or acute change in alcohol level could interfere with either, perhaps directly or through an intermediary process or processes. Fish cannot learn a simple maze problem at levels over 750 mg per 100 ml and it is obvious that there are comparable levels for humans with comparable tasks.

Storm and Smart (20) also suggested that the larger the dosages reached, the greater the dissociation. This seems plausible in view of the second experiment

[3] Or more specifically, a short-term memory deficit.

in which performance actually increased under lower levels of alcohol (400 mg per 100 ml) while dissociation occurred only when going from alcohol to water (AN) and not when going from water to alcohol (NA).

State-dependent learning may also offer an explanation of why the degree of impairment of several tests at the same blood levels decreased in the order: abstemious > moderate drinkers > heavy drinkers (16). Perhaps the alcoholic has learned to function in the intoxicated state and is able to retrieve necessary information from his central nervous system when the same state is again imposed, while the abstemious or moderate drinker must adapt to the unfamiliar intoxication. It is therefore not surprising that impairment in function is not found until almost toxic doses are given to the alcoholic (27). Furthermore, Mendelson (28) has recently reported that there is no significant difference in the ability of the alcoholic and the nonalcoholic to metabolize alcohol. Nevertheless, for the alcoholic and nonalcoholic, the idea of being able to put oneself in another state may indeed have a seductive appeal.

## REFERENCES

1. Lashley, K. S. The effect of strychnine and caffeine upon rate of learning. *Psychobiology* **1**: 141–170, 1917.
2. Girden, E., and Culler, E. A. Conditioned responses in curarized striate muscle in dogs. *J. comp. Psychol.* **23**: 261–274, 1937.
3. Gardner, L., and McCullogh, C. A. A reinvestigation of the dissociative effect of curareform drugs. *Amer. Psychologist* **17**: 398, 1962.
4. Overton, D. A. State-dependent or "dissociated" learning produced with pentobarbital. *J. comp. physiol. Psychol.* **57**: 3–12, 1964.
5. Sachs, E., Weingarten, M., and Klein, N. W., Jr. Effects of chlordiazepoxide on the acquisition of avoidance learning and its transfer to the normal state and to other drug conditions. *Psychopharmacologia,* Berl. **9**: 17–30, 1966.
6. Otis, L. S. Dissociation and recovery of a response learned under the influence of chlorpromazine or saline. *Science* **143**: 1347–1348, 1964.
7. Belleville, R. E. Control of behavior by drug-produced internal stimuli. *Psychopharmacologia,* Berl. **5**: 95–105, 1964.
8. Overton, D. A. State-dependent learning produced by depressant and atropinelike drugs. *Psychopharmacologia,* Berl. **10**: 6–31, 1966.
9. Crow, L. T. Effects of alcohol on conditioned avoidance responding. *Physiol. & Behav.,* N.Y. **1**: 89–91, 1966.
10. Ryback, R. S., Percarpio, B., and Vitale, J. Equilibration and metabolism of ethanol in the goldfish. *Nature,* Lond. **222**: 1068–1070, 1969.
11. Nicloux, M. L'eau des tissus: Possibilité de mettre en évidence une eau imperméable à l'alcool éthylique; sa fixation par les protéides; sa mesure, ses variations. *Bull. Soc. Chim. biol.,* Paris **16**: 822–864, 1934.
12. Boeri, E., Bonnichsen, R. K., and Tosi, L. Alcohol dehydrogenase from fish liver. *Publ. Staz. zool. Napoli* **25**: 427–437, 1954.
13. Robbins, S. L. Textbook of pathology. 2d ed. Philadelphia; Saunders; 1962.
14. Widmark, E. M. P. Die theoretischen Grundlagen und die praktische Ver-

wendbarkeit der gerichtlich-medizinischen Alkoholbestimmung. *Fortschr. naturw. Forsch.*, No. 11, 1932.

15. MELLANBY, E. Alcohol; its absorption into and disappearance from the blood under different conditions. (Medical Research Committee, Special Report Series No. 31.) London; H.M. Stat. Off.; 1919.
16. GOLDBERG, L. Quantitative studies on alcohol tolerance in man: The influence of ethyl alcohol on sensory, motor and psychological functions referred to blood alcohol in normal and habituated individuals. *Acta physiol. Scand.* **5** (Suppl. 16): 7–128, 1943.
17. INGLE, D. The use of fish in neuropsychology. *Perspectives Biol. Med.* 8: 241–260, 1965.
18. RYBACK, R. The use of goldfish as a model for alcohol amnesia in man. *Quart. J. Stud. Alc.* **30**: 598–608, 1969.
19. REYNOLDS, G. S., and VAN SOMMERS, P. Effects of ethyl alcohol on avoidance behavior. *Science* **132**: 42–43, 1960.
20. STORM, T., and SMART, R. Dissociation; a possible explanation of some features of alcoholism, and implication for its treatment. *Quart J. Stud. Alc.* **26**: 111–115, 1965.
21. STORM, T., and CAIRD, W. K. The effects of alcohol on serial verbal learning in chronic alcoholics. *Psychonom. Sci.* **9**: 43–44, 1967.
22. DIETHELM, O., and BARR, R. Psychotherapeutic interviews and alcohol intoxication. *Quart. J. Stud. Alc.* **23**: 243–251, 1962.
23. BRAZIER, M. A. B. The action of anesthetics on the nervous system. In: ADRIAN, E. D., BREMER, F., and JASPER, H. H., eds. *Brain mechanisms and consciousness.* Oxford; Blackwell; 1954.
24. LAJTHA, A. Alteration and pathology of cerebral protein metabolism. *Int. Rev. Neurobiol.* 7: 40, 1964.
25. AGRANOFF, B. W., DAVIS, R. E., CASOLA, L., and LIM, R. Actinomycin D blocks formation of memory of shock-avoidance in goldfish. *Science* **158**: 1600–1601, 1967.
26. WASHBURNE, C. Alcohol, amnesia and awareness. *Quart. J. Stud. Alc.* **19**: 471–481, 1958.
27. TALLAND, G. A., MENDELSON, J. H., and RYACK, P. Experimentally induced chronic intoxication and withdrawal in alcoholics. *Pt. 4.* Tests of motor skills. *Quart. J. Stud. Alc.*, Suppl. No. 2, pp. 53–73, 1964.
28. MENDELSON, J. H. Ethanol-1-$C^{14}$ metabolism in alcoholics and nonalcoholics. *Science* **159**: 319–320, 1968.

# 7

# Discriminated Aversive Control in the Moderation of Alcoholics' Drinking Behavior*

S. H. LOVIBOND and G. CADDY

In the field of treatment of alcoholism, it is assumed almost universally that the alcoholic can never become a controlled or social drinker. Consequently, the usual goal of treatment is total abstinence. In the treatment to be described, however, the therapeutic goal is to train the alcoholic to drink in moderation.

The treatment procedure consists essentially of two phases. In the first phase, the subject is trained to discriminate his own blood alcohol concentration (BAC) within the range zero to 0.08%. In the second, or aversive conditioning phase, the consumption of alcohol is followed by strong electric shock if the subject's BAC is above 0.065%,[1] but is allowed to occur with impunity if the BAC is below this value.

## METHOD

### Discrimination Training

At the beginning of discrimination training, the subject is provided with a very general scale of the behavioral effects which typically accompany different BACs. For example, he is told that at a BAC of about 0.04–.05%, drinkers usually experience the first feelings of warmth and relaxation, and that between 0.05 and 0.08% they become aware of a progressive loss of social inhibitions. The subject is then asked to consume pure alcohol in fruit juice, and to examine his subjective experience and behavior as a basis for estimating his BAC. Every 15–20 min a Breathalyzer reading is taken, and the subject is required to make an estimate of his BAC. Immediately an estimate is given, the subject's actual BAC is fed back to him in the form of an adjustment to the reading of a large meter in front of him. Each time a BAC is presented to the subject, he is encouraged to associate his present subjective state with the meter reading and to construct his own BAC symptom scale.

From *Behavior Therapy*, Vol. 1, 1970, pp. 437–444. 

* This investigation was supported by Research Grant 65/15863 from the Australian Research Grants Committee. The authors wish to express their gratitude to Tooheys Ltd. who supplied a Breathalyzer unit and alcoholic beverages, and Penfold Wines Pty. Ltd. who also supplied alcoholic beverages.

[1] A BAC of 0.065% represents a concentration of ethanol in the blood of 65 mg/100 ml of blood volume, and is the approximate level typically reached when 2–3 double martinis are consumed within an hour at a cocktail party.

During discrimination training a personal history is obtained, and the subject is given a detailed account of the nature and aims of the treatment procedure to follow. A training session lasts 1½–2 hr, during which time the subject's BAC rises to about 0.08% and then declines. One training session only is given prior to conditioning.

## Conditioning Procedure

During the conditioning or treatment phase, a 1½-in. square stainless-steel shock electrode is attached by adhesive tape to a point approximately 1 in. below chin level, and a similar electrode is positioned on various areas of the face and neck. The subject is required to drink his preferred alcoholic beverage at a steady rate designed to raise his BAC to 0.065% in approximately 1½ hr. As in the first phase, estimates of BAC are required every 15–20 min, followed by feedback of actual BAC on the meter. The subject is told that he may drink with impunity as long as his BAC remains below 0.065%, the "red-line" on the meter. As soon as his BAC rises above this value, however, he must expect to be shocked when he drinks. The subject is required to continue drinking after the BAC reaches 0.065%, and shocks are administered according to a prearranged schedule. The shock schedule is designed to maximize uncertainty (Lovibond, 1968, 1970[a]). First, drinking is shocked on only 80% of occasions, and, on nonshock trials, the subject is allowed to swallow a small quantity of alcohol. Second, the duration of the shock is varied from 1–6 sec. Third, shock intensity is varied from intense to very intense (4–7 mA). Fourth, the point in the drinking sequence when the shock occurs is varied from trial to trial. Occasionally, the shock occurs when the subject picks up his glass, but on most trials the shock is delayed until the subject is in the act of swallowing the alcohol.

The treatment is conducted on an outpatient basis, and the subject is encouraged to pursue his normal occupation and social activities.

The first three sessions are spaced approximately 5–7 days apart, and some 8–10 shocks are administered if the subject can tolerate this number. The duration of the conditioning sessions is approximately 2 hr. Later sessions are spaced more widely, and the number of shocks per session is reduced to 3–4. After some 6–12 sessions and 30–70 shocks, depending on the progress of the subject, treatment is discontinued.

When possible, a member of the subject's family attends at least some of the treatment sessions, and the importance of the supporting role of the family member is stressed. The involvement of a family member also enables a check to be made on the subject's reports concerning his drinking behavior.

Throughout the program, the subject is treated as a person with a particular problem, and a set of associated problems, to be overcome. It is pointed out to the subject that the treatment alone cannot ensure control of his drinking behavior. He is told that the purpose of the treatment is to provide him with an inbuilt stop mechanism which will assist his own efforts at self-control. His self-control, however, is ultimately decisive. In short, the general therapeutic goal is to assist the subject to regain self-respect by exerting the self-control necessary to maintain a pattern of moderate social drinking.

## Control Procedure

As a control procedure, a group of subjects has been given a period of treatment identical to that of the experimental subjects, except for the removal of the contingencies between the shock and BAC and drinking behavior. Control subjects receive initial training in BAC discrimination, the support of a family member, and self-control instructions. In the conditioning sessions they drink the same amount of alcohol as experimental subjects, and receive equivalent shocks. The shocks begin, however, before the BAC reaches 0.065%, and thereafter occur at random intervals, with the restriction that no shock is given during the 2-min period prior to drinking, or the 3-min period after drinking. The control subjects receive random shocks during the first three conditioning sessions only. In the remaining sessions, shocks are made contingent on BAC and drinking as in the case of experimental subjects.

## Apparatus

Blood alcohol concentration is measured by a Breathalyzer Model 900. (It is unlikely that the high degree of precision of this instrument is essential to the treatment process, and the possibility of developing a cheaper instrument of sufficient precision deserves investigation.)

A modified milliammeter with an 8-in. dial is used to feed back actual BACs to the subject. The milliammeter scale is replaced by a BAC scale reading from zero to 0.10%, with a red band extending from 0.065–0.10%. The meter is in circuit with dry cells and a potentiometer under the manual control of the experimenter.

The stimulator in current use is a Grason Stadler Model E1064 modified to give an output of 7 mA. (As there is no evidence to suggest that type of shock is an important variable in the present type of therapy, any AC stimulator with the necessary output should be equally satisfactory.)

## Subjects

The only criteria used for selection of subjects have been willingness to accept the electric shocks and absence of obvious psychoticism. Only one volunteer has so far been refused entry into the program. To date 44 subjects, with an age range of 22–56 years, have been accepted. Of this number, 31 (25 males and six females) have been allocated to the treatment group, and 13 (10 males and three females) have been selected at random for control treatment.

Some subjects were referred by general medical practitioners or psychiatric hospitals, but most were self-referred after publicity given the project by the news media. On the average, subjects were found to have had a history of alcoholism extending over a period of 10 years prior to acceptance, and most had been hospitalized for alcoholism on numerous occasions. Many subjects were found to have additional psychological problems, such as depression and character disorder.

Twenty-eight of the 31 treatment subjects have completed the full treatment course. Three subjects failed to return after the first or second session. Five of the 13 control subjects have completed the three sessions of the control treatment procedure. Three control subjects dropped out after the first session, and a further five did not return after the second session.

Follow-up information has been obtained from all subjects at regular intervals since treatment. Contact has been maintained by telephone and occasional interviews. In all cases, subjects' reports have been corroborated by a member of the family or other informant, e.g., foreman or employer. The follow-up period has extended over 16–60 weeks.

## RESULTS AND DISCUSSION

It has been found that most nonalcoholics and alcoholics can learn to estimate their BACs with a high degree of accuracy. After a single training session, errors in excess of ± 0.01% rarely occur (Lovibond, 1970 [b]). Most subjects are able to find symptoms corresponding to different BACs, particularly when the BAC is rising. For example, a subject may note that, at about the 0.03% concentration, the skin on his cheeks tightens slightly, and at 0.06%; his ears seem to pop.

Table 1 presents a summary of treatment outcome derived from follow-up data obtained from the 28 experimental subjects who have completed treatment. Twenty-one of the 28 subjects are regarded tentatively as complete successes in that they are drinking in a controlled fashion, and exceeding the 0.07% BAC only rarely. Three subjects have been categorized as considerably improved. These subjects are drinking considerably less, but are still exceeding a BAC of 0.07% once or twice per week. Four subjects are considered to be only slightly improved. They are not getting drunk as often as before, but they are drinking only a little less than previously, and they are not at all satisfied with their progress.

Figure 1 shows the mean weekly alcohol intake of experimental and control subjects before treatment, during treatment, and at follow-up. It can be seen that in the experimental group there is a marked drop in alcohol intake after the first treatment session. There is a suggestion of a slow recovery in alcohol intake subsequent to treatment, but the intake means in the later stages of follow-up are based on very small numbers. It should be noted also that the mean intake of the three subjects who have been followed for 50 weeks is not in excess of the weekly alcohol consumption of the average Australian drinker (Rankin, 1970; Sargent, 1968). The alcohol consumption of the control subjects also drops sharply during the initial period of control treatment. Unlike the experimental subjects, however, the controls rapidly return to intakes approaching their pre-treatment levels. The divergence between the two groups is such that by the end of the third week of treatment, the intake of control subjects is significantly higher than that of the

**TABLE 1. Outcome of Completed Treatment of 28 Experimental Subjects**

| *Category* | *Definition* | *No. of Cases* |
|---|---|---|
| Complete success | Drinking in controlled fashion, exceeding 0.07 only rarely | 21 |
| Considerably improved | Drinking less but exceeding 0.07 once or twice per week | 3 |
| Slightly improved | Drinking only slightly less | 4 |

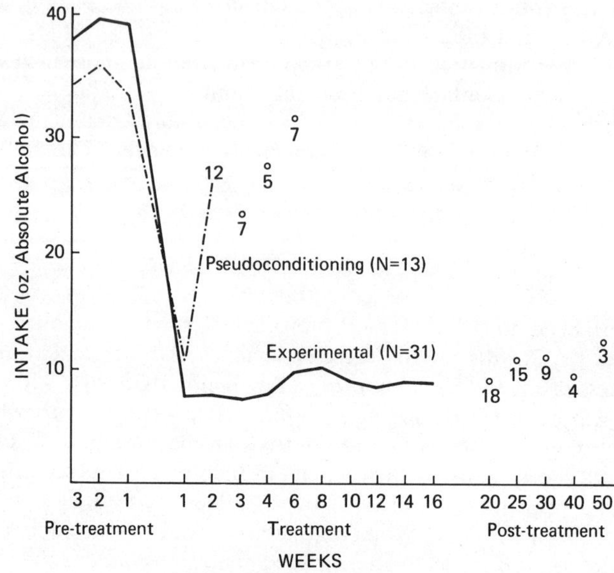


**Figure 1** Mean weekly alcohol intake, expressed in ounces of pure alcohol, of experimental and control subjects before, during, and after treatment. (Numbers by data points indicate reduced number of subjects at those points.)

experimentals (Mann–Whitney $U = 192.5$, $z = 3.169$, $p < .008$). (Subjects who dropped out during the first 3 weeks of treatment were followed whenever possible, and the data from these subjects are included in the graph.)

The dropout rates of the experimentals (10%) and controls (61%) after the second session also differ significantly ($X^2 = 13.14$, $df = p < .001$).

It seems likely that the control group's initial reduction in alcohol intake is largely a function of commitment to treatment, but some generalized effect of the shock might also be present. It seems probable also, that a substantial dropout rate will continue to be observed in the control subjects, because these subjects fail to detect any substantial benefits from the treatment. By contrast, the treatment subjects are positively reinforced by observing the therapeutic effects of the first treatment session, and this feedback seems to be sufficient to sustain most subjects through the highly unpleasant treatment procedure. It is in order to maximize the subject's perception of immediate therapeutic benefit that as many shocks as the subject can tolerate are administered in the first treatment session.

Figure 2 shows the estimated mean number of times subjects' BACs have exceeded 0.07%, before, during, and after treatment. In general, the changes occurring in this measure are similar to those observed in the measure of weekly intake of alcohol, with a significant difference between the two groups emerging by the end of the third week of the program (Mann–Whitney $U = 163.5$, $z = 3.70$, $p < .0001$).

It should be noted that in the experimental group there is typically a sharp difference between the pre- and post-treatment episodes of drinking in excess of

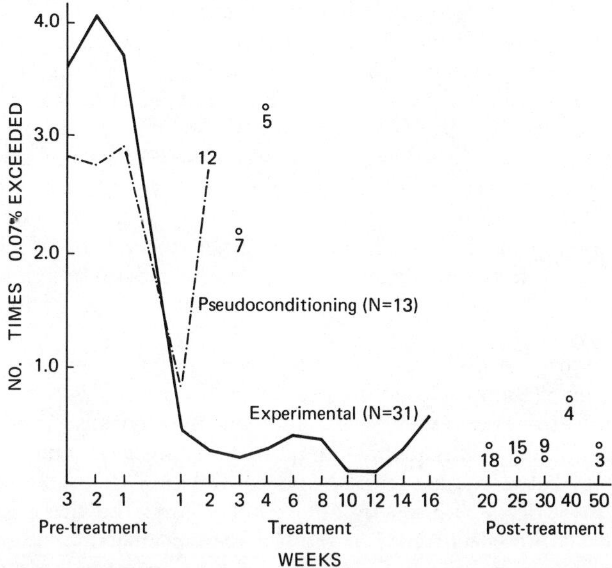


**Figure 2** Mean number of times per week subject's blood alcohol concentration has exceeded 0.07% before, during, and after treatment. (Numbers by data points indicate reduced numbers of subjects at those points.)

0.07%. Unlike those prior to treatment, post-treatment episodes rarely involve levels much higher than 0.07%, and, in addition, they are of short duration.

In addition to the reduction in alcohol intake, there has been a dramatic improvement in the general health, well-being, and self-respect of most subjects in the experimental group. Perhaps the most interesting change observed, however, has been in the desire to drink. It is usually believed that conditioning treatment of alcoholism produces its effect by developing in the subject a conditioned aversion to alcohol, and indeed, when the present work was begun, the aim was to produce a discriminated conditioned aversion. In other words, an attempt was made to render drinking aversive, if, and only if, the BAC was above 0.065% It has been found, however, that a marked conditioned aversion develops in only about 20% of the subjects. The more common outcome is simply a loss of desire to continue drinking beyond three or four glasses, with little evidence of a conditioned aversive reaction. In other words, the treatment typically produces a motivational change rather than merely a conditioned fear reaction. Although the control subjects report some loss of desire to drink, the change in the treatment subjects is much more dramatic.

It is clear that a much longer follow-up period is required to evaluate fully the therapeutic procedure outlined. It can be argued, however, that there are good reasons for optimism regarding the outcome of long-term follow-up. First, in other areas of behavior therapy it has been found that the majority of relapses occur rather early, so that it is possible to estimate the ultimate relapse rate from the number of early relapses. Second, the emphasis placed throughout on self-control means that the subject is not passively relying on a conditioning mechanism, but has an active participatory role in limiting his consumption of alcohol. Consequently, his ability to maintain a pattern of controlled drinking is inherently reinforcing. Third, it is emphasized to the subject during treatment, that it is quite normal to exceed a BAC of 0.06% occasionally. Consequently, the patient does not experience a sense of complete therapeutic failure if he occasionally drinks in excess of the 0.06% level. It seems not unreasonable to believe that under these conditions the probability of relapse is reduced.

On the other hand, it is possible to question the validity of the follow-up data obtained. Despite the insistence on corroborative reports from a family member or a close associate, it is conceivable that, in some cases, optimistic reports have been received.

The adequacy of the control procedure used in the present study might also be questioned on the grounds that a therapist with a psychological investment in the outcome treated both experimental subjects and controls. It is difficult to believe, however, that unintentional interpersonal influences could produce outcome differences between experimental and control subjects as marked as those observed. In any case, replication by other workers must be the final arbiter. If replication affirms the effectiveness of the therapeutic program, the obvious next step is to carry out an experimental analysis of the treatment procedure.

In choosing 0.065% as the BAC to be discriminated in training, it was assumed that this concentration would not significantly impair learning capacity, and would not unduly restrict the subsequent use of alcohol as a social relaxant. It is now believed that 0.065% is an unnecessarily liberal training concentration, and in current work the concentration has been lowered to 0.05%.

One of the possible fields of application of the present method is the treatment of problem drinkers who have been convicted of driving under the influence of liquor. It is now well documented that problem drinkers are responsible for a disproportionate share of serious road accidents. Hence, any procedure which reduces the excessive use of alcohol by such persons, particularly the younger ones, will help to reduce the severity of two problems simultaneously—alcoholism and road accidents. It is unlikely that young incipient alcoholics who are convicted of drinking-driving offenses will be willing to undergo treatment aimed at making them total abstainers. On the other hand, treatment designed to moderate the drinking habits of such persons might be an acceptable alternative to the usual statutory punishments for drinking-driving offenses.

Finally, the method would appear to merit a trial in the treatment of other types of positively motivated behavior disorders providing a reduction in the frequency of the behavior in question is an acceptable therapeutic goal.

## REFERENCES

Lovibond, S. H. The aversiveness of uncertainty: an analysis in terms of activation and information theory. *Australian Journal of Psychology*, 1968, **20**, 85–91.

Lovibond, S. H. Aversive control of behavior. *Behavior Therapy*, 1970, **1**, 80–91. (a)

LOVIBOND, S. H. Pure and applied psychology: towards a significant interaction. *Australian Psychologist,* 1970, 5, 120–140. (b)

RANKIN, J. G. The size and nature of the use and misuse of alcohol and drugs in Australia. Paper presented at the 29th International Congress on Alcoholism and Drug Dependence, Sydney, Australia, 1970.

SARGENT, M. J. Heavy drinking and its relation to alcoholism—with special reference to Australia. *Australian and New Zealand Journal of Sociology,* 1968, 4, 146–157.

# 8

## A Behaviorally Oriented Treatment Program for Alcoholism

JOHN F. McBREARTY, MARVIN DICHTER,
ZALMON GARFIELD, GLEN HEATH

In a recent critical review of psychotherapy with alcoholics, Hill and Blane (1967) made the following comment: "We are unable to form any conclusive opinion as to the value of psychotherapeutic methods in the treatment of alcoholism," at least from the point of existent controlled studies. Their review represented an exhaustive coverage of the literature from 1952 through 1963, and their conclusion is similar to that of Voegtlin and Lemere (1942) who reported a review of all studies published between 1909 and 1941 that evaluated any form of treatment for alcoholics. Gerard, Saenger, and Wile (1962) followed up some 399 patients treated in a variety of clinics and found that fewer than 19% were able to maintain a period of abstinence for even one year following treatment. The picture which emerges from even a cursory review of studies of the efficacy of treatment maneuvers with alcoholics is not very optimistic, and the time is at hand for investment of effort in newer ideas, newer approaches to the problem of alcoholism.

The overall concerns and interests here are in the presentation of a program which is based on the application of the principles of behavior modification to the myriad behavioral problems presented by alcoholics. Occurring with increasing frequency on the national and international scene today are numerous demonstrations of the possible efficacy of behaviorally oriented treatment procedures in the alleviation and elimination of maladaptive behaviors (Eysenck, 1960, 1964; Franks, 1964; Ullmann & Krasner, 1965; Krasner & Ullmann, 1965). Such behavioral problem areas as anxiety states, impotence, frigidity, phobias, psychotic

From *Psychological Reports,* Vol. 22, 1968, pp. 287–298. Reprinted by permission of authors and publisher.

manifestations, to mention a few, have been demonstrated to be responsive to behaviorally oriented techniques. While Franks (1966) has already presented an exhaustive survey of the literature in this area, nevertheless some citations seem necessary in order to provide perspective.

Early work in the application of conditioning principles to the problem of alcoholism was initiated by Voegtlin (1940), who used emetine in order to induce an aversive reaction (nausea) following ingestion of alcohol. A number of studies, reviewed by Miller, et al. (1960) followed, using for the most part either apomorphine or emetine as an unconditioned stimulus (UCS) and alcohol as the conditioned stimulus (CS). Earlier, Kantorovich (1930) made use of faradic stimulation as the UCS, pairing this with suggestions of an actual appearance of liquor (CS). Other early workers in the use of a chemical stimulus as a UCS were Thimann (1949a, 1949b), Kant (1945), and Wallerstein et al. (1957). The latter studied the effects of four different treatment approaches to alcoholism and found the conditioning approach to be least effective. Franks (1966), in his review of the work of this early period, concluded that the claims made were virtually impossible to evaluate because of inadequacy in reporting procedures, controls and follow-up.

More recently, the use of pharmacologically based aversive conditioning has seen modifications. For example, Raymond (1964) developed a program which, among other things, allows for a careful determination of "nausea time." Miller and his co-workers (1960) have adapted this procedure for use with groups of Ss. Sanderson, et al. (1962, 1963) in a series of studies have worked with the drug succinylcholine chloride dihydrate in traumatic conditioning. These researchers, following several studies using this methodology, conclude "Using traumatic conditioning as part of a more complete treatment is more promising" (Madill, et al., 1966, p. 505).

Another technique used in aversion therapy is that of faradic stimulation, an example being the work of Hsu (1965). Aversion-Relief Therapy, developed by Thorpe, et al. (1964), involves the use of aversive conditioning and reciprocal inhibition, and while used by Thorpe and associates in dealing with sexual problems, is adaptable to alcoholism, as will be brought out in the program to be presented. Similarly, the work of Cautela (1967), involving the technique of covert sensitization, shows promise as an aversive conditioning method. The aversion here is established by means of fantasy-induced nausea.

The work cited above has for the most part been concerned with aversive conditioning. Aversive conditioning, of course, represents but a single facet of the spectrum of behavioral techniques which could be applied to the problem of alcoholism. To our knowledge, except for this program, no such broadly based behavioral program for treating alcoholics has been established. The Willmar State Hospital group has made suggestions for such a program, but to date nothing very palpable has developed. Our plans and current efforts include, for example, the use of the principles and techniques of an operant ward (Ayllon & Michael, 1959; Krasner & Ullmann, 1965) in treatment of alcoholism; but, except for Narrol's (1967) pilot project, no reports of controlled environments with simulated economies in treating alcoholism have been found. The beginnings of operant analysis of drinking behavior are, however, noted in the work of Mendelson (1964,

1966) and Mello & Mendelson (1965). The suggestions of several writers [Narrol (1967): "An amalgam of operant personality reshaping and aversion therapy might well be an effective combination for coping with alcoholism"; Madill, et al. (1966): "In short, an aversive conditioning therapy could be employed in conjunction with other learning therapies"; Franks (1966): "To this end, McBrearty (1965) has developed a promising program which combines many procedures"] lend credence to the notion that the program outlined here has promise.

## THE RATIONALE OF THE BEHAVIORAL PROGRAM

The distinguishing and unique characteristic of the program is the utilization of a variety of procedures for behavioral modification. The fundamental desideratum is that alcoholism represents a learned behavioral excess the functions of which can be isolated and described and the modification of which will follow the principles of behavior modification. The program here delineated makes use of aversive conditioning, but as will be seen shortly, the distinguishing and unique characteristic is the utilization of a variety of conditioning procedures.

Basic considerations in the approach to this problem are several. For one, the point of view is adopted that the drinking response is only one facet of a complex process which includes a series of closely linked or chained antedating responses that are essential to the appearance of the culminating event, *viz.*, drinking. It is further maintained that the efficiency of any treatment maneuvers will be directly a function of the degree to which not only the consummatory response (drinking) is interfered with but also the degree to which the fractional antedating responses are successfully manipulated or corrected. One of the difficulties here, of course, is in determining the crucial elements in the behavioral chain; and identifying these elements involves considerable efforts in behavioral monitoring, i.e., observing and discovering the important functional components of the response sequence that leads to drinking alcohol.

The behavioral excess of alcoholism, defined, following Kanfer and Saslow (1965) in terms of its frequency, intensity, and duration, is manifestly the problem and is quite likely maintained because of its consequences. Its continuation, once the sequence has started and continued to the point of inebriation and "hangover" effects, is apparently a function of immediately positive reinforcing effects, i.e., certain discomforting or aversive physiological effects are alleviated; thus the "eye-opener" or "hair-of-the-dog" phenomena. Closer scrutiny of the behavioral process, i.e., monitoring for functional components, however, leads to the suggestion that other behavioral excesses and deficits occur as antedating responses. One example of such a behavioral excess is anxiety, which is defined as a painful emotional experience which the person will attempt to avoid or escape. For instance, we observed in some of our male alcoholic patients that an anxiety reaction was a response to heterosexual stimulation, and consumption of alcohol resulted in alleviation of the anxiety and consequent sexual response. Treatment maneuvers, therefore, would call for interruption of alcohol as a positive reinforcing stimulus, and manipulation of events antecedent to the alcohol response, i.e., eliminating the anxiety. Following the example, with the alleviation of anxiety the male alcoholic could then work toward the development of a repertoire of behaviors which would lead to effective sexual experiences in the absence of alcohol.

Another important consideration concerns the point that adequate monitoring requires that the situation under observation resemble as closely as possible in essential detail, the usual drinking situation; and such a consideration makes it mandatory that alcohol be available in the relearning situation.

A fourth consideration involves the point of view that alcohol drinking behavior is maintained in part by virtue of the consequences of the behavior. While it may be difficult to come to a consensus as to the specific consequences of drinking behavior, or at least those which serve to maintain the behavior, nevertheless, there is a sufficient body of information from psychology to warrant presuming that this is the case with the alcohol drinking response. Whatever these consequences may be, it seems obvious that the stimulus of alcohol cannot be characterized as aversive, or at least it is not effectively or immediately aversive. If this reasoning is correct, the application of an aversive-relief technique for modifying the drinking response is indicated. In essence this would involve the use of an aversive stimulus presented simultaneously with the ingestion of alcohol, so that the latter may take on the aversive qualities of the former. Such a juxtaposition of stimuli would lead to a state where alcohol would result in immediately aversive consequences and thus would be avoided; and the avoidance behavior would be associated with relief and thus because of positive consequences the avoidance behavior would be strengthened.

Another consideration is the choice of the aversive stimulus. To date most of the aversion therapy reported in the literature has made use of a chemical stimulus, with perhaps the use of nausea-producing drugs in the treatment of alcoholism as the best example. While Voegtlin and Lemere (1942) report a 51% abstinence rate with their patients, several other investigators have seriously challenged the effectiveness of apomorphine and emetine hydrochloride in aversion therapy. More recently there is increased stress being placed on the use of electrical stimulation as an unconditioned stimulus in aversion therapy, and it is thought that many of the disadvantages of drugs are eliminated (e.g., temporal interval between the stimulus being presented and the nausea being produced is uncertain; the patient may not even feel nausea). For these reasons, therefore, it is intended to use electric shock (non-convulsive) as the aversive stimulus.

It might be argued that the association of shock with direct and immediate ingestion of alcohol is utilizing a rather trivial noxious stimulus when compared to the often catastrophic events in real life which result from alcoholism, e.g., loss of home, family, job, etc. Our point here is that these "real life" effects have questionable efficacy as being functionally related to drinking alcohol. In the eyes of many they seem related to "alcoholism," but our aim here is bringing the effects (shock) of drinking into closer temporal relationship with the immediate drinking response. It is our contention that "loss of home" is rather remote in time to operate as an aversive consequence for drinking.

In similar fashion, one may question our supposition that alcohol serves to reduce anxiety, and recent findings (Mendelson, 1964) seem to suggest the contrary. Actually, the anxiety construct is not crucial to our thinking, our major emphasis being to remain close to empirical relationships. We certainly have considerable reservations about uncritical acceptance of the hypothesis that alcohol neutralizes anxiety, a point of view attributed to psychiatrists by Mendelson and Stein (Mendelson, 1966, p. 13). On the other hand, recent findings (Boe & Church, 1966) from comparative research, in contrast to the early findings of Skinner (1938) and Estes (1944), suggest that shock leads to a permanent reduction in responses during extinction training. Further, we find most interesting Mendelson's observation (1964, p. 49) that the alcoholic is correct in perceiving that alcohol permits him to operate more efficiently and effectively in a variety of social and cognitive tasks. Our aim would be in the interruption of this process by establishing alcohol as an aversive event to which avoidance behavior is established, and it is here that alternate modes of behavior can be learned in order to achieve the same degree of efficiency and effectiveness without the intervening event of alcohol intake. Our position, therefore, is that anxiety is as much in need of research as the data for which it is used as an explanatory principle. We might also indicate that polygraphic studies are planned in the near future that will address themselves to operationalize the concept of anxiety and its role, if any, as an explanatory concept in the treatment process.

While it may appear up to this point that aversive techniques alone are dictated by our reasoning, such is not the case. It should be recalled that the view here is that the drinking behavior is but a facet of a complex process which includes antedating responses that are tied to the consummatory (drinking) behavior. We would say, therefore, that our approach to interruption of this behavior would be a *broad band* or *broad spectrum* approach, focusing not only on the specific target behavior of drinking excess, but also those behaviors or conditions which represent fractional components of a complex series. To illustrate what is meant by a broad spectrum approach, the following work with an alcoholic patient can be cited. In monitoring the drinking behavior of this patient it was noted that the frequency and intensity of the drinking increased in situations (stimulus complex) involving travel and sexual stimulation. Depending upon other considerations, e.g., problem-solving ability and tolerance for frustration, one might choose to block off (make lower in the hierarchy of probable responses) the alcohol drinking response by use of aversive conditioning; but when a primary drive such as sex is concerned, i.e., intimately tied in the chain of responses, working directly with the sexual problem would also be indicated. With this patient anxiety or fear was associated with the female and also was built up especially in railroad stations. We have therefore two sets of overly sensitized stimulus complexes associated with drinking. The treatment called for was desensitization to the frequently recurring stimulus situations (travel and sex) and sensitization to the alcohol. For example, following the procedures outlined by Wolpe and Lazarus (1966), the patient was trained to establish a state of deep muscle relaxation, and at the same time a hierarchy of progressively more anxiety-stimulating sexual scenes was set up. The conditioning of the relaxation response to the sexual scenes was then carried out. With these therapeutic procedures the patient is then in a position to develop more adaptive behaviors in areas of previous deficit, i.e., develops a repertoire of sexual behavior and travel behavior, in the absence of alcohol. The notion is suggested here that earlier use of aversion techniques failed in many instances to take into account those antecedent conditions which were the original controlling stimuli for drinking behavior. As a result, when the drinking was modified or temporarily eliminated, those antedating conditions became operational again as stimuli which inevitably produced a response of drinking behavior.

We have referred to antecedent behaviors or "conditions," and we mean by the latter term to include such antecedent possibilities as physiological state, recognizing for example that blood-sugar ratio for some alcoholics may well represent an essential element in the alcohol-drinking chain. Research in this area, however, remains equivocal; and following Mendelson (1964), our position is that the functional relationships of these physiological states to alcoholism remain to be more fully investigated. It may well be that for purposes of further exploration of the efficacy of the learning model in the therapeutic situation, physiological characteristics should be considered as predispositional in character. To the extent they are present, they may heighten the probability or indeed make certain a drinking response in appropriate environmental circumstances. Dichotomizing alcoholism as "process" and "reactive" in terms of physiological components at this stage seems premature. While it may be dichotomized at some future time, an interim approach seems more suitable for the present, especially in an empirical approach to determine effective treatment conditions.

## THE BEHAVIOR THERAPY PROGRAM

### Didactic Training for Behavioral Change

This phase of the program consists of regularly scheduled meetings, three times a week, in small groups of 10 patients, during which patients discuss and practice with a trained counselor the various principles of behavior modification. Such topics as shaping, reinforcement, extinction, stimulus generalization, etc., are discussed. Each patient is given a copy of the Mertens and Fuller "Manual for Alcoholics" (1964) for his personal use. This manual is a presentation of the principles of behavioral change, and assignments are made each therapy session for the patients to read. The counselor in charge of each group functions as the person responsible for all behavioral treatment procedures with the patients in this group. These group meetings take place for the duration of the patient's stay at the hospital. While this process is more apparently didactic than other aspects of the program, it is intended also to utilize operant techniques with the group directly. Individual problems are discussed as a matter of course in exemplifying the methods described for counseling and modifying behavior. "Homework assignments" involve developing and presenting such application to the group. "In situ" applications are then attempted by group members. The remainder of the group and the therapist serve as social reinforcing agents in relation to the results. Within the context of this didactic behavior group-therapy, the following topics, in addition to others, are covered and discussed as they bear on the problem of alcohol and its control: Basic principles of a learning approach to alcoholism, reinforcement and extinction, shaping of behavior, deprivation and satiation, and incompatible responses. The final test of the efficacy of this knowledge in controlling alcohol-drinking behavior must await the accumulation of data, but we have found the teaching of such material quite manageable and apparently meaningful to the patients, especially when principles are related to tangible, personal behaviors.

## Aversive Conditioning Procedures

### *Visual-Verbal Sequence*

This involves the projection of verbal symbols to which the patient responds. Such words as beer, gin, alcohol, etc., are projected on a screen, and electric shock (nonconvulsive but aversive) is delivered through electrodes attached to the fingers when the patient speaks the word. What we refer to as an aversive-relief model is used here, i.e., nine alcohol-related words appear in a series and shock is administered. Following the nine alcoholic words, a "relief" word appears, such as "relax," and no shock is delivered. Concomitant with this "relief" word the patient also engages in the instrumental act of drinking juice or soda from an available glass. In addition, it should be noted, the shock is delivered on what is called a variable ratio schedule of reinforcement, i.e., in one series of nine words, all will be shocked, but on another series only 50% or 25% will be shocked.

The reasoning for the use of words is as follows: It is assumed that some of the antecedent events in the chained sequence leading to drinking are the thoughts related to drinking and that thoughts involve words. The goal here, therefore, is to create an aversion for thoughts of alcohol, the expectation being that, if such thoughts do in fact become aversive, the individual will develop avoidant behavior, i.e., try to avoid such thoughts. Thus a first step in breaking up a drinking response sequence. Of further value in such a process may be early inter-therapeutic session use of thought-stopping techniques by the patient (Wolpe-Lazarus). This method consists of a sharp cessation by S of a particular pattern of rumination in areas productive of anxiety or depressive reaction. Immediately after doing so, S is instructed to engage in behavior producing positive reinforcement (cup of coffee, favorite TV show, calling a good friend). The object here is to create a "set" for sharply breaking an undesired chaining process in the thought area. Used in conjunction with aversive conditioning, thought stopping may (a) keep the patient "dry" until aversive training becomes effective, or (b) accelerate the conditioning process itself. Its adaptability to the alcoholic problem is sufficient to justify its inclusion in the conditioning process. Small portable shock boxes have been developed and successfully utilized in assisting patients in controlling thoughts about drinking. Some controlled observations of this self-directed aversion conditioning are being executed at the present time.

The choice of the aversive-relief model is based on the following considerations. Shock renders the patient highly activated or anxious, and with successive exposures the activation should crescendo so that by the appearance of the ninth stimulus word, the patient should be most anxious and such a state should be associated with the alcoholic stimulation. The variable ratio schedule also adds to this effect. The tenth verbal stimulus (thought) then becomes associated with a tremendous deactivation and in view of the juxtaposition of stimuli should acquire the capacity to bring forth such behavior in the future.

### *Sip and Sniff Sequence*

This technique involves the actual use of alcohol in the conditioning procedures and again utilizes the aversive-relief model. Placed before the patient are nine shot glasses containing one or all of the following: whiskey, gin, wine. Some of the glasses contain 1.5 cc of the alcoholic beverage and are for oral consumption, while the remaining contain a small piece of cotton saturated with 3 cc of alcohol and are for olfactory stimulation. As the procedures are carried out the patient either drinks or smells the contents, at which time an aversive electric strong shock is administered, again on a variable ratio schedule. At the end of a series of nine, a glass of orange juice is presented with no shock. The rationale for this procedure is essentially the same as with that involved in the visual-verbal sequence: build-up of tension or activation with the alcohol stimulation, and sudden release and comfort associated with a nonalcoholic beverage. Additionally, however, is the added emphasis on the direct engagement of olfactory and gustatory stimulation.

### *Complex Sequence*

This represents an attempt to combine the various elements of the drinking response. Here a word associated with alcohol is flashed on the screen and the patient is instructed to say the word. At the same time patient says the word he is required to press a lever. Prior to this he has been told that if he completed this operation of saying the word and pressing the lever, he could sometimes avoid being shocked because these responses would lead to something else. When the patient presses the bar, three things can happen: (a) After a 7-sec. delay the word "take" would be flashed on the screen and patient would be required to take one of the shot glasses before him and drink its contents (gin, whiskey, wine). Shock would be delivered with this. (b) After a 7-sec. delay patient is shocked directly. (c) The word "relax" appears on the screen. This is an absolute guarantee that no shock will occur. Concomitantly, patient consumes juice as word "relax" remains projected on screen. The patient experiences a sequence of 14 of these randomly arranged events: 5 sips of alcohol, 5 presentations of "relax," and 4 presentations of shock alone.

In addition to involving greater complexity of events, this sequence involves the use of an instrumental action which leads to a scheduled positive reinforcement. The attempt here, as with the previous variable ratio schedule, is to obtain greater resistance to extinction of the instrumental action.

### *Covert Sensitization*

This procedure necessitates training the patient in relaxation (a part of the program which is explained below). The attempt here is to condition an aversive reaction to alcohol by means of inducing the response of nausea. This latter response is induced through suggestion. In brief, alcohol-drinking behavior is associated with feelings of nausea, while relaxation and nonnausea behavior become associated with avoidance or rejection of alcohol drinking. The patient is treated individually by the therapist with this technique. It is considered, however, possible to develop a group approach to this technique. Obvious advantages accrue to the method of applying this aversion-relief model. No apparatus is required. Danger of injury to the patient is minimized. Actual drinking of or sniffing alcohol is not required. While the problem of adaptation to the situation remains, it is perhaps more readily controlled by varying frequency of presentation than by the continuous process of adjusting shock level. As with the use of portable shocks, but once again without the requirement of equipment, inter-therapy sessions training can be carried on by the patient. It is here the therapist must seek to avoid adaptation effects.

## Relaxation Procedures

### *Individual Setting*

Here the patient is taught by the counselor various exercises designed to facilitate the patient's acquiring increased control over relaxation. The patient works individually with the counselor here. Actually, this phase of the program is most effectively used in combination with other phases and is so intended to be used in this program.

### *Group Setting*

This phase merely represents an extension and modification of the Individual Setting. In essence, three or four patients work in a group, each reclining on a couch and listening to a taped presentation of the various instructions for inducing a relaxation response.

## Desensitization Procedures

This phase is designed to operate in behavioral areas thought to be involved in the chain of behaviors leading to drinking. If anxiety occurs as an integral part of the chain, the counselor first establishes relaxation training with the patient and then proceeds to fractionate the feared stimulus situation (anxiety producing) into its most and least feared components, arranging these situations hierarchically (e.g., a fear of heterosexual expression for a male might be a situation of seducing the female as the most anxiety producing, with a situation of simply chatting with her as the least fear producing). Situations of intermediate intensities of anxiety are arranged appropriately between these anchor points. The counselor starts off with the patient relaxed and has him imagine the various scenes, being sure to take the patient only as far as he can imagine the scenes while maintaining relaxation. This procedure is often called the "method of successive approximations" or "fading in" a response. With most alcoholic patients there are quite likely several sensitized areas, and desensitization in each would be indicated.

## Training in Areas of Behavioral Deficit

Since the entire program is based on a broad-band approach, other facets of the patient's total behavioral repertoire are worked with if they are considered currently conducive to the alcoholism or are seen as potential obstacles in later rehabilitation. One most important consideration would be in the area of gainful employment, and here collaboration with other professionals is sought. Very frequently vocational training will be sought. Other areas frequently exhibiting deficit are areas involving husband behavior, or father behavior, etc. Work in these areas very often will involve treatment with the family.

### *Behaviorodrama*

As the term suggests this approach springs from the work of Moreno in psychodrama, but unlike the latter, the rationale is based on the principles of learning. In essence it involves the rehearsal by S of behaviors for which there is demonstrable deficit. If, for example, there is deficit in the area of assertive behavior, the patient (after exposure to some of the methods outlined above, e.g., relaxation training) is exposed to fabricated scenes and required to practice adaptive behavior. In learning theory terms, this procedure increases the probability that such adaptive behavior will appear when the appropriate circumstances (complex of stimulus events) appear.

### *In Vivo Training*

This procedure involves the graduated exposure of the patient to situations which originally elicited maladaptive behavior. An example should clarify the procedure. For many of our patients a barroom represents a stimulus complex associated with behaviors of high probability of occurrence, viz., approach and consumption; the desired behavior, avoiding or walking by is highly improbable, but it is the latter which is desired and which must occur to some degree in the presence of the stimulus complex. What we utilize, therefore, are "therapeutic" passes, i.e., after some exposure to training in behavioral control, the patient is told to go downtown and walk by two or three bars.

### Controlling Behavioral Excesses and Deficits by Systematic Application of Contingent Reinforcement Procedures

In essence this represents an adaptation of the work of Ayllon and Michael (1959), Krasner and Ullmann (1965) and others to the problem of alcoholism. It could be thought of as extending the pilot work so recently reported by Narrol (1967) and involves the establishment of an operant ward for alcoholics. Preliminary thinking has led us to envisage a self-contained living arrangement unit, such as one of our cottages, where male alcoholic patients would live. Initially drinking patterns would be baselined, perhaps in a manner similar to that of Mello and Mendelson (1965), following which the broad spectrum behavioral treatment, including operant-ward exposure, would be introduced. This latter would be an attempt to approximate a real-world situation where what the patient receives is contingent upon what he does. For example, in order to eat, one must pay (points), and in order to pay, one must work in order to accumulate points. General target behaviors would be set up along with more idiosyncratic areas reflecting individual needs.

## CONCLUDING COMMENTS

The program outlined above is based upon the early formulations and therapeutic work with alcoholics of the senior author, and the current efforts of the first three authors at the Eagleville Hospital and Rehabilitation Center. The program is currently being carried out at the Eagleville Center and will be researched over the coming year. Approximately 50 patients are exposed to the program at any given time, and it is expected that approximately 300 alcoholic patients will have received such exposure over the year. Research will include how much of the total "package" or program is needed for effecting more adaptive behavior for the alcoholic.

## REFERENCES


Ayllon, T., & Michael, J. The psychiatric nurse as a behavioral engineer. *J. exp. Anal. Behav.*, 1959, 2, 323–334.

Boe, E. E., & Church, R. M. The permanent effect of punishment during extinction. Paper read at Eastern Psychological Association, New York City, April, 1966.

Cautela, J. R. Covert sensitization. *Psychol. Rep.*, 1967, 20, 459–468.

Estes, W. K. An experimental study of punishment. *Psychol. Monogr.*, 1944, 57, No. 3 (Whole No. 263).

Eysenck, H. J. (Ed.) *Behavior therapy and the neuroses.* London: Pergamon, 1960.

Eysenck, H. J. (Ed.) *Experiments in behavior therapy*. London: Pergamon, 1964.

Franks, C. M. (Ed.) *Conditioning techniques in clinical practice and research.* New York: Springer, 1964.

Franks, C. M. Conditioning and conditional aversion therapies in the treatment of the alcoholic. *Int. J. Addictions*, 1966, 1, 61–98.

Gerard, D. L., Saenger, G., & Wile, R. The abstinent alcoholic. *Arch. gen. Psychiat.*, 1962, 6, 83–95.

Hill, M. J., & Blane, H. T. Evaluation of psychotherapy with alcoholics. *Quart. J. Stud. Alcohol.*, 1967, 28, 76–104.

Hsu, J. J. Electroconditioning therapy of alcoholics: a preliminary report. *Quart J. Stud. Alcohol*, 1965, 26, 449–459.

Kanfer, F. H., & Saslow, G. Behavioral analysis: an alternative to diagnostic classification. *Arch. Gen. Psychiat.*, 1965, 12, 529–538.

Kant, F. The use of conditioned reflex in the treatment of alcohol addicts. *Wis. Med. J.*, 1945, 44, 217–221.

Kantorovich, N. V. An attempt at associative-reflex therapy in alcoholism. *Psychol. Abstr.*, 1930, 4, 493. (Abstract)

Krasner, L., & Ullmann, L. P. (Eds.) *Research in behavior modification.* New York: Holt, Rinehart and Winston, 1965.

Madill, M., Campbell, D., Laverty, S. G., Sanderson, R. E., & Vandewater, S. L. Aversion treatment of alcoholics by succinyl-choline-induced apneic paralyses. *Quart. J. Stud. Alcohol*, 1966, 27, 483–509.

McBrearty, J. F. Modification of the alcohol drinking response: a preliminary study. Paper read at the workshop in Behavior Therapy, Haverford State Hospital, 1965.

Mello, N. K., & Mendelson, J. Operant analysis of drinking patterns of chronic alcoholics. *Nature*, 1965, 206, 43.

Mendelson, J. H. (Ed.) Experimentally induced chronic intoxication and withdrawal in alcoholic subjects. *Quart J. Stud. Alcohol*, 1964, Suppl. 2.

Mendelson, J. H. Research on alcoholism. Paper presented at a symposium, 133rd AAAS annual meeting, Washington, D. C., Dec., 1966.

MENDELSON, J. H., & STEIN, S. The definition of alcoholism. *Int. Psychiat. Clinica*, 1966, 3, 13–19.

MERTENS, G. C., & FULLER. G. B. *The manual for the alcoholic*. Willmar, Minn.: Willmar State Hospital, 1964.

MILLER, E. C., DVORAK, B. A., & TURNER, D. W. A method of creating aversion to alcohol by reflex conditioning in a group setting. *Quart. J. Stud. Alcohol*, 1960, 21, 424–431.

NARROL, H. G. Experimental application of reinforcement principles to the analysis and treatment of hospitalized alcoholics. *Quart J. Stud. Alcohol*, 1967, 28, 105–115.

RAYMOND, M. J. The treatment of addiction by aversion conditioning by apomorphine. *Behav. Res. Ther.*, 1964, 1, 287–291.

SANDERSON, R. E., CAMPBELL, D., & LAVERTY, S. G. Therapeutically conditioned responses acquired during respiratory paralysis. *Nature*, 1962, 196, 1235–1236.

SANDERSON, R. E., CAMPBELL, D., & LAVERTY, S. G. An investigation of a new aversive conditioning treatment for alcoholism. *Quart. J. Stud. Alcohol*, 1963, 24, 261–275.

SKINNER, B. F. *The behavior of organisms*. New York: Appleton-Century, 1938.

THIMANN, J. Conditioned reflex treatment of alcoholism: I. Its rationale and technic. *New England J. Med.*, 1949, 241, 368–370. (a)

THIMANN, J. Conditioned reflex treatment of alcoholism: II. The risks of its application, its indications, contraindications, and psychotherapeutic aspects. *New England J. Med.*, 1949, 241, 408–410. (b)

THORPE, J. G., SCHMIDT, E., BROWN, P., & CARTELL, D. Aversion therapy: a new method for general application. *Behav. Res. Therapy*, 1964, 1, 71–82.

ULLMANN, L. P., & KRASNER, L. (Eds.) *Case studies in behavior modification*. New York: Holt, Rinehart and Winston, 1965.

VOEGTLIN, W. L. The treatment of alcoholism by establishing a conditioned reflex. *Amer. J. Med. Sci.*, 1940, 199, 802–809.

VOEGTLIN, W. L., & LEMERE, F. The treatment of alcohol addiction: a review of the literature. *Quart. J. Stud. Alcohol*, 1942, 2, 717–803.

WALLERSTEIN, R. S. *Hospital treatment of alcoholism: a comparative experimental study*. New York: Basic Books, 1957.

WOLPE, J., & LAZARUS, A. *Behavior therapy techniques*. New York: Pergamon, 1966.

# 9

## *Toward a Medical Understanding of Marihuana*

CONRAD J. SCHWARZ

The current controversy around the subject of *marihuana* is complicated by the fact that it involves many aspects of life other than medical knowledge of the

Paper read at the Western Regional Meeting of the Canadian Psychiatric Association, Vancouver, B.C., January 23, 1969. Reprinted by permission of author and publisher.

effects of the drug. Individuals prominent in the fields of anthropology, sociology, philosophy, psychology, religion, law and politics have assumed rigid positions for or against *marihuana*, based on their own individual attitudes and professional development, with comparatively little attention given to what medical information is available. On the other hand, professionals in the field of medicine have been inclined to use their status as experts on drugs to advise society on its moral, ethical and philosophical attitudes toward the use of such drugs.

The purpose of this paper is to present the major medical observations made on *marihuana* and related derivatives of the Indian Hemp plant, and to avoid moralizing about what society should decide to do about these substances. This approach is based on the assumption that even if, as has been recently suggested (31), society is moving toward greater individual freedom in relation to drug usage, humanitarian principles will require that permitted drugs do not carry actual or potential dangers which would outweigh any benefits (41).

The observations noted in this paper have been made by a number of researchers in many parts of the world and relate to various preparations of the Indian Hemp plant. Whenever a particular observation appeared to refer only to a definable substance this has been stated in the text. If such clarification does not appear it is the author's interpretation that the observation can, but does not necessarily always, occur with most of the preparations available from the plant. A more specific guide to the nature of a particular study can be found in the accompanying table, but here again in a few instances the author has had to use his own discretion in interpreting which type of preparation is being studied.

The review covers the English language literature for the past thirty-five years and, although the studies on *cannabis* users cover several thousand subjects, direct experimental administration to human beings refers to only about two hundred Eastern subjects and about one hundred and forty Western subjects.

## THE NATURE OF THE SUBSTANCE

The Indian Hemp plant *Cannabis sativa* is a universal weed which is thought to have originated sometime prior to the 8th Century B.C. in Northern

**TABLE 1. References on Cannabis Effects on Humans**

| | *Eastern Subjects* | *Western Subjects* |
|---|---|---|
| Studies on human users | | |
| Marihuana | 3, 4, 6, 9, 10, 15, 30, 43, 49 | 5, 11, 12, 13, 14, 17, 19, 20, 21, 25, 27, 28, 31, 32, 37, 39, 42, 44, 45 |
| Hashish | 3, 4, 6, 9, 10, 15, 18, 30, 43, 48, 49 | 20, 33, 35 |
| Experimental observations on humans | | |
| Marihuana (smoked) | 30 | 1, 17, 42, 44 |
| Hashish | 15 | |
| Cannabis extract | | 1, 2, 16, 44 |
| Synthetic substance | | 23 |

Syria, from whence it spread to become indigenous to the Middle East, North Africa, India and Pakistan (10). In more recent centuries it found its way into most parts of the world by natural dissemination or by human cultivation, either because of its value in the production of textiles, rope and birdseed, or because of its ability to produce intoxication.

The major botanical feature of the plant is the extreme variability in its appearance, characteristics and properties when grown in different geographical and climatic conditions (1, 8, 10, 15, 17, 20, 35, 47), so much so that for many years it was believed that plants grown in different regions were of different species (10). When grown in warm, moist climates the plant usually produces a strong trunk and stems with fibrous qualities suitable for the textile industry but with little intoxicating potency; in hot, dry climates textile properties are poor but the intoxicating principle is stronger, presumably due to the increased amount of resin which the plant secretes as a defence against heat, and which is thought to be the main source of the active psychic ingredients (10).

The psychic potency varies further with a number of factors related to cultivation. Even when grown in the same field individual plants show differences in potency (17). If the male plants are not removed and fertilization occurs, the female plants which carry the main intoxicating properties are considerably weakened in that respect (15, 42). In addition, unless harvesting is carried out immediately before the blossoming of the flowers there is further weakening and variation in the potency of the produce (10, 38).

The fact that there is no standard *cannabis* plant available for experimental study has had to be obviated to some extent by the development of the United Nations Reference Sample, which consists of a common mixture of plants grown in different parts of the world (24).

The Indian Hemp plant yields three rough grades of intoxicating substances, but without any clear boundaries between them:

1. The pure resin which is scraped from the leaves and flowering tops of the female plant is referred to as *charas*. Because of its deleterious effects this substance is universally banned (38), even in India where it used to have some spiritual significance (15), and its illicit use seems to be restricted to a few small areas there.
2. A medium range preparation consisting of an agglomeration of the female flowering tops and stems with whatever resin is attached to their surfaces, has varying names in different countries, the two most common being *hashish* and *ganja*. It is thought to contain about 40% of resin (47).
3. A low potency preparation consisting of the dried matured leaves and flowering tops of both male and female plants, which also has a variety of names, the two most common being *bhang* and *marihuana*. It is thought to contain from 5% to 8% of resin (47).

The intoxicating preparations may be used in their natural state or may be mixed with spices or sweetmeats (10), tobacco (15), alcohol (10, 15), tincture of camphor (46), morphine, heroin (12) or opium (4, 10, 15). Regardless of storage procedures the potency of these preparations deteriorates with time (15, 17).

Medicinal extracts of *cannabis* which had a vogue in Western methods of treatment of a wide range of disorders in the latter half of the 19th century fell into disuse in the early part of the 20th century because they were unreliable and variable in potency (18, 42, 47), and also deteriorated with time (15).

Although the elucidation of the chemical nature of the active ingredients of *cannabis* has received considerable attention, knowledge in this area is still in the primitive stage. After a number of years of assuming that substances such as *cannabinol, cannabidiol,* and "*cannabol*" were the potent ingredients, these have more recently been shown to be pharmacologically inactive (17, 22, 29). Attention is currently focused on the tetrahydrocannabinol group of substances, of which about eighty have so far been postulated, but only a few of these have known chemical structures and fewer have been synthesized (7, 23). These tetrahydrocannabinols are very unstable (35). The identification of the active ingredients is even further complicated by the fact that the potency of *cannabis* seems to depend on the ongoing biological interaction of tetrahydrocannabinol substances in the plant or in its resin (22).

Finally, as regards the general properties of the plant and its derivatives, when these substances are burned they produce a heavy, acrid odor which is similar to burning hay and which clings to the environs if smoked indoors. Both for æsthetic purposes and for concealment the odor may have to be masked by the use of incense.

Given the above variations in the plant and in its products and extracts, together with the continuing ignorance of its chemistry, it is not surprising that it is virtually impossible to make direct comparisons between the various studies on the effects of *cannabis* on human beings who are even more individually variable.

It is obvious from the literature that there are wide individual variations in response to different *cannabis* preparations, but it is equally clear that even when the same substance is administered experimentally to a number of people there are significant differences in response from subject to subject and in the same subject at varying times. The effects of *cannabis* have a wave-like quality and fluctuations occur in the same person during any single episode of intoxication (2). While, in general, the stronger the preparation the greater the response, idiosyncratic psychotic states have been precipitated in experimental subjects even with low doses of a pure synthetic tetrahydrocannabinol (23). One recent observer, finding a number of psychological tests unreliable in assessing the effects of a *cannabis* extract on individuals, likened its unpredictability to that of LSD (16). While the duration of effects is generally reported as being from one-half to four hours, in some subjects the intoxicated state may last up to twelve hours (1) with residual effects of varying degrees persisting for several days (2, 12) or even weeks (28).

## ACUTE PHYSICAL EFFECTS

Whether ingested or inhaled the initial physical effects of *cannabis* have been described as unpleasant or ambiguous (5, 43, 49) and it has been stated that "before the smoker can derive agreeable sensations from *cannabis,* he must first go through the discomforts of habituation" (10, page 27). If he is to become a regular user of *marihuana* the initiate must learn to ignore these symptoms or to excuse them as the necessary tribulations of getting "high" (5).

Among the general effects of *cannabis* preparations the more commonly described ones are increased appetite (1, 15, 42, 44, 47), headache (2, 20, 39), dizziness (35, 44), vertigo (6, 20), fainting (20, 44) and perspiration (10, 15). In addition to any residual effects described previously, and contrary to popular belief, hangover effects have been described (1, 13).

The cardiovascular system is generally reported as showing an increased pulse rate (1, 15, 23, 35, 42, 44), and an increased blood pressure (1, 15, 44), although some reports indicate no change in this (23, 42). Palpitations have been reported (2, 20), as have tightness of the chest (44) and severe precordial discomfort with slight EEG changes (2). Injection of the conjunctival blood vessels is regarded as pathognomonic (1, 2, 8, 23, 44, 46, 47), and edema of the eyelids has also been reported (2).

As regards the gastrointestinal system, dryness of the mouth is common (1, 2, 10, 15, 44), and thirst may become intense (10, 15). Nausea is sufficiently common (8, 20, 39, 44, 46) to be regarded as usual (10, 15). Vomiting is not uncommon (2, 8, 10, 20, 44) and less frequently diarrhea (8, 44) and constipation (6) occur.

The effects on the respiratory system can be experienced by anyone who cares to inhale an ordinary cigarette in the manner necessary for proper *marihuana* usage. Take some smoke into the mouth, open the mouth wide, and inhale as quickly and as deeply as possible. *Marihuana* is an irritant inhalant (10) and inhaled in this way will not infrequently produce a spasm of coughing (8, 10, 39), expiratory dyspnoea (2), a dry throat, (1, 39, 44) and acute bronchitis (10, 15).

On the genito-urinary system, frequency and urgency of micturition have been reported (2, 44, 46, 47) and diuresis has been sufficiently pronounced to suggest a therapeutic potential (2). It is generally agreed that there is no physical aphrodisiac effect (10, 19, 44, 48), and in some individuals impotence (6) may be precipitated.

Neurological signs are not infrequently evident. Incoordination (2, 11, 44, 46), ataxia (1, 20, 44), tremors (1, 6, 20, 44), involuntary twitching (1, 2), choreic movements (11) and catalepsy (11) have been reported. Dilatation of the pupils (1, 8, 10, 15, 44, 46, 47) is generally described and other effects on the eyes have included nystagmus (1), conjugate deviation of the eyes persisting for six weeks (36), blurred vision (44) and photophobia (1). Parathesia of the extremities has been reported (2, 10). Complex psychomotor functioning is affected (16, 44), and it is not surprising that driving competence is considered to be impaired (4, 31).

## ACUTE PSYCHOLOGICAL EFFECTS

The predominant emotional effect of *cannabis* preparations is euphoria (1, 2, 10, 11, 15, 20, 24, 31, 44), which may or may not be accompanied by feelings of well-being (10, 20), confidence (20), and adequacy (44). On the other hand there are reports of apprehension (1), more frequently described as anxiety (2, 11, 12, 14, 15, 27, 32, 44), reaching a degree of panic (11, 25, 38) even in experienced users (31). In fact some observers consider anxiety so common that they regard it as a necessary part of the intoxication syndrome (12, 14), and depression has also been reported (15, 17, 27). The acute state shows wave-like undulations in mood and behavior (35).

On an intellectual level distortions of the sense of time (2, 10, 11, 20, 24, 43) and space (10, 11) are sufficiently common to be pathognomonic. Perception of color and sound may be intensified (2, 24). Fragmentation of thought (2), 43), difficulty in immediate recall (43), loss of contact with reality (2) and confusion (10, 11) may occur, interspersed with episodes of subjective clarity which are not objectively substantiated (2, 11). Somato-sensory distortions (1, 15, 47), body image disintegration (2, 11), and depersonalization (2, 10, 24) may occur. Illusions (2, 10, 11) and even frank hallucinations (10, 15, 24, 31) have been described. Suspiciousness (1, 2) may reach paranoid proportions (17, 27) and judgment is considered to be impaired (20). The individual may become significantly intoxicated without being aware of his condition (6).

On the behavioral level the subject may experience lassitude (1) to the point of sedation (31). On the other hand he may be hyperactive (1), hyperresponsive (1, 10, 17), and irritable (17) to the point of being resistive, assaultive, or combative (3, 4, 6, 10, 11, 15, 17, 18, 20, 35, 37, 38, 42, 47). Suicide attempts have been reported by several observers (10, 12, 32).

The sensational attention given to the complex subject of *cannabis* and crime has ignored the multifactorial etiology of criminal behavior. Even those observers from both East and West who insist on a close relationship between *cannabis* and crime (6, 10, 20, 21, 30, 35, 37, 48) clearly qualify this statement by placing major emphasis on the personality of the individual and his social, economic and cultural attributes. Some Western observers (4, 12, 14, 19, 31, 32) tend to minimize any significant relationship but admit that anti-social and criminal behavior can occur in people who have lost their inhibitions under the influence of *marihuana*. There are a number of reports that individuals in different cultures use *cannabis* to give themselves courage to carry out criminal activity (2, 4, 17, 20, 31, 48).

Other features of behavior in the acute intoxicated state are rapid (1, 11), disjointed (10), and incoherent (10) speech, silly laughter (2, 10, 11, 42), and increased suggestibility (10).

A psychotic state is clearly described by a number of observers (4, 6, 9, 10, 12, 15, 18, 19, 20, 27, 30, 32) but heavy emphasis is placed on the pre-existing personality of the users, and *cannabis* is generally regarded as a precipitant rather than as a primary cause of this. The incidence of such psychotic reactions among the multitude of users is generally thought to be low (6, 15), but in some areas of the world *cannabis* use has been related to a significant portion of admissions to mental hospitals, reaching as many as 26 percent of cases (6, 9, 15, 30).

In direct human experimentation with *cannabis* products, psychotic references have also been noted (1, 2, 23, 44) and the largest Western group so far studied included nine psychotic reactions in seventy-two subjects—an incidence of 12.5 percent (44).

## CHRONIC PHYSICAL EFFECTS

Usually the reports of chronic physical ill effects are to be found in Eastern studies of individuals using the stronger *hashish* or pure resinous substances over prolonged periods of time and are complicated by the immeasurable effects of many other social, economic, personality and cultural factors.

In one survey of 1,238 *cannabis* users (15), the individuals themselves reported that they felt major ill effects from the use of the drug in 15 percent of the cases, minor ill effects in 25 percent, improved health in 10 percent, with the remainder reporting no change. In a study of 253 *hashish* users in Egypt (43) about 67 percent reported that they would like to stop using the drug, giving finance as the first reason and the ill effects on physical health as the second reason.

Nonspecific chronic physical effects reportedly associated with *cannabis* include insomnia (28), headaches (10, 32) and persistent chronic injection of the blood vessels of the conjunctiva (15, 45). Loss of weight leading to cachexia (6, 10, 15), increased susceptibility to infection (10), high incidence of tuberculosis (15) and premature death (15) have been noted.

One careful study of sixty-six regular *hashish* users aged 22–37 observed over a five-year period reported five known deaths in the group—two from cardiac arrest, one each from suicide, automobile accident, and fighting (35).

Chronic gastrointestinal effects include anorexia (6, 10, 15), dyspepsia, and very commonly chronic diarrhea with or without alternating constipation (15).

As regards the respiratory system, chronic laryngitis (15), chronic bronchitis (15, 45), bronchopneumonia (10), and emphysema (15) have been observed in chronic users.

Epileptic seizures have been precipitated in known epileptics (26, 44).

In the area of human reproduction, impotence (6, 10) and a lower fecundity rate (15) have been reported.

Inevitably, with this last kind of report, possible teratogenic properties of *cannabis* would be studied. While an oral form of *cannabis* resin administered to female rats over a period of five months caused a reduction in reproductive activity and a higher incidence of death among the mothers, no fetal abnormalities were demonstrated (34). More recently, the use of an intraperitoneal *cannabis* resin has been shown to have teratogenic effects in rats and to a lesser degree in mice (40). There is no way in which this finding can be applied to humans except inasmuch as it should stimulate active investigation.

In addition to the subject of crime, the other sensational aspect of *cannabis* which frequently receives uninformed attention is the subject of addiction.

It is generally agreed by both Eastern and Western observers that *cannabis* is not physically addicting in the sense that opium and heroin are (3, 9, 10, 12, 15, 30, 42, 47). This is not quite the same as saying there is no physical addiction at all. Most observers state that there is no tolerance developed to the drug, and there is no need to increase the dose with continued use, but this statement is questioned by a few observers (1, 13, 33, 35, 44). The nonaddicting position is supported by the general observation that there is no physical withdrawal syndrome when the drug is not available (6, 12, 15, 20, 44, 47), but the occurrence of a physical withdrawal syndrome has been suggested by two observers (10, 32).

The argument about physical addiction tends to obscure the fact that few observers (20, 42) claim there is no psychological dependence. After prolonged use it is considered difficult to give up the use of *cannabis* (43, 47) and severe psychological dependence is stated by a number of observers to be present in chronic users (4, 12, 14, 19, 38, 47). In addition to this severe psychological withdrawal, symptoms are described including anxiety, restlessness, irritability, depression, self-mutilation, suicide fantasy and suicide attempts (10, 15, 32), aggressive outbursts, and psychotic episodes (18). It has been noted that regular *cannabis* users resent deprivation (20, 39) and are intent on returning to its use (13, 25), despite unpleasant reactions. It has been pointed out that while some may be able to use *cannabis* products purely for the purposes of pleasure, other individuals show the major characteristic of psychological dependence in that they are unable to feel well or to function adequately without regular use of the drug (13, 14, 32, 43).

Progression to the use of other drugs including the so-called "hard narcotics" is thought to be rare by some observers (14, 19, 44) and a serious danger by others (10, 13, 37, 39). Factors involved in such a development are seen as complex, involving the personality of the user, the exposure to criminal elements in obtaining the drug, the resorting to available heroin when *cannabis* has not been at hand, the use of heroin as a sedating antidote to terminate unpleasant effects of *cannabis* or as a less disturbing alternative to *cannabis* and a tendency to become indifferent to possible dangers once a drug usage orientation has been developed (13, 39).

## CHRONIC PSYCHOLOGICAL EFFECTS

The occurrence of psychotic illnesses sufficient to require medical attention has already been mentioned. The period of hospitalization when required for the treatment of these conditions is usually brief, but *cannabis*-precipitated psychosis may be associated with prolonged hospitalization in individuals whose predisposition is unstable (4, 6, 10, 15). A *cannabis*-associated form of dementia has been noted in Eastern reports (10, 15).

Personality changes have been observed by a number of workers, but again pre-existing defects in the individual are generally emphasized. Among the more significant alterations, attention has been drawn to fluctuations in behavior and mood (10), tendencies to irritability and violent outbursts (18, 35), general inadequacy (30, 35), reduced work capacity (35, 43), tendencies to disrupt family life (4, 10, 30), and the adoption of an amotivational (31) or apathetic way of life (10, 25).

## PERSONALITY CHARACTERISTICS OF USERS

As has already been indicated most observers regard primary personality characteristics of users as much more important than the drug itself in producing adverse effects in keeping with the old Moroccan proverb, "You are a *kef* addict long before you smoke your first pipe" (6, page 8).

From the references on the predisposing personality characteristics of regular users there are suggestions of correlations even in individuals in different cultures. The use of *cannabis* as an intoxicant is overwhelmingly found in males (8, 10, 12, 15, 25, 30, 39). Basic personalities have been described as inadequate (6, 30), insecure (44), and emotionally immature (6, 44), with tendencies to passivity (44) and feelings of inferiority (15). Users have been described as lonely (44) and socially ill at ease (44) and as alienated, distrustful, and even paranoid (32). Pre-existing delinquency has been noted (32), as have neurotic tendencies (15, 30), hypochondriasis (14, 15, 19), psychopathic tendencies (14), and prodromal schizophrenic conditions (6). They have been regarded as having a low frustration tolerance level (18, 32) and to be chronic complainers (14, 32) and resentful towards society (14, 32). They have been described as having poor heterosexual adjustment (14, 32, 44) and strong homosexual tendencies (14). Despite all this they are regarded as intense proselytizers in favor of the use of the drug (6, 32).

## FACTORS IN CAUSATION

Among the extraneous factors which have been reported as contributing towards the use of *cannabis*, have been broken-home situations (4, 32) and varying degrees of deprived family backgrounds (14, 19, 32). More immediately, problems of unemployment and malnutrition together with pressures of industrialization (6), have been regarded as contributing. An interesting theme which is mentioned by a number of observers in different parts of the world is the feature of mobility and the associated transition changes involved. In some areas the drug is most commonly used by wandering religious mendicants (15), truck drivers (4, 6), migrating workers, (48) and even wandering youth (39). The stresses involved in moving from a rural to an urban society with the associated disintegration of kinship ties and standards has been noted (4, 6, 9, 30).

## CONCLUSION

From the above review the following points emerge relative to the current level of medical understanding of *marihuana*:

1. *Marihuana* is a poorly defined intoxicant derived from the Indian Hemp plant (*Cannabis sativa*). It is qualitatively similar to, but quantitatively weaker than *hashish*, the other commonly used natural intoxicant derived from the plant.
2. The Indian Hemp plant varies widely in its botanical properties.
3. *Marihuana, hashish* and chemical extracts of *cannabis* vary widely in potency and deteriorate with time.
4. The chemical composition of these substances is largely unknown at this time.
5. There are wide variations in human response to these substances, and variations may also occur in the same individual using the same substance at different times.

6. The acute intoxicated state is of variable duration, and the individual is not necessarily aware that he is intoxicated.
7. The acute intoxicated state characteristically involves a feeling of euphoria, distortions of the sense of time and space, heightened sensory perceptions, and impairment of complex psychomotor activity. However, fluctuations in mood and behavior may occur and a state of toxic psychosis may result, which is not necessarily related to high dosage.
8. In order to achieve the state of intoxication the individual may have to accept some degree of unpleasant physical and psychological experiences.
9. Depending on the complex interaction of a number of variables of which the drug is only one, *hashish* and to a lesser extent *marihuana* can be associated with acute psychological distress requiring medical attention, intoxicated behavior dangerous to the individual himself or to others, drug dependency, personality deterioration and chronic physical ill-health.
10. The incidence of acute side effects is unknown, but it is generally considered that chronic side effects are more likely to occur with *hashish* when used regularly over a period of time.
11. Regular users of both *marihuana* and *hashish* so far studied tend to show basic defects in personality.

## SUMMARY

This paper is based on a review of the English language medical literature over the past 35 years on Indian Hemp, with direct reference being made to the more significant articles published during that time. The paucity of direct experimental observation is noted and the difficulties in experimental studies are highlighted by descriptions of the wide variations in the potency of Indian Hemp derivatives. Specific references are provided for the wide range of observations made in relation to acute and chronic physical and psychological effects, personal characteristics of the users, and possible factors in causation. It is concluded that *marihuana* is a poorly defined intoxicant which varies in potency, deteriorates with time, and whose chemical composition is largely unknown at present. There are wide variations in human response and the state of intoxication itself carries with it varying degrees of unpleasant physical and psychological experiences. The association between *hashish* and, to a lesser extent, *marihuana* and short-term and long-term complications is discussed in relation to complex variables, of which the drug is but one factor.

## REFERENCES

1. ALLENTUCK, S., and BOWMAN, W. M.: The psychiatric aspects of *marihuana* intoxication. *Amer. J. Psychiat.*, 99, 248–251, 1942.
2. AMES, F.: A clinical and metabolic study of acute intoxication with *Cannabis sativa* and its role in the model psychoses. *J. Ment. Sci.*, *104*, 972–999, 1958.

3. ANDRADE, O. M.: The criminogenic action of *cannabis* (*marihuana*) and narcotics. *Bull. Narcotics, 16, 4*, 23–28, 1964.
4. ASUNI, T.: Socio-psychiatric problems of *cannabis* in Nigeria. *Bull. Narcotics, 16*, 2, 17–28, 1964.
5. BECKER, H. S.: Marihuana use and social control. *Social Problems*, 3, 35–44, 1955.
6. BENABUD, A.: Psycho-pathological aspects of the *cannabis* situation in Morocco: Statistical data for 1956. *Bull. Narcotics*, 9, *4*, 1–16, 1957.
7. BICHER, H. L., and MECHOULAM, R.: Pharmacological effects of two active constituents of *marihuana. Arch. Int. Pharmacodyn.*, *172*, 24–31, 1968.
8. BLOOMQUIST, E. R.: *Marihuana*. Beverley Hills, Calif., Glencoe Press, 1968.
9. BOROFFKA, A.: Mental illness and Indian Hemp in Lagos. *East Afr. Med. J.*, *43*, 377–384, 1966.
10. BOUQUET, R. J.: *Cannabis. Bull. Narcotics*, 2, *4*, 14–30, 1950 (Part I) and 3, *1*, 22–45, 1951 (Part II).
11. BROMBERG, W.: *Marihuana* intoxication. A clinical study of *Cannabis sativa* Intoxication. *Amer. J. Psychiat.*, *91*, 303–330, 1934.
12. BROMBERG, W.: *Marihuana*: A psychiatric study. *J.A.M.A.*, *113*, 4–12, 1939.
13. CHAPPLE, P. A. L.: *Cannabis*—a toxic and dangerous substance—a study of eighty takers. *Brit. J. Addict*, *61*, 269–282, 1966.
14. CHAREN, S., and PERELMAN, L.: Personality studies of *marihuana* addicts. *Amer. J. Psychiat.*, *102*, 674–682, 1946.
15. CHOPRA, I. C., and CHOPRA, R. N.: The use of *cannabis* drugs in India. *Bull. Narcotics*, 9, *1*, 4–29, 1957.
16. CLARK, L. D., and NAKASHIMA, E. N.: Experimental studies of *marihuana. Amer. J. Psychiat.*, *125*, 379–384, 1968.
17. DE FARIAS, R. C.: Use of maconha (*cannabis sativa 1*) in Brazil. Control by health and police authorities. *Bull. Narcotics*, 7, 2, 5–19, 1955.
18. FRASER, J. D.: Withdrawal symptoms in *Cannabis indica* addicts. *Lancet*, *49*, 257, 747–748, 1949.
19. FREEDMAN, H. L., and ROCKMORE, M. J.: *Marihuana*: a factor in personality evaluation and army maladjustment. *J. Clin Psychopathol.*, 7, 765–782, 1946 (Part I) and *8*, 221–236, 1946 (Part II).
20. GASKILL, H. S.: *Marihuana*, an intoxicant. *Amer. J. Psychiat.*, *102*, 202–204, 1945.
21. GOMILA, F. R., and LAMBOU, G. L.: Present Status of the Marihuana Vice in the United States, in *Marihuana: America's New Drug Problem*. Walton, R. P., New York, J. B. Lippincott Co., 1938, pp. 27–39.
22. GRLIC, L.: Recent advances in the chemical research of *cannabis. Bull. Narcotics*, *16*, *4*, 29–38, 1964.
23. ISBELL, H. et al.: Effects of (−) delta-9-transtetrahydrocannabinol in man. *Psychopharmacol.*, *11*, 184–188, 1967.
24. JOACHIMOGLU, G., KIBURIS, J., and MIRAS, C.: Studies with the U.N. *cannabis* reference sample. *Bull. Narcotics*, *19*, *1*, 21–22, 1967.
25. KEELER, M. H.: Adverse reaction to *marihuana. Amer. J. Psychiat.*, *124*, 674–677, 1967.
26. KEELER, M. H., and REIFLER, C. B.: Grand mal convulsions subsequent to *marihuana* use. *Dis. Nerv. Sys.* 28, 474–475, 1967.
27. KEELER, M. H.: Motivation for *marihuana* use: a correlate of adverse reaction. *Amer. J. Psychiat.*, *125*, 386–390, 1968.

28. KEELER, M. H., REIFLER, C. B., and LIPTZIN, M. B.: Spontaneous recurrence of *marihuana* effect. *Amer. J. Psychiat.*, *125*, 384–386, 1968.
29. KORTE, F., and SIEPER, H.: Recent results of *hashish* analysis in, *Hashish*: Its chemistry and pharmacology. *Ciba Foundation Study Group No. 21*, 1965, pp. 15–36.
30. LAMBO, T. A.: Medical and social problems of drug addiction in West Africa. *Bull. Narcotics*, *17*, *1*, 3–13, 1965.
31. McGLOTHLIN, W. H., and WEST, L.: The *marihuana* problem: an overview. *Amer. J. Psychiat.*, *125*, 370–378, 1968.
32. MARCOVITZ, E., and MYERS, H. J.: The *marihuana* addict in the army. *War Medicine*, *6*, 382–391, 1945.
33. MIRAS, C. J.: *Hashish Smokers and Metabolic Disturbances*. Report II (Final) April, 1957. From the Department of Biological Chemistry, Univ. of Athens, Greece, April, 1957.
34. MIRAS, C. J.: Some aspects of *cannabis* action in *Hashish*: Its chemistry and *pharmacology*. *Ciba Foundation Study Group No. 21*, 1965, pp. 37–53.
35. MIRAS, C. J.: *Marihuana* and *hashish*. Paper based on seminar delivered at the Department of Pharmacology, U.C.L.A., on September 11, 1967. From the Department of Biological Chemistry, Univ. of Athens, Greece.
36. MOHAN, H., and SOOD, G. C.: Conjugate deviation of the eyes following *cannabis indica* intoxication. *Brit. J. Ophth.*, *48*, 160–161, 1964.
37. MUNCH, J. C.: *Marihuana* and crime. *Bull. Narcotics*, *18*, 2, 15–22, 1966.
38. MURPHY, J. B. M.: The *cannabis* habit: A review of recent psychiatric literature. *Bull. Narcotics*, *15*, *1*, 15–23, 1963.
39. PAULUS, I., and WILLIAMS, H. R.: *Marihuana* and young adults. *Brit. Col. Med. J.*, *8*, 240–244, 1966.
40. PERSAUD, T. V. N., and ELLINGTON, A. C.: Teratogenic activity of *cannabis* resin. *Lancet*, 2, 406–407, 1968.
41. SCHWARZ, C. J.: LSD, *marihuana* and the law. *Brit. Col. Med. J.*, 9, 274–285, 1967.
42. SILER, J. F., et al.: *Marihuana* smoking in Panama. *Military Surgeon*, *73*, 269–280, 1933.
43. SOUIEF, M. I.: *Hashish* consumption in Egypt with special reference to psychosocial aspects. *Bull. Narcotics*, *19*, 2, 1–12, 1967.
44. *The Marihuana Problem in the City of New York*. Lancaster, Pa., Jacques Cattell Press, 1944.
45. TYLDEN, E.: A case for *Cannabis*? *B.M.J.*, 3, 556, 1967.
46. UNWIN, J. R.: Illicit drug use among Canadian youth 1968. *C.M.A.J.*, 98, 402–407, 1968 (Part I) and TR, 449–454 (Part II).
47. WALTON, R. P.: *Marihuana*: *America's New Drug Problem*. New York, J. B. Lippincott Co., 1938.
48. WATT, J. M.: *Dagga* in South Africa. *Bull. Narcotics*, *13*, 3, 9–14, 1961.
49. WATT, J. M.: Drug dependence of *hashish type*. in *Hashish*: Its chemistry and pharmacology. *Ciba Foundation Study Group No. 21*, 1965, pp. 54–69.

# 10

## *Clinical and Psychological Effects of Marihuana in Man**

ANDREW T. WEIL, NORMAN E. ZINBERG, JUDITH M. NELSEN

In the spring of 1968 we conducted a series of pilot experiments on acute marihuana intoxication in human subjects. The study was not undertaken to prove or disprove popularly held convictions about marihuana as an intoxicant, to compare it with other drugs, or to introduce our own opinions. Our concern was simply to collect some long overdue pharmacological data. In this article we describe the primitive state of knowledge of the drug, the research problems encountered in designing a replicable study, and the results of our investigations.

Marihuana is a crude preparation of flowering tops, leaves, seeds, and stems of female plants of Indian hemp *Cannabis sativa* L.; it is usually smoked. The intoxicating constituents of hemp are found in the sticky resin exuded by the tops of the plants, particularly the females. Male plants produce some resin but are grown mainly for hemp fiber, not for marihuana. The resin itself, when prepared for smoking or eating, is known as "hashish." Various *Cannabis* preparations are used as intoxicants throughout the world; their potency varies directly with the amount of resin present (1). Samples of American marihuana differ greatly in pharmacological activity, depending on their composition (tops contain most resin; stems, seeds, and lower leaves least) and on the conditions under which the plants were grown. In addition, different varieties of *Cannabis* probably produce resins with different proportions of constituents (2). Botanists feel that only one species of hemp exists, but work on the phytochemistry of the varieties of this species is incomplete (3). Chronic users claim that samples of marihuana differ in quality of effects as well as in potency; that some types cause a preponderance of physical symptoms, and that other types tend to cause greater distortions of perception or of thought.

Pharmacological studies of *Cannabis* indicate that the tetrahydrocannabinol fraction of the resin is the active portion. In 1965, Mechoulam and Gaoni (4) reported the first total synthesis of (—)-$\Delta^1$-*trans*-tetrahydrocannabinol (THC), which they called "the psychotomimetically active constituent of hashish (marihuana)." Synthetic THC is now available for research in very limited supply.

In the United States, the use of *Cannabis* extracts as therapeutics goes back to the 19th century, but it was not until the 1920s that use of marihuana as an intoxicant by migrant Mexican laborers, urban Negroes, and certain Bohemian

From *Science*, Vol. 162, December 13, 1968, pp. 1234–1242. 

* This work was conducted in the Behavioral Pharmacology Laboratory of the Boston University School of Medicine, sponsored and supported by its division of psychiatry, and at the Boston University Medical Center, Boston, Mass.

groups caused public concern (3). Despite increasingly severe legal penalties imposed during the 1930s, use of marihuana continued in these relatively small populations without great public uproar or apparent changes in numbers or types of users until the last few years. The fact that almost none of the studies devoted to the physiological and psychological effects of *Cannabis* in man was based on controlled laboratory experimentation escaped general notice. But with the explosion of use in the 1960s, at first on college campuses followed by a spread downward to a portion of the established middle class, controversy over the dangers of marihuana generated a desire for more objective information about the drug.

Of the three known studies on human subjects performed by Americans, the first (see 5) was done in the Canal Zone with 34 soldiers; the consequences reported were hunger and hyperphagia, loss of inhibitions, increased pulse rate with unchanged blood pressure, a tendency to sleep, and unchanged performance of psychological and neurological tests. Doses and type of marihuana were not specified.

The second study, known as the 1944 LaGuardia Report (6), noted that 72 prisoners, 48 of whom were previous *Cannabis* users, showed minimum physiological responses, but suffered impaired intellectual functioning and decreased body steadiness, especially well demonstrated by nonusers after high doses. Basic personality structures remained unchanged as subjects reported feelings of relaxation, disinhibition, and self-confidence. In that study, the drug was administered orally as an extract. No controls were described, and doses and quality of marihuana were unspecified.

Williams et al. in 1946 (7) studied a small number of prisoners who were chronic users; they were chiefly interested in effects of long-term smoking on psychological functioning. They found an initial exhilaration and euphoria which gave way after a few days of smoking to indifference and lassitude that somewhat impaired performance requiring concentration and manual dexterity. Again, no controls were provided.

Predictably, these studies, each deficient in design for obtaining reliable physiological and psychological data, contributed no dramatic or conclusive results. The 1967 President's Commission on Law Enforcement and the Administration of Justice described the present state of knowledge by concluding (3): ". . . no careful and detailed analysis of the American experience [with marihuana] seems to have been attempted. Basic research has been almost nonexistent. . . ." Since then, no other studies with marihuana itself have been reported, but in 1967 Isbell (8) administered synthetic THC to chronic users. At doses of 120 $\mu$g/kg orally or 50 $\mu$g/kg by smoking, subjects reported this drug to be similar to marihuana. At higher doses (300 to 400 $\mu$g/kg orally or 200 to 250 $\mu$g/kg by smoking), psychotomimetic effects occurred in most subjects. This synthetic has not yet been compared with marihuana in nonusers or given to any subjects along with marihuana in double-blind fashion.

Investigations outside the United States have been scientifically deficient, and for the most part have been limited to anecdotal and sociological approaches (9–12). So far as we know, our study is the first attempt to investigate marihuana in a formal double-blind experiment with the appropriate controls. It is also the first attempt to collect basic clinical and psychological information on the drug by observing its effects on marihuana-naive human subjects in a neutral laboratory setting.

## RESEARCH PROBLEMS

That valid basic research on marihuana is almost nonexistent is not entirely accounted for by legislation which restricts even legitimate laboratory investigations or by public reaction sometimes verging on hysteria. A number of obstacles are intrinsic to the study of this drug. We now present a detailed description of our specific experimental approach, but must comment separately on six general problems confronting the investigator who contemplates marihuana research.

1. Concerning the route of administration, many pharmacologists dismiss the possibility of giving marihuana by smoking because, they say, the dose cannot be standardized (13). We consider it not only possible, but important to administer the drug to humans by smoking rather than by the oral route for the following reasons. (i) Smoking is the way nearly all Americans use marihuana. (ii) It is possible to have subjects smoke marihuana cigarettes in such a way that drug dosage is reasonably uniform for all subjects. (iii) Standardization of dose is not assured by giving the drug orally because little is known about gastrointestinal absorption of the highly water-insoluble cannabinols in man. (iv) There is considerable indirect evidence from users that the quality of the intoxication is different when marihuana or preparations of it are ingested rather than smoked. In particular, ingestion seems to cause more powerful effects, more "LSD-like" effects, longer-lasting effects, and more hangovers (12, 14). Further, marihuana smokers are accustomed to a very rapid onset of action due to efficient absorption through the lungs, whereas the latency for onset of effects may be 45 or 60 minutes after ingestion. (v) There is reported evidence from experiments with rats and mice that the pharmacological activities of natural hashish (not subjected to combustion) and hashish sublimate (the combustion products) are different (14).

2. Until quite recently, it was extremely difficult to estimate the relative potencies of different samples of marihuana by the techniques of analytical chemistry. For this study, we were able to have the marihuana samples assayed spectrophotometrically (15) for THC content. However, since THC has not been established as the sole determinant of marihuana's activity, we still feel it is important to have chronic users sample and rate marihuana used in research. Therefore, we assayed our material by this method as well.

3. One of the major deficiencies in previous studies has been the absence of negative control or placebo treatments, which we consider essential to the design of this kind of investigation. Because marihuana smoke has a distinctive odor and taste, it is difficult to find an effective placebo for use with chronic users. The problem is much less difficult with nonusers. Our solution to this dilemma was the use of portions of male hemp stalks (16), devoid of THC, in the placebo cigarettes.

4. In view of the primitive state of knowledge about marihuana, it is difficult to predict which psychological tests will be sensitive to the effects of the drug. The tests we chose were selected because, in addition to being likely to demon-

strate effects, they have been used to evaluate many other psychoactive drugs. Of the various physiological parameters available, we chose to measure (i) heart rate, because previous studies have consistently reported increases in heart rate after administration of marihuana (for example, 5); (ii) respiratory rate, because it is an easily measured vital sign, and depression has been reported (11, 17); (iii) pupil size, because folklore on effects of marihuana consistently includes reports of pupillary dilatation, although objective experimental evidence of an effect of the drug on pupils has not been sought; (iv) conjunctival appearance, because both marihuana smokers and eaters are said to develop red eyes (11); and (v) blood sugar, because hypoglycemia has been invoked as a cause of the hunger and hyperphagia commonly reported by marihuana users, but animal and human evidence of this effect is contradictory (6, 10, 11). [The LaGuardia Report, quoted by Jaffe in Goodman and Gilman (18) described hyperglycemia as an effect of acute intoxication.] We did not measure blood pressure because previous studies have failed to demonstrate any consistent effect on blood pressure in man, and we were unwilling to subject our volunteers to a nonessential annoyance.

5. It is necessary to control set and setting. "Set" refers to the subject's psychological expectations of what a drug will do to him in relation to his general personality structure. The total environment in which the drug is taken is the setting. All indications are that the form of marihuana intoxication is particularly dependent on the interaction of drug, set, and setting. Because of recent increases in the extent of use and in attention given this use by the mass media, it is difficult to find subjects with a neutral set toward marihuana. Our method of selecting subjects (described below), at the least, enabled us to identify the subjects' attitudes. Unfortunately, too many researchers have succumbed to the temptation to have subjects take drugs in "psychedelic" environments or have influenced the response to the drug by asking questions that disturb the setting. Even a question as simple as, "How do you feel?" contains an element of suggestion that alters the drug-set-setting interaction. We took great pains to keep our laboratory setting neutral by strict adherence to an experimental timetable and to a prearranged set of conventions governing interactions between subjects and experimenters.

6. Medical, social, ethical, and legal concerns about the welfare of subjects are a major problem in a project of this kind. Is it ethical to introduce people to marihuana? When can subjects safely be sent home from the laboratory? What kind of follow-up care, if any, should be given? These are only a few specific questions with which the investigator must wrestle. Examples of some of the precautions we took are as follows. (i) All subjects were volunteers. All were given psychiatric screening interviews and were clearly informed that they might be asked to smoke marihuana. All nonusers tested were persons who had reported that they had been planning to try marihuana. (ii) All subjects were driven home by an experimenter; they agreed not to engage in unusual activity or operate machinery until the next morning and to report any unusual, delayed effects. (iii) All subjects agreed to report for follow-up interviews 6 months after the experiment. Among other things, the check at 6 months should answer the question whether participation in the experiment encouraged further drug use. (iv) All subjects were protected from possible legal repercussions of their participation in these experiments by specific agreements with the Federal Bureau of Narcotics, the Office of the

Attorney General of Massachusetts, and the Massachusetts Bureau of Drug Abuse and Drug Control (19).

## SUBJECTS

The central group of subjects consisted of nine healthy, male volunteers, 21 to 26 years of age, all of whom smoked tobacco cigarettes regularly but had never tried marihuana previously. Eight chronic users of marihuana also participated, both to "assay" the quality of marihuana received from the Federal Bureau of Narcotics and to enable the experimenters to standardize the protocol, using subjects familiar with their responses to the drug. The age range for users was also 21 to 26 years. They all smoked marihuana regularly, most of them every day or every other day.

The nine "naive" subjects were selected after a careful screening process. An initial pool of prospective subjects was obtained by placing advertisements in the student newspapers of a number of universities in the Boston area. These advertisements sought "male volunteers, at least 21 years old, for psychological experiments." After nonsmokers were eliminated from this pool, the remaining volunteers were interviewed individually by a psychiatrist who determined their histories of use of alcohol and other intoxicants as well as their general personality types. In addition to serving as a potential screening technique to eliminate volunteers with evidence of psychosis, or of serious mental or personality disorder, these interviews served as the basis for the psychiatrist's prediction of the type of response an individual subject might have after smoking marihuana. (It should be noted that no marihuana-naive volunteer had to be disqualified on psychiatric grounds.) Only after a prospective subject passed the interview was he informed that the "psychological experiment" for which he had volunteered was a marihuana study. If he consented to participate, he was asked to sign a release, informing him that he would be "expected to smoke cigarettes containing marihuana or an inert substance." He was also required to agree to a number of conditions, among them that he would "during the course of the experiment take no psychoactive drugs, including alcohol, other than those drugs administered in the course of the experiment."

It proved extremely difficult to find marihuana-naive persons in the student population of Boston, and nearly two months of inverviewing were required to obtain nine men. All those interviewed who had already tried marihuana volunteered this information quite freely and were delighted to discuss their use of drugs with the psychiatrist. Nearly all persons encountered who had not tried marihuana admitted this somewhat apologetically. Several said they had been meaning to try the drug but had not got around to it. A few said they had no access to it. Only one person cited the current laws as his reason for not having experimented with marihuana. It seemed clear in the interviews that many of these persons were actually afraid of how they might react to marihuana; they therefore welcomed a chance to smoke it under medical supervision. Only one person (an Indian exchange student) who passed the screening interview refused to participate after learning the nature of the experiment.

The eight heavy users of marihuana were obtained with much less difficulty. They were interviewed in the same manner as the other subjects and were instructed not to smoke any marihuana on the day of their appointment in the laboratory.

Subjects were questioned during screening interviews and at the conclusion of the experiments to determine their knowledge of marihuana effects. None of the nine naive subjects had ever watched anyone smoke marihuana or observed anyone high on marihuana. Most of them knew of the effects of the drug only through reports in the popular press. Two subjects had friends who used marihuana frequently; one of these (No. 4) announced his intention to "prove" in the experiments that marihuana really did not do anything; the other (No. 3) was extremely eager to get high because "everyone I know is always talking about it very positively."

## SETTING

Greatest effort was made to create a neutral setting. That is, subjects were made comfortable and secure in a pleasant suite of laboratories and offices, but the experimental staff carefully avoided encouraging any person to have an enjoyable experience. Subjects were never asked how they felt, and no subject was permitted to discuss the experiment with the staff until he had completed all four sessions. Verbal interactions between staff and subjects were minimum and formal. At the end of each session, subjects were asked to complete a brief form asking whether they thought they had smoked marihuana that night; if so, whether a high dose or a low dose; and how confident they were of their answers. The experimenters completed similar forms on each subject.

## MARIHUANA

Marihuana used in these experiments was of Mexican origin, supplied by the Federal Bureau of Narcotics (20). It consisted of finely chopped leaves of *Cannabis*, largely free of seeds and stems. An initial batch, which was judged to be of low potency by the experimenters on the basis of the doses needed to produce symptoms of intoxication in the chronic users, was subsequently found to contain only 0.3 percent of THC by weight. A second batch, assayed at 0.9 percent THC, was rated by the chronic users to be "good, average" marihuana, neither exceptionally strong nor exceptionally weak compared to their usual supplies. Users consistently reported symptoms of intoxication after smoking about 0.5 gram of the material with a variation of only a few puffs from subject to subject. This second batch of marihuana was used in the experiments described below; the low dose was 0.5 gram, and the high dose was 2.0 grams.

TABLE 1. Composition of the Dose

| Dose | Marihuana in Each Cigarette (g) | Total Dose Marihuana (2 cigarettes) (g) | Approximate Dose THC |
|---|---|---|---|
| Placebo | | | |
| Low | 0.25 | 0.5 | 4.5 mg |
| High | 1.0 | 2.0 | 18 mg |

The placebo cigarette consisted of placebo material, tobacco filler, and mint leaves for masking flavor. The low dose was made up of marihuana, tobacco filler, and mint leaves. The high dose consisted of marihuana and mint leaves.

All marihuana was administered in the form of cigarettes of standard size made with a hand-operated rolling machine. In any given experimental session, each person was required to smoke two cigarettes in succession (Table 1).

Placebo material consisted of the chopped outer covering of mature stalks of male hemp plants; it contained no THC. All cigarettes had a tiny plug of tobacco at one end and a plug of paper at the other end so that the contents were not visible. The length to which each cigarette was to be smoked was indicated by an ink line. Marihuana and placebos were administered to the naive subjects in double-blind fashion. Scented aerosols were sprayed in the laboratory before smoking, to mask the odor of marihuana. The protocol during an experimental session was as shown below. The sessions began at approximately 5.30 p.m.

## EXPERIMENTAL SESSIONS

Chronic users were tested only on high doses of marihuana with no practice sessions. Each naive subject was required to come to four sessions, spaced about a week apart. The first was always a practice session, in which the subject learned the proper smoking technique and during which he became thoroughly acquainted with the tests and the protocol. In the practice session, each subject completed the entire protocol, smoking two hand-rolled tobacco cigarettes. He was instructed to take a long puff, to inhale deeply, and to maintain inspiration for 20 seconds, as

| Time | Procedure |
|---|---|
| 0:00 | Physiological measurements: blood sample drawn |
| 0:05 | Psychological test battery No. 1 (base line) |
| 0:35 | Verbal sample No. 1 |
| 0:40 | Cigarette smoking |
| 1:00 | Rest period |
| 1:15 | Physiological measurements: blood sample drawn |
| 1:20 | Psychological test battery No. 2 |
| 1:50 | Verbal sample No. 2 |
| 1:55 | Rest period (supper) |
| 2:30 | Physiological measurements |
| 2:35 | Psychological test battery No. 3 |
| 3:05 | End of testing |

timed by an experimenter with a stopwatch. Subjects were allowed 8 to 12 minutes to smoke each of the two cigarettes. One purpose of this practice smoking was to identify and eliminate individuals who were not tolerant to high doses of nicotine, thus reducing the effect of nicotine on the variables measured during subsequent drug sessions (21). A surprising number (five) of volunteers who had described themselves in screening interviews as heavy cigarette smokers, "inhaling" up to two packs of cigarettes a day, developed acute nicotine reactions when they smoked two tobacco cigarettes by the required method. Occurrence of such a reaction disqualified a subject from participation in the experiments.

In subsequent sessions, when cigarettes contained either drug or placebo, all smoking was similarly supervised by an experimenter with a stopwatch. Subjects were not permitted to smoke tobacco cigarettes while the experiment was in progress. They were assigned to one of the three treatment groups listed in Table 2.

## PHYSIOLOGICAL AND PSYCHOLOGICAL MEASURES

The physiological parameters measured were heart rate, respiratory rate, pupil size, blood glucose level, and conjunctival vascular state. Pupil size was measured with a millimeter rule under constant illumination with eyes focused on an object at constant distance. Conjunctival appearance was rated by an experienced experimenter for dilation of blood vessels on a 0 to 4 scale with ratings of 3 and 4 indicating "significant" vasodilatation. Blood samples were collected for immediate determinations of serum glucose and for the serum to be frozen and stored for possible future biochemical studies. Subjects were asked not to eat and not to imbibe a beverage containing sugar or caffeine during the four hours preceding a session. They were given supper after the second blood sample was drawn.

The psychological test battery consisted of (i) the Continuous Performance Test (CPT)—5 minutes; (ii) the Digit Symbol Substitution Test (DSST)—90 seconds; (iii), CPT with strobe light distraction—5 minutes; (iv) self-rating bipolar mood scale—3 minutes; and (v) pursuit rotor—10 minutes.

The Continuous Performance Test was designed to measure a subject's capacity for sustained attention (22). The subject was placed in a darkened room and directed to watch a small screen upon which six letters of the alphabet were flashed rapidly and in random order. The subject was instructed to press a button whenever a specified critical letter appeared. The number of letters presented, correct responses, and errors of commission and omission were counted over the 5-minute period. The test was also done with a strobe light flickering at 50 cycles per second. Normal subjects make no or nearly no errors on this test either with or without strobe distraction; but sleep deprivation, organic brain disease, and

**TABLE 2. Order of Treatment**

| | *Drug Session* | | |
|---|---|---|---|
| *Group* | *1* | *2* | *3* |
| I | High | Placebo | Low |
| II | Low | High | Placebo |
| III | Placebo | Low | High |

certain drugs like chlorpromazine adversely affect performance. Presence or absence of previous exposure to the task has no effect on performance.

The Digit Symbol Substitution Test is a simple test of cognitive function (see Figure 1). A subject's score was the number of correct answers in a 90-second period. As in the case of the CPT, practice should have little or no effect on performance.

The self-rating bipolar mood scale used in these experiments was one developed by Smith and Beecher (23) to evaluate subjective effects of morphine. By allowing subjects to rate themselves within a given category of moods, on an arbitrary scale from +3 to −3, it minimizes suggestion and is thus more neutral than the checklists often employed in drug testing.

The pursuit rotor measures muscular coordination and attention. The subject's task was to keep a stylus in contact with a small spot on a moving turntable. In these experiments, subjects were given ten 30-second trials in each battery. The score for each trial was total time in contact with the spot. There is a marked practice effect on this test, but naive subjects were brought to high levels of performance during their practice session, so that the changes due to practice were reduced during the actual drug sessions. In addition, since there was a different order of treatments for each of the three groups of naive subjects, any session-to-session practice effects were minimized in the statistical analysis of the pooled data.

At the end of the psychological test battery, a verbal sample was collected from each subject. The subject was left alone in a room with a tape recorder and instructions to describe "an interesting or dramatic experience" in his life until he was stopped. After exactly 5 minutes he was interrupted and asked how long he had

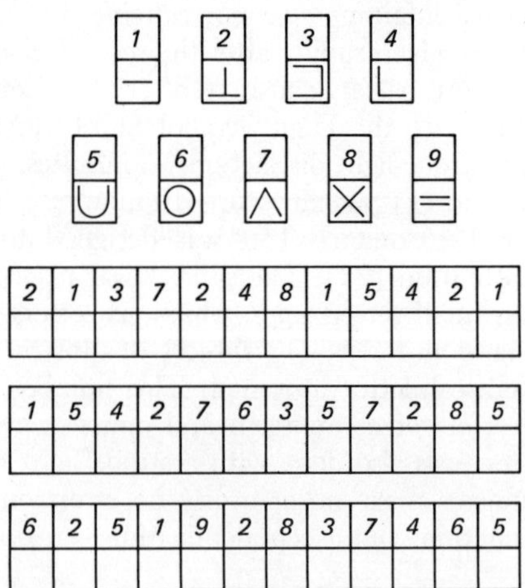


**Figure 1.** This is a sample of the Digit Symbol Substitution Test as used in these studies. On a signal from the examiner the subject was required to fill as many of the empty spaces as possible with the appropriate symbols. The code was always available to the subject during the 90-second administration of the test. [This figure appeared originally in *Psychopharmacologia* **5,** 164 (1964).]

been in the recording room. In this way, an estimate of the subject's ability to judge time was also obtained.

## RESULTS

1. *Safety of marihuana in human volunteers.* In view of the apprehension expressed by many persons over the safety of administering marihuana to research subjects, we wish to emphasize that no adverse marihuana reactions occurred in any of our subjects. In fact, the five acute nicotine reactions mentioned earlier were far more spectacular than any effects produced by marihuana.

In these experiments, observable effects of marihuana were maximum at 15 minutes after smoking. They were diminished between 30 minutes and 1 hour, and they were largely dissipated 3 hours after the end of smoking. No delayed or persistent effects beyond 3 hours were observed or reported.

2. *Intoxicating properties of marihuana in a neutral setting.* With the high dose of marihuana (2.0 grams), all chronic users became "high" (24) by their own accounts and in the judgment of experimenters who had observed many persons under the influence of marihuana. The effect was consistent even though prior to the session some of these subjects expressed anxiety about smoking marihuana and submitting to tests in a laboratory.

On the other hand, only one of the nine naive subjects (No. 3) had a definite "marihuana reaction" on the same high dose. He became markedly euphoric and laughed continuously during his first battery of tests after taking the drug. Interestingly, he was the one subject who had expressed his desire to get high.

3. *Comparison of naive and chronic user subjects.* Throughout the experiments it was apparent that the two groups of subjects reacted differently to identical doses of marihuana. We must caution, however, that our study was designed to allow rigorous statistical analysis of data from the naive group—it was not designed to permit formal comparison between chronic users and naive subjects. The conditions of the experiment were not the same for both groups: the chronic users were tested with the drug on their first visit to the laboratory with no practice and were informed that they were to receive high doses of marihuana. Therefore, differences between the chronic and naive groups reported below—although statistically valid—must be regarded as trends to be confirmed or rejected by additional experiments.

4. *Recognition of marihuana versus placebo.* All nine naive subjects reported that they had not been able to identify the taste or smell of marihuana in the experimental cigarettes. A few subjects remarked that they noticed differences in the taste of the three sets of cigarettes but could not interpret the differences. Most subjects found the pure marihuana cigarettes (high dose) more mild than the low dose or placebo cigarettes, both of which contained tobacco.

The subjects' guesses of the contents of cigarettes for their three sessions are presented in Table 3. It is noteworthy that one of the two subjects who called the high dose a placebo was the subject (No. 4) who had told us he wanted to prove that marihuana really did nothing. There were three outstanding findings: (i) most subjects receiving marihuana in either high or low dose recognized that they

**TABLE 3. Subjects' Appraisal of the Dose**

| *Actual Dose* | *Guessed Dose* Placebo | Low | High | *Fraction Correct* |
|---|---|---|---|---|
| Placebo | 8 | 1 | | 8/9 |
| Low | 3 | 6 | | 6/9 |
| High | 2 | 6 | 1 | 1/9 |

were getting a drug; (ii) most subjects receiving placebos recognized that they were receiving placebos; (iii) most subjects called their high dose a low dose, but none called his low dose a high dose, emphasizing the unimpressiveness of their subjective reactions.

5. *Effect of marihuana on heart rate.* The mean changes in heart rate from base-line rates before smoking the drug to rates at 15 and 90 minutes after smoking marihuana and placebo (Table 4) were tested for significance at the .05 level by an analysis of variance; Tukey's method was applied for all possible comparisons (Table 5). In the naive subjects, marihuana in low dose or high dose was followed by increased heart rate 15 minutes after smoking, but the effect was not demonstrated to be dose-dependent. The high dose caused a statistically greater increase

**TABLE 4. Change in Heart Rate (Beat/Min) after Smoking the Best Material (Results are recorded as a change from the base line 15 minutes and 90 minutes after the smoking session)**

| | *15 Minutes* | | | *90 Minutes* | | |
|---|---|---|---|---|---|---|
| *Subject* | *Placebo* | *Low* | *High* | *Placebo* | *Low* | *High* |
| | | | *Naive subjects* | | | |
| 1 | + 16 | + 20 | + 16 | + 20 | − 6 | − 4 |
| 2 | + 12 | + 24 | + 12 | − 6 | + 4 | − 8 |
| 3 | + 8 | + 8 | + 26 | − 4 | + 4 | + 8 |
| 4 | + 20 | + 8 | | | + 20 | − 4 |
| 5 | + 8 | + 4 | − 8 | | + 22 | − 8 |
| 6 | + 10 | + 20 | + 28 | − 20 | − 4 | − 4 |
| 7 | + 4 | + 28 | + 24 | + 12 | + 8 | + 18 |
| 8 | − 8 | + 20 | + 24 | − 3 | + 8 | − 24 |
| 9 | | + 20 | + 24 | + 8 | + 12 | |
| Mean | + 7.8 | + 16.9 | + 16.2 | + 0.8 | + 7.6 | − 2.9 |
| S.E. | 2.8 | 2.7 | 4.2 | 3.8 | 3.2 | 3.8 |
| | | | *Chronic subjects* | | | |
| 10 | | + 32 | | | + 4 | |
| 11 | | + 36 | | | + 36 | |
| 12 | | + 20 | | | + 12 | |
| 13 | | + 8 | | | + 4 | |
| 14 | | + 32 | | | + 12 | |
| 15 | | + 54 | | | + 22 | |
| 16 | | + 24 | | | | |
| 17 | | + 60 | | | | |
| Mean | | + 33.2 | | | + 15.0 | |
| S.E. | | 6.0 | | | 5.0 | |

**TABLE 5. Significance of Differences (at the .05 Level) in Heart Rate (Results of Tukey's test for all possible comparisons)**

| *Comparison* | *15 Minutes* | *90 Minutes* |
|---|---|---|
| Low dose versus placebo | Significant | Significant |
| High dose versus placebo | Significant | Not significant |
| Low dose versus high dose | Not significant | Significant |
| Chronic users versus high dose | Significant | Significant |

in the heart rates of chronic users than in those of the naive subjects 15 minutes after smoking.

Two of the chronic users had unusually low resting pulse rates (56 and 42), but deletion of these two subjects (No. 11 and No. 15) still gave a significant difference in mean pulse rise of chronic users compared to naives. Because the conditions of the sessions and experimental design were not identical for the two groups, we prefer to report this difference as a trend that must be confirmed by further studies.

6. *Effect of marihuana on respiratory rate.* In the naive group, there was no change in respiratory rate before and after smoking marihuana. Chronic users showed a small but statistically significant increase in respiratory rate after smoking, but we do not regard the change as clinically significant.

7. *Effect of marihuana on pupil size.* There was no change in pupil size before and after smoking marihuana in either group.

8. *Effect of marihuana on conjunctival appearance.* Significant reddening of conjunctivae due to dilatation of blood vessels occurred in one of nine subjects receiving placebo, three of nine receiving the low dose of marihuana, and eight of nine receiving the high dose. It occurred in all eight of the chronic users receiving the high dose and was rated as more prominent in them. The effect was more pronounced 15 minutes after the smoking period than 90 minutes after it.

9. *Effect of marihuana on blood sugar.* There was no significant change in blood sugar levels after smoking marihuana in either group.

10. *Effect of marihuana on the Continuous Performance Test.* Performance on the CPT and on the CPT with strobe distraction was unaffected by marihuana for both groups of subjects.

11. *Effect of marihuana on the Digit Symbol Substitution Test.* The significance of the differences in mean changes of scores at the .05 level was determined by an analysis of variance by means of Tukey's method for all possible comparisons. Results of these tests are summarized in Tables 6 and 7.

The results indicate that: (i) Decrements in performance of naive subjects

**TABLE 6. Significance of Differences (at the .05 Level) for the Digit Symbol Substitution Test (Results of Tukey's test for all possible comparisons)**

| *Comparison* | *15 Minutes* | *90 Minutes* |
|---|---|---|
| Low dose versus placebo | Significant | Significant |
| High dose versus placebo | Significant | Significant |
| Low dose versus high dose | Significant | Not significant |
| Chronic users versus high dose | Significant | Significant |

**TABLE 7. Digit Symbol Substitution Test**
**(Change in scores from base line [number correct] 15 and 90 minutes after the smoking session)**

| Subject | *15 Minutes* Placebo | *15 Minutes* Low | *15 Minutes* High | *90 Minutes* Placebo | *90 Minutes* Low | *90 Minutes* High |
|---|---|---|---|---|---|---|
| | | | *Naive subjects* | | | |
| 1 | − 3 | | + 5 | − 7 | + 4 | + 8 |
| 2 | + 10 | − 8 | − 17 | − 1 | − 15 | − 5 |
| 3 | − 3 | + 6 | − 7 | − 10 | + 2 | − 1 |
| 4 | + 3 | − 4 | − 3 | | − 7 | |
| 5 | + 4 | + 1 | − 7 | + 6 | | − 8 |
| 6 | − 3 | − 1 | − 9 | + 3 | − 5 | − 12 |
| 7 | + 2 | − 4 | − 6 | + 3 | − 5 | − 4 |
| 8 | − 1 | + 3 | + 1 | + 4 | + 4 | − 3 |
| 9 | − 1 | − 4 | − 3 | + 6 | − 1 | − 10 |
| Mean | + 0.9 | − 1.2 | − 5.1 | + 0.4 | − 2.6 | − 3.9 |
| S.E. | 1.4 | 1.4 | 2.1 | 1.9 | 2.0 | 2.0 |
| | | | *Chronic users* | | | |
| 10 | | | − 4 | | | − 16 |
| 11 | | | + 1 | | | + 6 |
| 12 | | | + 11 | | | + 18 |
| 13 | | | + 3 | | | + 4 |
| 14 | | | − 2 | | | − 3 |
| 15 | | | − 6 | | | + 8 |
| 16 | | | − 4 | | | |
| 17 | | | + 3 | | | |
| Mean | | | + 0.25 | | | + 2.8 |
| S.E. | | | 1.9 | | | 4.7 |

following low and high doses of marihuana were significant at 15 and 90 minutes after smoking. (ii) The decrement following marihuana was greater after high dose than after low dose at 15 minutes after taking the drug, giving preliminary evidence of a dose-response relationship. (iii) Chronic users started with good base-line performance and improved slightly on the DSST after smoking 2.0 grams of marihuana, whereas performance of the naive subjects was grossly impaired. Experience with the DSST suggests that absence of impairment in chronic users cannot be accounted for solely by a practice effect. Still, because of the different procedures employed, we prefer to report this difference as a trend.

12. *Effect of marihuana on pursuit rotor performance.* This result is presented in Table 8. Again applying Tukey's method in an analysis of variance, we tested differences in mean changes in scores (Table 9). Decrements in performance of naive subjects after both low and high doses of marihuana were significant at 15 and 90 minutes. This effect on performance followed a dose-response relation on testing batteries conducted at both 15 minutes and 90 minutes after the drug was smoked.

All chronic users started from good baselines and improved on the pursuit rotor after smoking marihuana. These data are not presented, however, because it is probable that the improvement was largely a practice effect.

13. *Effect of marihuana on time estimation.* Before smoking, all nine naive

**TABLE 8. Pursuit Rotor (Naive Subjects)**
**(Changes in scores [averages of ten trials] from base line [seconds])**

| | 15 Minutes | | | 90 Minutes | | |
|---|---|---|---|---|---|---|
| *Subject* | *Placebo* | *Low* | *High* | *Placebo* | *Low* | *High* |
| 1 | + 1.20 | − 1.04 | − 4.01 | + 1.87 | − 1.54 | − 6.54 |
| 2 | + 0.89 | − 1.43 | − 0.12 | + 0.52 | + 0.44 | − 0.68 |
| 3 | + 0.50 | − 0.60 | − 6.56 | + 0.84 | − 0.96 | − 4.34 |
| 4 | + 0.18 | − 0.11 | + 0.11 | + 0.06 | + 1.95 | − 1.37 |
| 5 | + 3.20 | + 0.39 | + 0.13 | + 2.64 | + 3.33 | + 0.34 |
| 6 | + 3.45 | − 0.32 | − 3.46 | + 2.93 | + 0.22 | − 2.26 |
| 7 | + 0.81 | + 0.48 | − 0.79 | + 0.63 | + 0.16 | − 0.52 |
| 8 | + 1.75 | − 0.39 | − 0.92 | + 2.13 | + 0.40 | + 1.02 |
| 9 | + 3.90 | − 1.94 | − 2.60 | + 3.11 | − 0.97 | − 3.09 |
| Mean | + 1.8 | − 0.6 | − 2.0 | + 1.6 | + 0.3 | − 1.9 |
| S.E. | 0.5 | 0.3 | 0.8 | 0.4 | 0.5 | 0.8 |

subjects estimated the 5-minute verbal sample to be 5 ± 2 minutes. After placebo, no subject changed his guess. After the low dose, three subjects raised their estimates to 10 ± 2 minutes, and after the high dose, four raised their estimates.

14. *Subjective effects of marihuana.* When questioned at the end of their participation in the experiment, persons who had never taken marihuana previously reported minimum subjective effects after smoking the drug, or, more precisely, few effects like those commonly reported by chronic users. Nonusers reported little euphoria, no distortion of visual or auditory perception, and no confusion. However, several subjects mentioned that "things seemed to take longer." Below are examples of comments by naive subjects after high doses.

> Subject 1: "It was stronger than the previous time (low dose) but I really didn't think it could be marihuana. Things seemed to go slower."
>
> Subject 2: "I think I realize why they took our watches. There was a sense of the past disappearing as happens when you're driving too long without sleeping. With a start you wake up to realize you were asleep for an instant; you discover yourself driving along the road. It was the same tonight with eating a sandwich. I'd look down to discover I'd just swallowed a bite but I hadn't noticed it at the time."
>
> Subject 6: "I felt a combination of being almost-drunk and tired, with occasional fits of silliness—not my normal reaction to smoking tobacco."
>
> Subject 8: "I felt faint briefly, but the dizziness went away, and I felt normal or slightly tired. I can't believe I had a high dose of marihuana."

**TABLE 9. Significance of Differences (at the .05 Level) for the Pursuit Rotor (Results of Tukey's test for all possible comparisons, 15 and 90 minutes after the smoking session)**

| *Comparison* | *15 Minutes* | *90 Minutes* |
|---|---|---|
| Low dose versus placebo | Significant | Significant |
| High dose versus placebo | Significant | Significant |
| Low dose versus high dose | Significant | Significant |

Subject 9: "Time seemed very drawn out. I would keep forgetting what I was doing, especially on the continuous performance test, but somehow every time an 'X' (the critical letter) came up, I found myself pushing the button."

After smoking their high dose, chronic users were asked to rate themselves on a scale of 1 to 10, 10 representing "the highest you've ever been." All subjects placed themselves between 7 and 10, most at 8 or 9. Many of these subjects expressed anxiety at the start of their first battery of tests after smoking the drug when they were feeling very high. Then they expressed surprise during and after the tests when they judged (correctly) that their performance was as good as or better than it had been before taking the drug.

15. The effect of marihuana on the self-rating mood scale, the effect of marihuana on a 5-minute verbal sample, and the correlation of personality type with subjective effects of marihuana will be reported separately.

## DISCUSSION

Several results from this study raise important questions about the action of marihuana and suggest directions for future research. Our finding that subjects who were naive to marihuana did not become subjectively "high" after a high dose of marihuana in a neutral setting is interesting when contrasted with the response of regular users who consistently reported and exhibited highs. It agrees with the reports of chronic users that many, if not most, people do not become high on their first exposure to marihuana even if they smoke it correctly. This puzzling phenomenon can be discussed from either a physiological or psychosocial point of view. Neither interpretation is entirely satisfactory. The physiological hypothesis suggests that getting high on marihuana occurs only after some sort of pharmacological sensitization takes place. The psychosocial interpretation is that repeated exposure to marihuana reduces psychological inhibition, as part of, or as the result of a learning process.

Indirect evidence makes the psychological hypothesis attractive. Anxiety about drug use in this country is sufficiently great to make worthy of careful consideration the possibility of an unconscious psychological inhibition or block on the part of naive drug takers. The subjective responses of our subjects indicate that they had imagined a marihuana effect to be much more profoundly disorganizing than what they experienced. For example, subject No. 4, who started with a bias against the possibility of becoming high on marihuana, was able to control subjectively the effect of the drug and report that he had received a placebo when he had actually gotten a high dose. As anxiety about the drug is lessened with experience, the block may decrease, and the subject may permit himself to notice the drug's effects.

It is well known that marihuana users, in introducing friends to the drug, do actually "teach" them to notice subtle effects of the drug on consciousness (25). The apparently enormous influence of set and setting on the form of the marihuana response is consistent with this hypothesis, as is the testimony of users that, as use becomes more frequent, the amount of drug required to produce intoxication decreases—a unique example of "reverse tolerance." (Regular use of many intoxicants is accompanied by the need for increasing doses to achieve the same effects.)

On the other hand, the suggestion arising from this study that users and nonusers react differently to the drug, not only subjectively but also physiologically, increases the plausibility of the pharmacological-sensitization hypothesis. Of course, reverse tolerance could equally well be a manifestation of this sensitization.

It would be useful to confirm the suggested differences between users and nonusers and then to test in a systematic manner the hypothetical explanations of the phenomenon. One possible approach would be to continue to administer high doses of marihuana to the naive subjects according to the protocol described. If subjects begin reporting high responses to the drug only after several exposures, in the absence of psychedelic settings, suggestions, or manipulations of mood, then the likelihood that marihuana induces a true physiological sensitization or that experience reduces psychological inhibitions, permitting real drug effects to appear, would be increased. If subjects fail to become high, we could conclude that learning to respond to marihuana requires some sort of teaching or suggestion.

An investigation of the literature of countries where anxieties over drug use are less prominent would be useful. If this difference between responses of users and nonusers is a uniquely American phenomenon, a psychological explanation would be indicated, although it would not account for greater effects with smaller doses after the initial, anxiety-reducing stage.

One impetus for reporting the finding of differences between chronic and naive subjects on some of the tests, despite the fact that the experimental designs were not the same, is that this finding agrees with the statements of many users. They say that the effects of marihuana are easily suppressed—much more so than those of alcohol. Our observation, that the chronic users after smoking marihuana performed on some tests as well as or better than they did before taking the drug, reinforced the argument advanced by chronic users that maintaining effective levels of performance for many tasks—driving, for example (26)—is much easier under the influence of marihuana than under that of other psychoactive drugs. Certainly the surprise that the chronic users expressed when they found they were performing more effectively on the CPT, DSST, and pursuit rotor tests than they thought they would is remarkable. It is quite the opposite of the false sense of improvement subjects have under some psychoactive drugs that actually impair performance.

What might be the basis of this suppressibility? Possibly, the actions of marihuana are confined to higher cortical functions without any general stimulatory or depressive effect on lower brain centers. The relative absence of neurological—as opposed to psychiatric—symptoms in marihuana intoxication suggests this possibility (7).

Our failure to detect any changes in blood sugar levels of subjects after they had smoked marihuana forces us to look elsewhere for an explanation of the hunger and hyperphagia commonly reported by users. A first step would be careful interviewing of users to determine whether they really become hungry after smoking marihuana or whether they simply find eating more pleasurable. Possibly, the basis of this effect is also central rather than due to some peripheral physiological change.

Lack of any change in pupil size of subjects after they had smoked marihuana is an enlightening finding especially because so many users and law-enforcement agents firmly believe that marihuana dilates pupils. (Since users generally observe each other in dim surroundings, it is not surprising that they see large pupils.) This negative finding emphasizes the need for data from carefully controlled investigations rather than from casual observation or anecdotal reports in the evaluation of marihuana. It also agrees with the findings of others that synthetic THC does not alter pupil size (8, 27).

Finally, we would like to comment on the fact that marihuana appears to be a relatively mild intoxicant in our studies. If these results seem to differ from those of earlier experiments, it must be remembered that other experimenters have given marihuana orally, have given doses much higher than those commonly smoked by users, have administered potent synthetics, and have not strictly controlled the laboratory setting. As noted in our introduction, more powerful effects are often reported by users who ingest preparations of marihuana. This may mean that some active constituents which enter the body when the drug is ingested are destroyed by combustion, a suggestion that must be investigated in man. Another priority consideration is the extent to which synthetic THC reproduces marihuana intoxication—a problem that must be resolved before marihuana research proceeds with THC instead of the natural resin of the whole plant.

The set, both of subjects and experimenters, and the setting must be recognized as critical variables in studies of marihuana. Drug, set, and setting interact to shape the form of a marihuana reaction. The researcher who sets out with prior conviction that hemp is psychotomimetic or a "mild hallucinogen" is likely to confirm his conviction experimentally (10), but he would probably confirm the opposite hypothesis if his bias were in the opposite direction. Precautions to insure neutrality of set and setting, including use of a double-blind procedure as an absolute minimum, are vitally important if the object of investigation is to measure real marihuana-induced responses.

## CONCLUSIONS

1. It is feasible and safe to study the effects of marihuana on human volunteers who smoke it in a laboratory.
2. In a neutral setting persons who are naive to marihuana do not have strong subjective experiences after smoking low or high doses of the drug, and the effects they do report are not the same as those described by regular users of marihuana who take the drug in the same neutral setting.
3. Marihuana-naive persons do demonstrate impaired performance on simple intellectual and psychomotor tests after smoking marihuana; the impairment is dose-related in some cases.
4. Regular users of marihuana do get high after smoking marihuana in a neutral setting but do not show the same degree of impairment of performance on the tests as do naive subjects. In some cases, their performance even appears to improve slightly after smoking marihuana.
5. Marihuana increases heart rate moderately.

6. No change in respiratory rate follows administration of marihuana by inhalation.
7. No change in pupil size occurs in short term exposure to marihuana.
8. Marihuana administration causes dilatation of conjunctival blood vessels.
9. Marihuana treatment produces no change in blood sugar levels.
10. In a neutral setting the physiological and psychological effects of a single, inhaled dose of marihuana appear to reach maximum intensity within one-half hour of inhalation, to be diminished after 1 hour, and to be completely dissipated by 3 hours.

## REFERENCES AND NOTES


1. R. J. Bouquet, *Bull. Narcotics* **2**, 14 (1950).
2. F. Korte and H. Sieper, in *Hashish: Its Chemistry and Pharmacology*, G. E. W. Wolstenholme and J. Knight, Eds. (Little, Brown, Boston, 1965), pp. 15–30.
3. Task Force on Narcotics and Drug Abuse, the President's Commission on Law Enforcement and the Administration of Justice, *Task Force Report: Narcotics and Drug Abuse* (1967), p. 14.
4. R. Mechoulam, and Y. Gaoni, *J. Amer. Chem. Soc.* **67**, 3273 (1965).
5. J. F. Siler, W. L. Sheep, L. B. Bates, G. F. Clark, G. W. Cook, W. A. Smith, *Mil. Surg.* (November 1933), pp. 269–280.
6. Mayor's Committee on Marihuana, *The Marihuana Problem in the City of New York*, 1944.
7. E. G. Williams, C. K. Himmelsbach, A. Winkler, D. C. Ruble, B. J. Lloyd, *Public Health Rep.* **61**, 1059 (1946).
8. H. Isbell, *Psychopharmacologia* **11**, 184 (1967).
9. I. C. Chopra and R. N. Chopra, *Bull. Narcotics* **9**, 4 (1957).
10. F. Ames, *J. Ment. Sci.* **104**, 972 (1958).
11. C. J. Miras, in *Hashish: Its Chemistry and Pharmacology*, G. E. W. Wolstenholme and J. Knight, Eds. (Little, Brown, Boston, 1965), pp. 37–47.
12. J. M. Watt, in *Hashish: Its Chemistry and Pharmacology*, G. E. W. Wolstenholme and J. Knight, Eds. (Little, Brown, Boston, 1965), pp. 54–66.
13. AMA Council on Mental Health, *J. Amer. Med. Ass.* **204**, 1181 (1968).
14. G. Joachimoglu, in *Hashish: Its Chemistry and Pharmacology*, G. E. W. Wolstenholme and J. Knight, Eds. (Little, Brown, Boston, 1965), pp. 2–10.
15. We thank M. Lerner and A. Bober of the U.S. Customs Laboratory, Baltimore, for performing this assay.
16. We thank R. H. Pace and E. H. Hall of the Peter J. Schweitzer Division of the Kimberly-Clark Corp. for supplying placebo material.
17. S. Garattini, in *Hashish: Its Chemistry and Pharmacology*, G. E. W. Wolstenholme and J. Knight, Eds. (Little, Brown, Boston, 1965), pp. 70–78.
18. J. H. Jaffe, in *The Pharmacological Basis of Therapeutics*, L. S. Goodman and A. Gilman, Eds. (Macmillan, New York, ed. 3, 1965), pp. 299–301.
19. We thank E. L. Richardson, Attorney General of the Commonwealth of Massachusetts for permitting these experiments to proceed and N. L. Chayet for legal assistance. We do not consider it appropriate to describe here the opposition we encountered from governmental agents and agencies and from university bureaucracies.

20. We thank D. Miller and M. Seifer of the Federal Bureau of Narcotics (now part of the Bureau of Narcotics and Dangerous Drugs, under the Department of Justice) for help in obtaining marihuana for this research.
21. The doses of tobacco in placebo and low-dose cigarettes were too small to cause physiological changes in subjects who qualified in the practice session.
22. K. E. Rosvold, A. F. Mirsky, I. Sarason, E. D. Bransome, L. H. Beck, *J. Consult. Psychol.* **20,** 343 (1956); A. F. Mirsky and P. V. Cardon, *Electroencephalogr. Clin. Neurophysiol.* **14,** 1 (1962); C. Kornetsky and G. Bain, *Psychopharmacologia* 8, 277 (1965).
23. G. M. Smith and H. K. Beecher, *J. Pharmacol.* **126,** 50 (1959).
24. We will attempt to define the complex nature of a marihuana high in a subsequent paper discussing the speech samples and interviews.
25. H. S. Becker, *Outsiders: Studies in the Sociology of Deviance* (Macmillan, New York, 1963), chap. 3.
26. Although the motor skills measured by the pursuit rotor are represented in driving ability, they are only components of that ability. The influence of marihuana on driving skill remains an open question of high medico-legal priority.
27. L. E. Hollister, R. K. Richards, H. K. Gillespie, in preparation.
28. Sponsored and supported by Boston University's division of psychiatry, in part through PHS grants MH12568, MH06795–06, MH7753–06, and MH33319 and the Boston University Medical Center. The authors thank Dr. P. H. Knapp and Dr. C. Kornetsky of the Boston University School of Medicine, Department of Psychiatry and Pharmacology, for consistent support and excellent advice, and J. Finkelstein of 650 Madison Avenue, New York City, for his support at a crucial time.

# 11

## *Comparison of the Effects of Marihuana and Alcohol on Simulated Driving Performance*

A. CRANCER, J. M. DILLE, J. C. DELAY,
J. E. WALLACE, M. HAYKIN

We have determined the effect of a "normal social marihuana high" on simulated driving performance among experienced marihuana smokers. We compared the degree of driving impairment due to smoking marihuana to the effect on driving of a recognized standard—that is, legally defined intoxication at the presumptive limit

From *Science,* Vol. 164, May 16, 1969, pp. 851–854. 

of 0.10 percent alcohol concentration in the blood. This study focused attention on the effect of smoking marihuana rather than on the effect of ingesting $\Delta^9$-tetrahydrocannabinol ($\Delta^9$-THC), the principal active component.

Weil et al. (1) have studied the clinical and psychological effects of smoking marihuana on both experienced and inexperienced subjects. They suggest, as do others (2), that experienced smokers when "high" show no significant impairment as judged by performance on selected tests; they also establish the existence of physiological changes that are useful in determining whether a subject smoking marihuana is "high." A review of the relation of alcohol to fatal accidents (3) showed that nearly half of the drivers fatally injured in an accident had an alcohol concentration in the blood of 0.05 percent or more.

Crancer (4) found a driving simulator test to be a valid indicator for distinguishing driving performance; this result was based on a 5-year driving record. Further studies (5) indicated that a behind-the-wheel road test is not significantly correlated to driving performance. We therefore chose the simulator test, which presents a programmed series of emergency situations that are impractical and dangerous in actual road tests.

Subjects were required to be (i) experienced marihuana smokers who had been smoking marihuana at least twice a month for the past 6 months, (ii) licensed as a motor vehicle operator, (iii) engaged in a generally accepted educational or vocational pursuit, and (iv) familiar with the effects of alcohol. The subjects were given (i) a physical examination to exclude persons currently in poor health or under medication, and (ii) a written personality inventory (Minnesota Multiphasic Personality Inventory) to exclude persons showing a combination of psychological stress and inflexible defense patterns. Seven of the subjects were females and 29 were males (mean age, 22.9).

We compared the effects of a marihuana "high," alcohol intoxication, and no treatment on simulated driving performance over a four-and-one-half-hour period. We used a Latin-square analysis of variance design (6) to account for the effects of treatments, subjects, days, and the order in which the treatments were given. To measure the time response effects of each treatment, simulator scores were obtained at three constant points in the course of each experimental period. A sample of 36 subjects was determined to be sufficient in size to meet the demands of this experimental design.

Three treatments were given to each subject. In treatment M (normal social marihuana "high"), the experimental subject stated that he experienced the physical and psychological effects of smoking marihuana in a social environment comparable to his previous experiences. This subjective evaluation of "high" was confirmed by requiring a minimum consumption of marihuana established with a separate test group, and by identifying an increase in pulse rate (1).

In treatment M, the subjects smoked two marihuana (7) cigarettes of approximately equal weight and totaling 1.7 g. They completed smoking in about 30 minutes and were given their first simulator test 30 minutes later.

Some confirmation that the amount of marihuana smoked was sufficient to produce a "high" is found in Weil's (1) study. His subjects smoked about 0.5 g of marihuana of 0.9 percent $\Delta^9$-THC.

In treatment A, subjects consumed two drinks containing equal amounts of 95 percent alcohol mixed in orange or tomato juice. Dosage was regulated according to subject's weight with the intended result of a 0.10 blood alcohol concentration as determined by a Breathalyzer reading (8). Thus, a subject weighing 120 pounds received 84 ml of 95 percent laboratory alcohol equally divided between two drinks. This was equivalent to about 6 ounces of 86 proof liquor. The dosage was increased 14 ml or ½ ounce for each additional 15 pounds of body weight. A Breathalyzer reading was obtained for each subject about 1 hour after drinking began; most subjects completed drinking in 30 minutes.

Treatment C consisted of waiting in the lounge with no treatment for the same period of time required for treatments M and A. The experimental subject stated that his physiological and psychological condition was normal. Subjects were requested to refrain from all drug or alcohol use during the time they were participating in the experiment.

A driver-training simulator was specially modified to obtain data on the effect of the treatments. The car unit was a console mockup of a recent model containing all the control and instrument equipment relevant to the driving task. The car unit faced a 6 by 18 foot screen upon which the test film was projected. The test film gave the subject a driver's eye view of the road as it led him through normal and emergency driving situations on freeways and urban and suburban streets. From the logic unit, located to the rear of the driver, the examiner started the automated test, observed the subject driving, and recorded the final scores.

A series of checks was placed on the 23-minute driving film which monitored driver reactions to a programmed series of driving stimuli. The test variables monitored were: accelerator (164 checks), brake (106 checks), turn signals (59 checks), steering (53 checks), and speedometer (23 checks). There was a total of 405 checks, allowing driver scores to range from zero to 405 errors per test. Errors were accumulated as follows.

1. Speedometer errors: Speedometer readings outside the range of 15 to 35 mile/hour for city portion of film and 45 to 65 mile/hour for freeways. The speed of the filmed presentation is not under the control of the driver. Therefore, speedometer errors are not an indication of speeding errors, but of the amount of time spent monitoring the speedometer.
2. Steering errors: Steering wheel in other than the appropriate position.
3. Brake errors: Not braking when the appropriate response is to brake, or braking at an inappropriate time.
4. Accelerator errors: Acceleration when the appropriate response is to decelerate, or deceleration when it is appropriate to accelerate.
5. Signal errors: Use of turn signal at an inappropriate time or position.
6. Total errors: An accumulation of the total number of errors on the five test variables.

Two rooms were used for the experiment. The lounge, designed to provide a familiar and comfortable environment for the subjects, was approximately 12 feet square and contained six casual chairs, a refrigerator, a desk, and several small movable tables. The room was lighted by a red lava lamp and one indirect red light, and contemporary rock music was played. Snacks, soft drinks, ashtrays, wastebaskets, and a supply of cigarettes were readily available. Subjects remained in this room except during simulator tests.

The driving simulator was located in a larger room about 50 feet from the lounge. The simulator room was approximately 20 by 30 feet and was kept in almost total darkness.

Each subject took three preliminary tests on the driving simulator to familiarize himself with the equipment and to minimize the effect of learning through practice during the experiment. Subjects whose error scores varied by more than 10 percent between the second and third tests were given subsequent tests until the stability criterion was met.

The experiment was conducted over a 6-week period. Six subjects were tested each week. On day 1, six subjects took a final test on the driving simulator to assure recent familiarity with the equipment. A "normal" pulse rate was recorded, and each was given two marihuana cigarettes of approximately 0.9 g each. Subjects smoked the marihuana in the lounge to become acquainted with the surroundings and other test subjects, and with the potency of the marihuana. A second pulse reading was recorded for each subject when he reported that he was "high" in order to obtain an indication of the expected rate increase during the experiment proper. They remained in the lounge for approximately 4 hours after they had started smoking.

Three of the subjects were scheduled for testing in the early evening on days 2, 4, and 6; the remaining three subjects for days 3, 5, and 7. A single treatment was given each evening. Within a given week, all subjects received treatments in the same order. Treatment order was changed from week to week to meet the requirements of a Latin-square design. Procedure for each evening was identical except for the specific treatment.

Subject 1 arrived at the laboratory and took the simulator warm-up test. Treatment A, M, or C was begun at zero hour and finished about ½ hour later. One hour after treatment began, subject 1 took simulator test 1, returning to the lounge when he was finished. He took simulator test 2 2½ hours after treatment began, and test 3 4 hours after treatment began. Pulse or Breathalyzer readings, depending on the treatment, were taken immediately before each simulator test.

Subject 2 followed the same schedule, beginning ½ hour after subject 1. Time used in testing one subject each evening was 4½ hours, with a total elapsed time of 5½ hours to test three subjects.

The three simulator tests taken after each treatment establish a time response effect for the treatment. For each treatment the total error scores for each time period were subjected to an analysis of variance. Table 1 presents the analysis of variance for period 1 scores; results comparable to these were obtained for scores in periods 2 and 3.

The simulated driving scores for subjects experiencing a normal social marihuana "high" and the same subjects under control conditions are not significantly different (Table 1). However, there are significantly more errors ($P < .01$) for intoxicated than for control subjects (difference of 15.4 percent). This finding is consistent with the mean error scores of the three treatments: control, 84.46 errors; marihuana, 84.49 errors; and alcohol, 97.44 errors.

The time response curves for "high" and control treatments are comparable (Fig. 1). In contrast, the curve for alcohol shows more total errors ($P < .01$). These higher error scores for alcohol persist across all three time periods with little evidence of the improvement shown under the other two treatments.

**TABLE 1. Analysis of Variance of Total Driving Simulator Error Scores for Three Treatments; Marihuana (M), Control (C), and Alcohol (A)**

| *Source of Variation* | *Sum of Squares* | *Degrees of Freedom* | *Mean Square* | *Mean Square Ratios* |
|---|---|---|---|---|
| Treatments | 2,595.1 | 2 | 1,297.5 | 6.7[a] |
| M versus C | (11.7) | (1) | 11.7 | 0.1 |
| A versus M and C | (2,583.4) | (1) | 2,583.4 | 13.3[b] |
| Days | 738.5 | 2 | 369.3 | 1.9 |
| Subjects | 40,872.5 | 24 | 1,703.0 | 9.7[b] |
| Squares | 13,708.5 | 11 | 1,247.2 | 6.4[b] |
| Pooled error | 13,253.8 | 68 | 194.9 | |
| Total | 71,168.4 | 107 | | |

[a] $P < .05$.
[b] $P < .01$.

A separate Latin-square analysis of variance was completed for each test variable to supplement the analysis of total errors (Table 2). In comparison of intoxicated and control subjects, significant differences ($P < .05$) were found for accelerator errors in periods 1 and 2, for signal errors in periods 1, 2, and 3, for braking errors in periods 2 and 3, and for speedometer errors in period 1. In the comparison of marihuana smokers and controls, a significant difference ($P < .05$) was found for speedometer errors in period 1. In all of these cases, the number of errors for the drug treatments exceeded the errors for the control treatment.

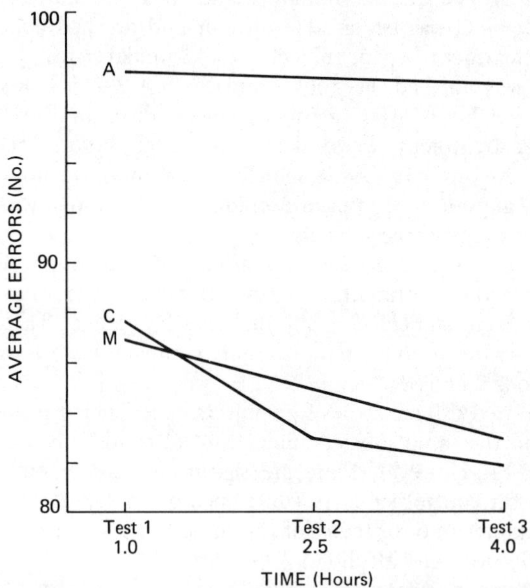


**Figure 1** Display of the effect of each treatment on simulator error scores over a 4-hour period. Alcohol (A), marihuana (M), and control (C).

**TABLE 2. Significant Treatment Differences from Latin-Square Analysis of Variance ($P < .05$)**

| *Simulator Test* | *Test variable errors* | | | | | |
|---|---|---|---|---|---|---|
| | *Accelerator* | *Signal* | *Total* | *Brake* | *Speedometer* | *Steering* |
| Period 1 | A > C | A > C | A > C | None | A > C<br>M > C | None |
| Period 2 | A > C | A > C | A > C | A > C | None | None |
| Period 3 | None | A > C | A > C | A > C | None | None |

Accelerator, signal, and total errors are significantly correlated with driving performance for normal drivers. No correlation was found for brake, speedometer, and steering errors; A > C, M > C indicate that error scores for alcohol (A) or marihuana (M) treatment are greater than control (C).

Other sources of variation are Latin squares, subjects, and days. In all of the analyses, the effect of subjects and Latin squares (representing groups of subjects) were significant ($P < .05$). In contrast, the effect of days was not significant, thus indicating that no significant amount of learning was associated with repeated exposure to the test material.

For normal drivers, Crancer (4) found a significant correlation ($P < .05$) between the three simulator test variables (signals, accelerator, and total errors) and driving performance. An increase in error scores was associated with an increase in number of accidents and violations on a driving record. In the same study, error scores for brake, speedometer, and steering were not correlated with driving performance.

It may not be valid to assume the same relationship for persons under the influence of alcohol or marihuana. However, we feel that, because the simulator task is a less complex but related task, deterioration in simulator performance implies deterioration in actual driving performance. We are less willing to assume that nondeterioration in simulator performance implies nondeterioration in actual driving. We therefore conclude that finding significantly more accelerator, signal, and total errors by intoxicated subjects implies a deterioration in actual driving performance.

Relating speedometer errors to actual driving performance is highly speculative because Crancer (4) found no correlation for normal drivers. This may be due in part to the fact that the speed of the filmed presentation is not under the control of the driver. However, speedometer errors are related to the amount of time spent monitoring the speedometer. The increase of speedometer errors by intoxicated or "high" subjects probably indicates that the subjects spent less time monitoring the speedometer than under control conditions.

This study could not determine if the drugs would alter the speed at which subjects normally drive. However, comments by marihuana users may be pertinent. They often report alteration of time and space perceptions, leading to a different sense of speed which generally results in driving more slowly.

Weil et al. (1) emphasize the importance and influence of both subject bias (set) and the experimental environment (setting). For this study, the environmental setting was conducive to good performance under all treatments.

Traditional methods for controlling potential subject bias by using placebos to disguise the form or effect of the marihuana treatment were not applicable. This is confirmed by Weil et al. (1); they showed that inexperienced subjects correctly appraised the presence or absence of a placebo in 21 of 27 trials.

The nature of selection probably resulted in subjects who preferred marihuana to alcohol and, therefore, had a set to perform better with marihuana. The main safeguard against bias was that subjects were not told how well they did on any of their driving tests, nor were they acquainted with the specific methods used to determine errors. Thus, it would have been very difficult intentionally and effectively to manipulate error scores on a given test or sequence of tests.

A further check on subject bias was made by comparing error scores on the warm-up tests given before each treatment. We found no significant difference in the mean error scores preceding the treatments of marihuana, alcohol, and control. This suggests that subjects were not "set" to perform better or worse on the day of a particular treatment.

In addition, an inspection of chance variation of individual error scores for treatment M shows about half the subjects doing worse and half better than under control conditions. This variability in direction is consistent with findings reviewed earlier, and we feel reasonably certain that a bias in favor of marihuana did not influence the results of this experiment.

A cursory investigation of dose response was made by retesting four subjects after they had smoked approximately three times the amount of marihuana used in the main experiment. None of the subjects showed a significant change in performance.

Four additional subjects who had never smoked marihuana before were pretested to obtain control scores, then given marihuana to smoke until they were subjectively "high" with an associated increase in pulse rate. All subjects smoked at least the minimum quantity established for the experiment. All subjects showed either no change or negligible improvement in their scores. These results suggest that impairment in simulated driving performance is not a function of increased marihuana dosage or inexperience with the drug.

A significant difference ($P < .01$) was found between pulse rates before and after the marihuana treatment. Similar results were reported (1) for both experienced and inexperienced marihuana subjects. We found no significant difference in pulse rates before and after drinking.

Thus, when subjects experienced a social marihuana "high," they accumulated significantly more speedometer errors on the simulator than under control conditions, but there were no significant differences in accelerator, brake, signal, steering, and total errors. The same subjects intoxicated from alcohol accumulated significantly more accelerator, brake, signal, speedometer, and total errors than under control conditions, but there was no significant difference in steering errors. Furthermore, impairment in simulated driving performance apparently is not a function of increased marihuana dosage or inexperience with the drug.

## REFERENCES AND NOTES

1. A. T. Weil, N. E. Zinberg, J. M. Nelsen, *Science* **162**, 1234 (1968).
2. Mayor's Committee on Marihuana, *The Marihuana Problem in the City of New York* (1944).

3. W. J. HADDON and V. A. BRADDESS, *J. Amer. Med. Ass.* **169**, No. 14, 127 (1959); J. R. McCarroll and W. J. Haddon, *J. Chronic Dis.* **15**, 811 (1962); J. H. W. Birell, *Med. J. Aust.* **2**, 949 (1965); R. A. Neilson, *Alcohol Involvement in Fatal Motor Vehicle Accidents in Twenty-Seven California Counties in 1964*, (California Traffic Safety Foundation, San Francisco, 1965).
4. A. CRANCER, *Predicting Driving Performance with a Driver Simulator Test* (Washington Department of Motor Vehicles, Olympia, 1968).
5. J. E. WALLACE and A. CRANCER, *Licensing Examinations and Their Relation to Subsequent Driving Record* (Washington Department of Motor Vehicles, Olympia, 1968).
6. A. E. EDWARDS, *Experimental Design in Psychological Research* (Holt, Rinehart and Winston, New York, 1968), pp. 173–174.
7. The marihuana was an assayed batch (1.312 percent $\Delta^9$-THC) from NIH through the cooperation of Dr. J. A. Scigliano.
8. L. A. GREENBERG, *Quart. J. Studies Alcohol* **29**, 252 (1968).

# 12

## *Marihuana and Simulated Driving*

HAROLD KALANT

The report by Crancer et al. (1) on the relative effects of alcohol and marihuana on a simulated driving task has limitations which seriously reduce the value of their work. They have designed their experiments carefully and have considered in detail the possible influence of subject bias on the results. They point out that all their subjects were favorably disposed toward marihuana, but that it would not have been easy for them to deliberately perform better during the marihuana trials. However, many marihuana users have a bias against alcohol, and Crancer et al. do not explain what safeguards were used to prevent this from influencing the results. Even if the subjects did not know the details of the scoring procedure, was it not possible for them to deliberately do badly on the simulated driving test in the alcohol trials? The finding of normal results in the trials before administration of the drug on alcohol days is of no help in this connection, since there would be no incentive for the subjects to do poorly before taking the alcohol. Since placebo controls are of little value in such a situation, it would have been desirable to include a second group of subjects who were experienced drinkers and probably biased in favor of alcohol.

My major criticism of the work of Crancer et al. is the arbitrary choice of a single dose of each substance for the comparison. The subjects, who were experienced marihuana users, smoked enough to achieve "a normal social marihuana 'high.'" In contrast, they consumed alcohol at a dosage of 112 ml of 95 percent ethanol (equivalent to 8 ounces of 86 proof liquor) for a 150-pound subject in a 30-minute period. This is far more than the amount required for a normal social alcohol "high" and would probably produce a peak blood ethanol concentration of about 0.15 percent (2). The objective was to achieve a concentration of 0.10 percent, but the authors do not indicate what values they actually observed. The finding that a heavy dose of alcohol caused more impairment than a mild dose of marihuana is neither surprising nor helpful in assessing the relative effects of the two drugs in the respective doses in which they are normally used.

If the authors had used three or more dosages of each drug with adequate numbers of subjects, the comparison of dose-response curves would have been a most satisfactory way of establishing the relative potencies of the two drugs; at the same time it would permit some inferences about the similarity or dissimilarity of their mechanisms of action. The studies by Goldberg (3) illustrate the sort of dose-response relations which are easily established for alcohol. Crancer et al. would have added greatly to our knowledge of *Cannabis* effects if they had obtained similar data with marihuana. They state that in four subjects the use of a tripled dose of marihuana did not result in any increase in error. They recognize that this was "a cursory investigation of dose response," and they do not indicate what measures were taken, if any, to ensure that the larger dose was effectively absorbed by their subjects. Therefore they would have been well advised not to draw from such limited observation the conclusion that "impairment in simulated driving performance is apparently not related to dose." Isbell et al. (4) have shown that changes in pulse rate as well as in subjective effects provided good dose-response curves for $\Delta^9$-tetrahydrocannabinol (THC) in man, and Dagirmanjian and Boyd (5) have observed dose-dependent impairment of polysynaptic reflexes by other THC derivatives. It is most likely, therefore, that the effects on complex performance tests in man will also prove to be dose-dependent when full studies are done.

A final note of caution must be sounded against making unwarranted extrapolations from this study. While performance on a simulated driving task may correlate well with actual driving performance, it does not follow automatically that lack of effect of a drug on the simulated task will correlate with lack of effect on the actual task. The simulation applies only to specific sensorimotor skills, and motivational factors may be quite dissimilar. Crancer et al. correctly drew no conclusion that use of marihuana will not impair driving or that it is safer than use of alcohol. It is to be hoped that their readers will also refrain from drawing unjustified conclusions.

## REFERENCES

1. A. Crancer, Jr., J. M. Dille, J. C. Delay, J. E. Wallace, M. D. Haykin *Science* **164**, 851 (1969).
2. L. A. Greenberg, *Quart. J. Stud. Alc.*, Suppl. 4, 252 (1968).

3. L. Goldberg, *Acta Physiol. Scand.* 5, Suppl. 16, 1 (1943).
4. H. Isbell, C. W. Gorodetzky, D. Jasinski, U. Claussen, F. von Spulak, F. Korte, *Psychopharmacologia* **11**, 184 (1967).
5. R. Dagirmanjian and E. S. Boyd, *J. Pharmacol. Exp. Ther.* **135**, 25 (1962).

# 3

# Uppers and Downers: The Psychotropic Drugs

The word *psychotropic* in the broadest sense means a turning or changing of consciousness or mood. Psychotropic drugs generally include the barbiturates, tranquilizers, and the stimulants. Originally developed for health purposes, these drugs are now abused by a variety of persons from the young child who drops "reds" (Seconal) in order to escape the "pain" associated with school to the chubby housewife who gets hooked on diet pills (amphetamines) because she thinks she is fat. The abuse of these drugs is an extremely serious problem because of the resultant behavioral (psychological) and physical factors. The following articles are included to point out some of the extreme dangers related to dependence and toxicity as well as the proper use of some new drugs.

Parry (1968) defines the problem of psychotropic drug use demographically and economically. Resnick (1968) reviews the effectiveness of psychotropic drugs in treatment of adolescent and adult criminal offenders. In an experimental study on children with behavior problems, Kenny et al. (1968) illustrate how new drugs may facilitate the treatment of aberrant behaviors. Knights and Hinton (1969) show how a stimulant (Ritalin) may be used to enhance the conditions for learning in children. Wikler (1968) describes a method for treatment of patients dependent on barbiturates and discusses drug dependence on nonbarbiturate sedatives and minor tranquilizers. In an excellent article on the effects of amphetamines, Cole (1967) reviews the literature on the depressant and facilitating action of the drug. Smith (1969a and 1969b) has written two dynamic articles on methamphetamine abuse. In the first study, Smith (1969a) characterizes the effects of high-dose methamphetamine use and describes the variability of response to the drug. The second article (Smith, 1969b) compares the drug subcultures of the "speed freak" and the "acid head" in the Haight-Ashbury district of San Francisco.

# 13

## *Use of Psychotropic Drugs by U.S. Adults**

HUGH J. PARRY

The mood-changing drugs can be divided into three broad categories—the hard drugs, such as opium derivatives and cocaine; the psychedelic drugs, such as LSD and the mescalin group, plus the older marijuana; and finally, the psychotropic drugs, namely, the sedatives, tranquilizers, and stimulants.

The first group is associated with urban slums, depressed minorities, and organized crime. The second group is usually visualized in terms of college campuses or hippy dropouts in little urban enclaves throughout the nation. It is associated with avant-gardism, alienation, and the revolt of youth. Both groups have been exhaustively analyzed in serious books and articles, magazine popularizations, and even in the comic strips. These two groups are—or can be made to appear—more exciting, glamorous, and dangerous or as representing a greater social problem than the third group. Thus the third group, psychotropic drugs, has been generally neglected by social researchers.

Yet the drug of choice for most adult Americans who use mood-changing drugs is a psychotrope. For every user of the "hard" narcotics or psychedelics, there are many times more users of the milder, generally medically prescribed psychotropes. (These psychotropic drugs, however, are by no means all medically prescribed. For example, a substantial proportion of the yearly production of stimulants traditionally moved in nonmedical channels before the passage of the Federal drug abuse control legislation of July 1966.)

In 1965, some 58 million new prescriptions and 108 million refills were written for psychotropes, and these 166 million prescriptions accounted for about 14 percent of the total prescriptions of all kinds written in the United States in that year. Indeed, for the years 1963–65, psychotropics accounted for a steady 14 percent of all prescriptions, at a yearly cost rising from $511 million in 1963 to $589 million in 1965 (1). Of every three prescriptions for psychotropic drugs, two are refills (1) compared with the normal 50–50 rate for other drugs—the preponderance of refills tending to operate against any sharp decline in consumption. Earlier research centered in the Metropolitan New York area suggests that on the order of three-fourths of the 166 million prescriptions for psychotropic drugs were written by general practitioners and about one in 20 by psychiatrists (2).

Despite the data on manufacture and sales and on prescriptions and costs of the psychotropic drugs, little material has been available on the prevalence of use.

From *Public Health Reports*, Vol. 83, October 1968, pp. 799–810. Reprinted by permission of the author.

* This research was conducted by the Social Research Group of George Washington University, Washington, D.C., in cooperation with the Family Research Center of the Langley Porter Institute, Berkeley, Calif., under National Institute of Mental Health Grant No. MH 12590-02.

We have not known what proportion of American adults had ever taken, or was currently taking, these drugs. However, now perhaps for the first time, fairly accurate figures are available to indicate the probable minimal prevalence of the use of psychotropic drugs.

Besides the surveys by the Opinion Research Corporation (ORC) of Princeton, N.J., and by the Social Research Group (SRG), on which my paper is based, research completed to date on psychotropic drug use includes an intensive pretest of an experimental questionnaire on several hundred adults in a Washington, D.C., suburb, an analysis of the answers to specific questions about the use of psychotropic drugs which were asked in a large national survey of American drinking behavior, and an intensive study of psychotropic drug use in a single California city by the Langley Porter Institute of Berkeley, Calif.

## SOURCES OF DATA

The research material from which my paper is derived represents the first wave in a series of sample surveys on the use of psychotropic drugs by U.S. adults. The 4-year project is designed to yield new data and fill in gaps on such subjects as the overall pattern of use, the frequency of use of specific types, the major stresses and stress symptoms that affect various subgroups in the U.S. population and the "copes"—the psychotropic drugs or other methods by which these subgroups handle such stresses, the types of personalities that seek out various kinds of copes, prevalent attitudes about use, and the sources of the psychotropic drugs—medical, quasi-medical, and extra-medical.

The first survey of a national sample for the Social Research Group was conducted by the Opinion Research Corporation. A few specific questions on the use of psychotropic drugs were added as "riders" to a questionnaire that the corporation administered in May 1967 to a national sample of Americans 18 years and over. The three questions added represented an attempt to obtain simple approximations of the current prevalence of psychotropic drug use among U.S. adults. Therefore data on dosage and frequency are lacking. For similar reasons, differential prevalence can only be analyzed in terms of relatively simple demographic factors. Also, there are compelling reasons to believe that the respondents' reports on use are underestimates (3). Experience with more refined methods of interviewing, such as a fairly elaborate approach to respondents' use of psychotropic drugs by collecting data on their health symptoms and their methods of coping with these symptoms and by the use of life-size color reproductions of the most common psychotropic pills, suggest that such techniques bring forth an increment of psychotropic drug users who are not reached by simple, conventional direct questioning (4). Thus, the prevalence figures cited in my report should be considered as minimal.

Despite these caveats, the data from the national survey are of interest and value, for they provide to a considerable degree what has been previously lacking, namely, reasonably accurate estimates of the minimal current prevalence of psychotropic drug use, plus a map of differential drug use by various subgroups in the population.

## PSYCHOTROPIC DRUG USE IN PAST 12 MONTHS

The results from two surveys of national samples, conducted independently by the Opinion Research Corporation and the Social Research Group, suggest that about one-fourth of the U.S. adult population currently uses one or another of the legal psychotropic drugs—sedatives, tranquilizers, and stimulants (Table 1).

Fieldwork for the Opinion Research Corporation study was conducted in May 1967 with a national sample of Americans 18 years and older. The respondents were asked the following questions:

> During the past 12 months, have you used any pills or medicines one or more times to help you sleep at night—pills that are often called sedatives, such as Seconal, Phenobarbital, Doriden, Sleep-Eze, and the like?
>
> . . . to help you calm down or keep you from getting nervous and upset—pills that are often called tranquilizers, such as Miltown, Equanil, Librium, Compoz, and the like?
>
> . . . that help you stay awake, pep you up, help you to lose weight or cheer you up—pills that are often called stimulants, such as Hexamyl, Dexedrine, Elavil, Preludin, No-Doz, and the like?

The respondents in the Social Research Group survey of April-October 1967 were instructed as follows:

> Here are three questions about the types of pills that people use. For each of the three types of pills listed below, please circle how recently you have used that type.
>
> A. Pills that help you sleep at night, like Sleep-Eze, Phenobarbital, and the like.
>
> B. Pills to calm you down and keep you from getting nervous and upset—pills that are often called tranquilizers, like Equanil, Compoz, and the like.
>
> C. Pills that pep you up, help you stay awake, make you more alert and less tired, that help you lose weight—pills that are often called stimulants, like Dexedrine, Dexamyl, No-Doz, Preludin, and the like.

For comparison, the ORC results for respondents under 21 years appear in a separate line in Table 1. All subsequent data from the ORC study, however, include this younger group.

**TABLE 1. Percent of Respondents in Two Surveys Who Used Psychotropic Drugs in Past 12 Months, by Type of Drug**

| Type of psychotrope | Social Research Group survey (N = 3,990) | Opinion Research Corporation surveys: Respondents 21 years and over (N = 2,531) | Respondents 18–20 years (N = 118) |
|---|---|---|---|
| Any type[a] | 25 | 24 | 25 |
| Sedatives | 13 | 11 | 4 |
| Tranquilizers | 14 | 15 | 12 |
| Stimulants | 7 | 6 | 14 |

[a]Less than the sum of the percents for the various types because many respondents used more than one type.

All differences to which I refer in this paper were found to be reliable at the 0.05 level or better; many of them were found to be reliable at the 0.01 level or better. Calculations of the reliability of differences are, of course, based on unweighted numbers. The percentages for drug use simply refer to the proportions of respondents in a subgroup who reported using one or more of the classes of psychotropic drugs at least once within the 12 months preceding the survey. Total ingestion is not considered, but it will be in the course of the 4-year project.

The evidence from the two surveys indicates that use of the "down" drugs (sedatives and tranquilizers) is markedly more common than use of the "up" drugs (stimulants). This pattern, however, does not appear to obtain among respondents aged 18, 19, and 20 years. Although use of any or all types of psychotropics is about the same for those 18–20 years old and 21 years and over, the pattern of use shows marked differences. The younger respondents apparently want to wake up rather than go to sleep; they are significantly more likely than their elders to use stimulants and are significantly less likely to use sedatives. Use of tranquilizers is about the same for both age groups. Only in this instance did a subgroup show any significant variation from the national pattern of using down drugs much more widely than up drugs. Incidentally, within the group 18–20 years old, men and women displayed similar patterns of psychotropic drug use—the young women being even slightly more likely to use stimulants than the young men. Probably the greater use among young women stems from a desire to lose weight.

## USE OF PSYCHOTROPIC DRUGS AT ANY TIME

The figures on use of psychotropic drugs at any time are approximately double those for use during the 12 months preceding the survey (Table 2). The prevalence of use at any time approaches a magnitude of about half of the U.S. population. As to the use of tranquilizers, available data suggest a 10-year trend. Research by several organizations indicates that the proportion of the adult population ever using tranquilizers has greatly increased over the decade 1957–1967 (Table 3).

**TABLE 2. Percent of Adult Respondents in Social Research Group Survey of October 1967 Who Had Used Psychotropic Drugs at Any Time, by Period of Use and Type**

| *Period of Use* | *Any Type* | *Sedatives* | *Tranquilizers* | *Stimulants* |
|---|---|---|---|---|
| Percent ever using[a] | 48 | 24 | 26 | 14 |
| Past 12 months | 25 | 13 | 14 | 7 |
| Previous 2 years | 10 | 5 | 5 | 2 |
| Earlier | 14 | 6 | 7 | 5 |

[a]The percents for the 3 periods of use may not add to the percent ever using since the individual percents have been independently rounded.

**TABLE 3. Increase in Use of Tranquilizers, 1957–67**

| *Surveys and Questions Posed* | *Date of Survey* | *Number Surveyed* | *Percent Using* |
|---|---|---|---|
| American Institute of Public Opinion: "Have you ever heard of pills called tranquilizers? (If YES) Have you ever tried them?" | March 1957 | 1,550 | 7 |
| Psychological Corporation: "By the way, have you yourself ever had occasion to take a tranquilizer?" (Asked of those who could define the word "tranquilizer.") | February 1960 | 3,885 | 14 |
| American Institute of Public Opinion: "Have you ever taken a tranquilizer?" | July 1960 | 1,440 | 25 |
| Social Research Group[a] | September 1967 | 3,390 | 26 |

[a]The questions posed in the SRG survey have been listed in the preceding section in connection with Table 1.

The rise in the proportions of adults reporting the use of tranquilizers at one time or another is reflected in the production and sales figures for tranquilizers reported over the decade (see chart). It can be seen that the steady growth in production and sales of tranquilizers, large though it is, by no means comes close to matching the growth in the proportion of adult Americans who report having used tranquilizers (5). Even if we take mean production and sales poundages for the 3-year periods 1957–59, 1960–62, and 1963–65 in order to minimize the effects of fluctuation in abnormal years, the same discrepancy remains. Several reasons for this discrepancy suggest themselves. Production and sales are year-by-year figures while percentages of the population who have ever used tranquilizers are in part cumulative; production and sales figures are given in thousands of pounds. Since 1957 there has been a tendency, partly caused by the development of newer and more powerful substances, to decrease the average psychotropic dose in milligrams and, consequently, to reduce the gross poundage. More people may be using smaller amounts of pills. This latter phenomenon has been observed in the case of alcohol consumption—in the last two decades the proportion of drinkers has grown much more rapidly than the total amount consumed.

## GROUP DIFFERENCES IN USE OF PSYCHOTROPIC DRUGS

A simple, first-order analysis of current psychotropic drug use among the major subgroups in the national population, based on the ORC survey, indicates relatively few and relatively small differences. Women were considerably more likely to have used psychotropics than men—an expected result which confirms earlier studies (2). The relatively well-to-do (those with family incomes of $10,000 and over) had slightly higher prevalence rates than poorer respondents. This pattern, however, did not prevail among the better-educated, though normally educa-

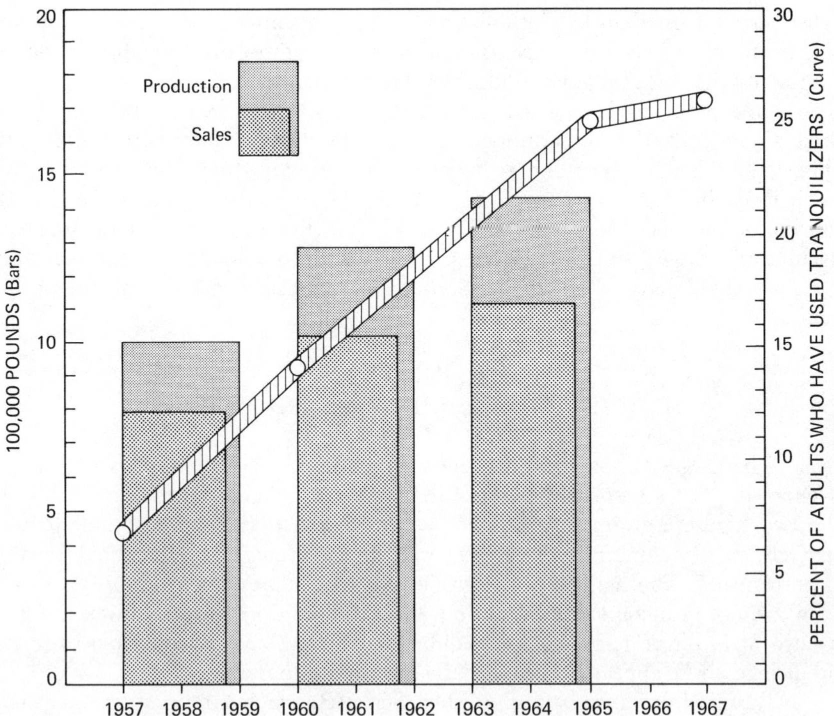


Comparison of pounds of tranquilizers produced and sold in the United States with the percentages of the adult population who reported ever using them. The figures on production and sales represent the means for the 3-year periods 1957–59, 1960–62, and 1963–65. The percentage ever using tranquilizers is derived from respondents' replies in surveys conducted in 1957, 1960, 1965, and 1967 (see Table 3).

tion and income closely correlate. Men in managerial positions (or their wives) showed a slightly higher level of prevalence of use than other occupational groups. Finally, race and religion (or other correlates associated with them) appeared to make a difference. Negro rates were lower than those of whites, while the reports of the small Jewish subsample indicated a particularly high prevalence of psychotropic drug use (Table 4).

For nearly all groups in the population, whatever the overall prevalence of use, the proportions using the down drugs were markedly larger than the proportions using the up drugs. The major exception is the small group of respondents aged 18–20, who have been discussed in relation to Table 1. The data in Table 4 suggest a continuing decline in the use of stimulants with increasing age. The proportion using stimulants tends to increase with a rising income, but this increase is matched by a similar increase in use of tranquilizers and psychotropic drugs in general.

The higher prevalence of psychotropic drug use by the small group of

Jewish respondents than by Catholics and Protestants appears to stem from a more widespread use of sedatives and tranquilizers. For stimulants, the figures on use reported by the three religious groups are comparable.

One proprietary drug which it is claimed exerts a psychotropic effect was listed along with the prescription drugs in the ORC survey. In general, the poorer and less educated tend to use more proprietary drugs than the wealthier and better educated and, conversely, to use prescription drugs less. Thus, if the wording of the question in the ORC survey had limited responses to prescribed psychotropic drugs, the differential prevalences of use by socioeconomic status probably would have been larger. Subsequent studies will take this point into account.

## RATES BY SEX, RELIGION, AND RACE

The largest apparent differences in current prevalence rates for use of psychotropic drugs seem to be associated with sex, religion, and race (Table 4). The two high-use groups are women (more than half the sample) and Jews (a relatively small subsample which was well above average in education, income, and urbanism). The major low-use group, Negroes, represents a minority which is below average in income and education. Education and urbanism, however, appear to have little direct relationship to differences in current psychotropic drug use, and income per se appears to be of relatively minor importance.

Results from a recently published Social Research Group study on American drinking practices shed some light on these three variations (6). In the two groups that I have mentioned as displaying a high prevalence of psychotropic drug use the proportions of escape drinkers—that is respondents who reported uisng alcohol primarily to change their moods—were below the national level (Table 5). In our society, taboos against drinking of any kind by women obtain among many subgroups. The widespread moderate use of alcohol in Jewish familial and religious settings, coupled with a traditional reprobation of heavy and escape drinking (7), also appears to inhibit the use of alcohol by Jews in stress situations. For neither group, however, are there similar well-structured and traditional objections to the use of psychotropics. In contrast, escape drinking seems to be relatively prevalent among Negro respondents and to be associated with what may be a consequent decrease in the prevalence of psychotropic drug use.

Other factors in the low prevalence rate among Negroes would probably also be less awareness of the existence of psychotropic drugs, less available medical care, and similar disadvantages associated with deprivation.

## PSYCHOTROPIC DRUG USE BY REGION

There is little variation among large geographic regions of the country in the current prevalence of psychotropic drug use (Table 6). The South appears to be a little higher than the other regions in overall prevalence, largely because of a more widespread use of tranquilizers in that region, but the differences do not

**TABLE 4. Proportions of Demographic Groups in a National Sample Who Used Psychotropic Drugs in Past 12 Months**

| Groups | Number of Respondents (unweighted) | Percent Using: Any Type | Sedatives | Tranquilizers | Stimulants |
|---|---|---|---|---|---|
| Total U.S. sample | 2,071 | 24 | 11 | 15 | 7 |
| *Sex* | | | | | |
| Men | 991 | 15 | 7 | 9 | 3 |
| Women | 1,080 | 31 | 13 | 20 | 9 |
| *Age (years)* | | | | | |
| 18–20 | 95 | 25 | 4 | 12 | 14 |
| 21–29 | 408 | 26 | 9 | 15 | 9 |
| 30–39 | 417 | 26 | 11 | 16 | 9 |
| 40–49 | 417 | 26 | 12 | 16 | 7 |
| 50–59 | 347 | 18 | 7 | 14 | 4 |
| 60 years or over | 452 | 23 | 14 | 14 | 2 |
| *Education* | | | | | |
| Less than high school completed | 899 | 23 | 10 | 15 | 5 |
| High school completed | 641 | 25 | 10 | 15 | 9 |
| Some college | 512 | 24 | 12 | 15 | 7 |
| *Occupation* | | | | | |
| Professional | 254 | 24 | 11 | 15 | 7 |
| Managerial | 215 | 31 | 12 | 15 | 10 |
| Clerical, sales | 208 | 25 | 9 | 15 | 7 |
| Craftsman, foreman | 391 | 25 | 9 | 17 | 9 |
| Other manual, service | 505 | 20 | 9 | 13 | 5 |
| Farmer, farm laborer | 134 | 19 | 8 | 10 | 4 |
| *Population of home town* | | | | | |
| Rural | 589 | 25 | 12 | 15 | 7 |
| 2,500–99,999 | 412 | 26 | 13 | 15 | 7 |
| 100,000–999,999 | 468 | 24 | 10 | 15 | 7 |
| 1,000,000 or over | 602 | 22 | 8 | 14 | 6 |
| *Region* | | | | | |
| Northeast | 510 | 21 | 11 | 13 | 5 |
| North Central | 651 | 24 | 11 | 12 | 8 |
| South | 602 | 27 | 12 | 19 | 5 |
| West | 308 | 23 | 7 | 14 | 9 |
| *Income* | | | | | |
| Under $5,000 | 640 | 22 | 12 | 14 | 4 |
| $5,000–$6,999 | 519 | 20 | 9 | 11 | 5 |
| $7,000–$9,999 | 437 | 24 | 11 | 14 | 7 |
| $10,000 or over | 445 | 31 | 10 | 20 | 11 |
| *Race* | | | | | |
| White | 1,703 | 26 | 11 | 16 | 7 |
| Negro | 211 | 13 | 7 | 8 | 2 |
| *Religion* | | | | | |
| Protestant | 1,294 | 23 | 10 | 15 | 6 |
| Catholic | 474 | 24 | 10 | 13 | 8 |
| Jewish | 43 | 47 | 21 | 36 | 8 |

Source: Unless otherwise indicated, all data here and from here on are derived from the ORC national study.

**TABLE 5. Comparison of Escape Drinkers with Users of Psychotropic Drugs, by Sex, Religion, and Race**

| *Demographic Group* | *Escape Drinkers in U.S. Population*[a] | | *Users of Psychotropic Drugs in Past 12 Months* | |
|---|---|---|---|---|
| | *Number* | *Percent* | *Number*[b] | *Percent* |
| Total in national sample | 2,746 | 20 | 2,071 | 24 |
| *Sex* | | | | |
| Men | 1,177 | 25 | 991 | 15 |
| Women | 1,569 | 16 | 1,080 | 31 |
| *Religion* | | | | |
| Jewish | 73 | 17 | 43 | 47 |
| Non-Jewish | 2,673 | 20 | 1,771 | 23 |
| *Race* | | | | |
| Negro | 200 | 30 | 157 | 13 |
| White | 2,511 | 19 | 1,703 | 26 |

[a]Source of data is reference 6.
[b]From Table 4.

appear to be reliable. However, when respondents in the four major regions are controlled for other demographic characteristics, considerably larger variations can be noted.

First of all, in two regions, as well as in the nation as a whole, persons with family incomes in the $10,000 and over category tended to show a higher prevalence of psychotropic drug use than did poorer respondents (Table 6). The contrast is particularly striking in the North Central States, notably in respect to

**TABLE 6. Proportions of Respondents in Major Geographic Regions Who Used Psychotropic Drugs in Past 12 Months, by Income**

| *Region and Income* | *Number of Respondents* | *Percent Using* | | | |
|---|---|---|---|---|---|
| | | *Any Type* | *Seda-tives* | *Tran-quilizers* | *Stimu-lants* |
| *Northeast* | | | | | |
| Under $10,000 | 373 | 19 | 11 | 11 | 5 |
| $10,000 and over | 137 | 25 | 10 | 18 | 5 |
| *North Central* | | | | | |
| Under $10,000 | 480 | 19 | 10 | 9 | 5 |
| $10,000 and over | 154 | 38 | 15 | 23 | 14 |
| *South* | | | | | |
| Under $10,000 | 517 | 27 | 13 | 19 | 4 |
| $10,000 and over | 79 | 29 | 9 | 17 | 9 |
| *West* | | | | | |
| Under $10,000 | 226 | 22 | 8 | 12 | 7 |
| $10,000 and over | 80 | 23 | 3 | 21 | 13 |

contrasting prevalences for use of tranquilizers and for use of stimulants. In the South and the West, in contrast, the overall use of psychotropic drugs is equally widespread within income groups both above and below the $10,000 level. In the South, there was a tendency for the poorer respondents to report higher rates for the down drugs, while the wealthier were more likely to report use of the up drugs.

Since nearly all southern Negroes in the sample fell into the "under $10,000" class, southern whites in the two income groups were compared separately. When this was done, there was little change in the percentages except to emphasize the pattern slightly more. In the West, the more well-to-do group reported higher prevalences for the newer drugs, whether tranquilizers or stimulants; the poorer group showed slightly higher use of the more old-fashioned sedatives.

Controlling the regional subsamples for age gives no revealing patterns in three of the four regions (Table 7). In the West, however, respondents under 30 were markedly higher than their elders in prevalence of overall psychotropic drug use—a variation that derives almost completely from a significantly more widespread use of the newer drugs (the tranquilizers and stimulants) by the younger group. Again, when it comes to education, there were notably larger differences in the West between the college-educated and the rest, manifested in particular by a much more widespread use of tranquilizers among the college graduates (Table 8). Even though the number of college-educated westerners in the sample was small, the differences are reliable.

**TABLE 7. Proportions of Respondents in Major Geographic Regions Who Used Psychotropic Drugs in Past 12 Months, by Age Group and Education**

| Region, Age, and Education | Number of Respondents | Percent Using: Any Type | Sedatives | Tranquilizers | Stimulants |
|---|---|---|---|---|---|
| *Northeast* | | | | | |
| Under 30 | 116 | 21 | 10 | 10 | 6 |
| 30 and over | 399 | 21 | 11 | 14 | 5 |
| Completed college | 80 | 23 | 10 | 15 | 7 |
| Less than college | 429 | 21 | 11 | 13 | 5 |
| *North Central* | | | | | |
| Under 30 | 155 | 28 | 11 | 12 | 13 |
| 30 and over | 494 | 23 | 11 | 13 | 7 |
| Completed college | 71 | 23 | 14 | 16 | 6 |
| Less than college | 576 | 24 | 10 | 12 | 8 |
| *South* | | | | | |
| Under 30 | 155 | 24 | 6 | 15 | 7 |
| 30 and over | 449 | 28 | 14 | 20 | 4 |
| Completed college | 62 | 26 | 16 | 9 | 4 |
| Less than college | 536 | 27 | 12 | 19 | 5 |
| *West* | | | | | |
| Under 30 | 84 | 31 | 7 | 22 | 15 |
| 30 and over | 221 | 19 | 6 | 11 | 6 |
| Completed college | 21 | 46 | 8 | 38 | 12 |
| Less than college | 280 | 21 | 7 | 13 | 8 |

**TABLE 8. Proportions of Respondents of Varying Economic Mobility Who Used Psychotropic Drugs in Past 12 Months, by Sex**

| | | *Percent Using* | | | |
|---|---|---|---|---|---|
| *Sex and Presumed Mobility* | *Number of Respondents* | *Any Type* | *Seda-tives* | *Tran-quilizers* | *Stimu-lants* |
| *Men* | | | | | |
| Upwardly mobile | 34 | 24 | 2 | 17 | 7 |
| Downwardly mobile | 63 | 13 | 9 | 6 | 1 |
| Higher stable | 67 | 24 | 10 | 16 | 4 |
| Lower stable | 379 | 16 | 9 | 10 | 2 |
| *Women* | | | | | |
| Upwardly mobile | 32 | 35 | 5 | 20 | 15 |
| Downwardly mobile | 56 | 35 | 22 | 17 | 10 |
| Higher stable | 42 | 38 | 12 | 29 | 13 |
| Lower stable | 417 | 28 | 13 | 18 | 7 |

Of the respondents interviewed in the West, most—about two-thirds—were located in California. It was impracticable to isolate a pure California sample, however, since the number of cases was too small and, more important, because no national sample is really designed for State-by-State comparisons. Comparable data based on an exclusively California sample are now being analyzed by Dean I. Manheimer and his colleagues at the Family Research Center at Berkeley. The data will be reported in a separate paper—"The Use of Psychoactive Drugs Among Adults in California" by Dean I. Manheimer and Glen D. Mellinger.

## PSYCHOTROPIC DRUGS AND ECONOMIC MOBILITY

Since the three questions on psychotropic drug use were "riders" on a national survey, analysis of the results except in terms of major demographic variables was generally not possible. However, by cross-analysis of the available data, we were able in some instances to isolate special groups. One such group consisted of respondents who appeared to be economically mobile, whether upwardly or downwardly. Part of these respondents had less than a high school education but a family income of $10,000 and over. The other part consisted of respondents with college or graduate education whose incomes were under $10,000. In Table 8, both groups are divided by sex and then compared with the corresponding higher stable and lower stable groups—that is, with the college graduates of higher income and the high school dropouts of lower income.

To account for younger college graduates whose careers (and incomes) were still in the early stage, the downwardly mobile group under 30 years was compared with the downwardly mobile groups 30 years and over. No important differences were found. In Table 8, the two age groups are combined for the sake of simplicity.

Some earlier research raised the possibility that both of the extremely mobile groups—the downwardly mobile and the abnormally upwardly mobile—

would be susceptible to some of the strains associated equally with failure and rapid success and would perhaps display a higher prevalence rate of psychotropic drug use than the other two groups (8). Although the number of persons in each cell is relatively small, a somewhat different pattern emerges. In prevalence of use of any class of psychotropic drugs, men of higher income, whether mobile or stable, tended to have a relatively high use, while use by lower income groups, whether mobile or stable, tended to be rather low. This result reflects the general contrast in usage found between the higher and lower income groups (Table 1). It suggests that mobile men of both kinds tend to move toward the patterns of psychotropic drug use characteristic of the economic level toward which they are either rising or falling. There is also a slight indication that the upwardly mobile men, as might be expected, tend to be low users of sedatives and high users of stimulants.

For female respondents (predominantly wives of wage earners), the pattern is less clear. The lower stable group reported low overall prevalence of psychotropic drug use. However, the downwardly mobile women had a rather high prevalence rate—basically because of a relatively more common use of sedatives. The upwardly mobile women, like the upwardly mobile men, also tended to report relatively low prevalence rates for the use of sedatives and relatively high rates for stimulants, although here the pattern is less clear than among the men. If we look at the men and women who fall into comparable cells, we note a generally higher prevalence for women whether in total use of psychotropic drugs or of specific classes. This contrast, however, is particularly great between downwardly mobile men and women. There is a suggestion here, which will be examined more systematically in future research, that the wives feel the strains of downward mobility more than their husbands, insofar as these strains manifest themselves in the use of psychotropic drugs.

## PATTERNS OF USE AMONG MEN AND WOMEN

As noted, the rates of prevalence of use of psychotropic drugs for women were about twice as high as for men for each of the three classes of psychotropic drugs and for any psychotropic drug (Table 4). Table 9 provides a detailed comparison by sex and income group and suggests that overall prevalence rates are highest for men and women at the $10,000 and over level—largely because of the richer group's more widespread use of tranquilizers. The variations for men are a little uneven and of small magnitude. In contrast, the differences for the women appear to be considerable.

To see whether prevalence rates continued to rise with income levels, the $10,000 and over" group was divided into subgroups "$10,000–$14,999" and "$15,000 and over." The overall rates for both sexes, and in particular the rates for tranquilizers, dropped back again somewhat for the richer of the two groups, suggesting that the progression may tail off in the higher income levels.

When the sexes are controlled for race, the sex differences among Negroes between rates for the three classes of drugs and for overall use are relatively small; for white persons, they are large. Among Negroes, sex does not appear to be an

**TABLE 9. Proportions of Male and Female Respondents Who Used Psychotropic Drugs in Past 12 Months, by Income and Race**

| | | Percent Using | | | |
|---|---|---|---|---|---|
| *Sex, Income, and Race* | *Number of Respondents* | *Any Type* | *Seda-tives* | *Tran-quilizers* | *Stimu-lants* |
| *Men* | | | | | |
| Under $5,000 | 258 | 15 | 11 | 10 | a |
| $5,000–$6,999 | 248 | 10 | 5 | 4 | 4 |
| $7,000–$9,999 | 222 | 14 | 5 | 8 | 3 |
| $10,000 and over | 233 | 22 | 8 | 14 | 6 |
| *Women* | | | | | |
| Under $5,000 | 379 | 26 | 13 | 17 | 7 |
| $5,000–$6,999 | 269 | 29 | 13 | 19 | 7 |
| $7,000–$9,999 | 220 | 33 | 16 | 20 | 10 |
| $10,000 and over | 215 | 42 | 13 | 26 | 16 |
| *Men* | | | | | |
| White | 796 | 17 | 8 | 10 | 4 |
| Negro | 87 | 12 | 4 | 7 | 1 |
| *Women* | | | | | |
| White | 898 | 34 | 14 | 21 | 10 |
| Negro | 92 | 13 | 8 | 8 | 4 |

[a]Less than 1 percent.

important factor in differing prevalence rates. To put it another way, the rates for Negro women are as low as—perhaps a little lower than—the rates for white men.

## YOUNG CHILDREN IN THE HOUSE AND DRUG USE

Among the strains to which women are subjected, a large number of children under 17 years in the house is by no means the least. Data on this point were collected in another section of the ORC questionnaire and made available to us. The figures suggest that among married men, who are usually away at work except on weekends, the number of children in the house has little connection with the use of psychotropic drugs. Among married women, in contrast, the data suggest that there is a small increase in the use of psychotropic drugs at the stages when the number of children in the home reaches three or four, but then a notable drop in the level of use once there are five or more children (Table 10). By and large, women with five children in the home tend to be from lower income groups in which psychotropic drug use (and for that matter medical care in general) is less frequent. Also, it may be that in a family with five or more children under 17 years, an older child can be detailed as a kind of noncommissioned officer to control the others.

One factor in the slightly higher prevalence rates among married women with three to four minor children in the house may be a higher income which, among women, is associated with higher use of psychotropic drugs (Table 5). Among women with three to four children, nearly one-third report family incomes

**TABLE 10. Proportions of Married Respondents Who Used Psychotropic Drugs in Past 12 Months, by Sex and Children under 17 Years in Home**

| | | *Percent Using* | | | |
|---|---|---|---|---|---|
| *Sex and children under 17* | *Number of Respondents* | *Any Type* | *Seda-tives* | *Tran-quilizers* | *Stimu-lants* |
| *Men* | | | | | |
| None | 314 | 16 | 8 | 9 | 3 |
| 1–2 | 319 | 16 | 6 | 10 | 3 |
| 3–4 | 105 | 15 | 8 | 6 | 4 |
| 5 or more | 45 | 16 | 5 | 11 | 5 |
| *Women* | | | | | |
| None | 317 | 31 | 15 | 19 | 7 |
| 1–2 | 285 | 33 | 12 | 20 | 13 |
| 3–4 | 140 | 39 | 15 | 22 | 14 |
| 5 or more | 57 | 22 | 13 | 16 | 10 |

of $10,000 or more—a considerably larger proportion than for married women in general. This factor, however, does not explain the rather sharp drop in use among women with five or more minor children in the house: among this subgroup, on the order of one in five reports a family income of $10,000 and over—about the same proportion as in the figures for all women. Age and race also do not appear to be involved.

## SUMMARY

Evidence from two current surveys of national samples suggests that about one of four U.S. adults uses one or more kinds of psychotropic drugs. Nearly half the U.S. adult population report the use of a psychotropic drug at some time. Stimulants are used by the smallest proportion, sedatives by a larger proportion, and tranquilizers by the largest group. Cumulative use of tranquilizers over a decade has shown a steady increase—from about 7 percent of the population in 1957 to about 27 percent in 1967.

There are relatively few significant differences in prevalence of use by major demographic groupings. Major differences appear to be related to sex, religion, and race. Women are markedly higher in use than men; Jews are higher than Protestants or Catholics in overall use and in sedatives and tranquilizers, but not in stimulants. Lower proportions of Negroes than of whites use these drugs; the pattern for both sexes among Negroes is fairly similar to that for white men. Among whites, in contrast, there are fairly large differences between the sexes. The two groups with high prevalence of psychotropic drug use (women and Jews) have low rates of escape drinking; the group with low prevalence (Negroes) displays high escape drinking rates.

Higher income seems to be associated with higher use in the Northeast and North Central regions, but not in the South and West. People apparently tend to adopt the drug use patterns of the economic groups that they are moving up or down into. The use by men in the highest income bracket differs only slightly from the use by men in the lowest; for women, the differences by income level are more substantial.

## REFERENCES

1. National prescription audits 1963, 1964, and 1965. R. A. Gosselin and Co., Dedham, Mass.
2. SHAPIRO, S., and BARON, S. H.: Prescriptions for psychotropic drugs in a noninstitutional population. Public Health Rep. 76: 483–485, June 1961.
3. Public information and attitudes concerning tranquilizers. Psychological Barometer Report. Psychological Corporation, New York, 1960, pp. 6–7.
4. MANHEIMER, D. I., and MELLINGER, G. D.: The psychotropic pilltaker—will he talk? *Public Opin. Quart.* 31:436–437, fall 1967.
5. U.S. TARIFF COMMISSION: Synthetic organic chemicals, U.S. production and sales. Statistical Abstract of the United States, 1967. U.S. Department of Commerce, Bureau of the Census, Washington, D.C., 1967, table 107, p. 82.
6. CAHALAN, D., CISIN, I. H., and CROSSLEY, H. M.: American drinking practices. Social Research Group, George Washington University, Washington, D.C., 1967, table A–96, pp. 326–328.
7. PLANT, T. A.: Alcohol problems—A report to the nation. Cooperative Commission on the Study of Alcoholism. Oxford University Press, Inc., New York, 1967, pp. 48–126.
8. BETTELHEIM, B., and JANOWITZ, M.: *Dynamics of prejudice*, Harper & Row, Publishers, New York, 1949, pp. 57–61.

# 14

# *The Use of Psychotropic Drugs with Criminals*

OSCAR RESNICK

The study of criminality is extremely complex and involves the many disciplines of sociology, psychology, and biomedicine. The topic assigned me is a discussion of *The Use of Psychotropic Drugs with Criminals.* Since the many different types of criminals of all ages exhibit a wide range of behavior patterns, such a discussion becomes very difficult indeed. Therefore, it becomes necessary to develop a simplified scheme to serve as a basis for the examination of the behavioral symptoma-

Paper presented at the Seventh Annual Meeting of the American College of Neuropsychopharmacology, San Juan, Puerto Rico, December 20, 1968. Reprinted by permission of the author.

tologies most frequently associated with criminality—thus allowing for a coherent and, hopefully, lucid discussion of the use of psychotropic drugs with criminals. This simplified scheme is based in large measure on the discussion by Dr. Adolph Jonas (1) in his classic book, *Ictal and Subictal Neurosis*.

Dr. Jonas states that there exists in the brain a continuum extending from the intense focal and generalized electrical discharges seen in grand mal states of epilepsy down to the normally firing brain. Occasionally, for one reason or another, there occur abnormal discharges, the symptom manifestations of which may either escape detection or may be quite dramatic and detectable. These symptoms have been given the various names, "ictal events," "subictal events," and "epileptic equivalents." It is further believed that most of the ictal and subictal events or epileptic equivalents are the result of functional or pathological changes in the temporal lobes, the rhinencephalon, and the hypothalamus. Ictal and subictal patients may experience an array of rapidly proliferating ideations, emotions, and sensations following spontaneous dysrhythmic discharges. Dr. Jonas further states that ictal and subictal phenomena may masquerade as hysteria, anxiety neurosis, or *psychopathy*. The ictally-afflicted person expresses an intense anxiety about the ego-alien happenings inside his own mind.

At this point, it might be of interest to present a partial list of symptoms which may be the result of ictal and subictal states (1):

1. Fibrillation or contraction of isolated muscle bundles or groups of muscles, e.g., twitching eyelids, a jumping muscle, an abrupt change in position (such as in nocturnal jactations during light sleep)
2. Paroxysmal or periodic attacks of vertigo, fainting spells, tachycardia, constriction of throat with sensation of suffocation, nausea, vasomotor changes, night sweats, night drooling, headaches, stabbing pains, neuralgia, pins and needles feeling, numbness, loss of feeling, prickly sensations, precordial pains, diarrhea, visual sensations including partial or complete loss of vision, auditory sensations including partial or complete deafness, olfactory and gustatory sensations (namely, a sensation of unpleasant odors and tastes), and the like

Such terms as "autonomic seizures," "abdominal migraine," and the like, exist in the literature to label the epileptic equivalents resulting from sympathetic and parasympathetic stimulation provoked by an ictal or dysrhythmic discharge. The term "psychic seizure" is used to label the following epileptic equivalents: delusion-illusions and hallucinations; micropsia; macropsia; feeling of shapes changing; déjà vu and déjà entendu; sudden familiarity and unfamiliarity; a sense of uncanniness; nightmares; somnambulism; fainting; day-dreaming; absentmindedness; automatism, that is, automatic acts followed by amnesia (e.g., a person driving his car for many miles without any memory of doing so); forced thinking; anxiety; depression (often with suicidal thoughts); hysteria; fear; agony; unexplainable and motiveless behavior; recurrent violent emotional upsets including violent temper tantrums and violent rage. Many authors have variously described individuals with these symptoms as aggressive, irritable, impulsive, unstable, egocentric, easily offended, obsessive, compulsive, and dependent (1).

The symptoms associated with the ictal or subictal events are widespread—

but are rarely if ever diagnosed as such (1). This is not surprising considering that the list of symptoms enumerated above is only a partial one. Another major reason for the difficulty in diagnosis is that abnormal EEG's may not be demonstrable in many individuals with epileptic equivalents or even with (frank) grand-mal epileptic seizures. The absence of a recognizable neurologic deficit or of an abnormal EEG does not rule out cerebral dysfunction. It only means that methods are not yet available to detect many, if not most, cases of abnormal brain function. The abnormal brain function may be the result of localized encephalitis, excessively high temperatures, hypoxic episodes, metabolic disorders, subdural hematoma, head trauma, genetic influences, and so on. In the aged, the abnormal brain function may be due to post-arteriosclerotic degenerative changes. Of special importance to this discussion is the observation that the above-mentioned descriptions of ictally and subictally afflicted individuals resemble very closely the descriptions in the literature of many prison inmates, psychopaths, and juvenile delinquents. The following is a very partial list of descriptions in the literature of emotionally disturbed children and juvenile delinquents:

1. periodically uncontrolled behavior
2. bizarre mannerisms and explosive violence
3. hyperactive, restless, unpredictable, destructive
4. episodic and violent outbursts of impulsive behavior
5. paroxysmal, unbridled aggression, rages, and temper tantrums
6. hostility, hypercritical attitudes, pathological lying, feeling of being pushed around, irritability, lack of self-control, and pronounced nonconformity
7. hyperreactivity, temper tantrums, fighting, lying, truancy, biting, cruelty to animals, firesetting, sexually acting out, homicidal and suicidal assaults

In each of the above cases, the authors felt that there was evidence of cerebral dysrhythmia and that the above symptoms were in fact ictal or subictal events. Several authors have found an extremely high incidence of abnormal EEG's, especially in the 14 and 6 positive spikes, in juveniles and adults who committed murder without any apparent motive. Many criminals charged with automotive manslaughter, robbery, and murder show evidence of having been in states of altered and clouded consciousness, fugue states, abnormal rages, automatism, and destructive behavior. Often there is a partial or complete amnesia to the criminal act. They will rarely attempt to flee or put up resistance when apprehended. They may show no emotions when questioned, thus appearing as hardened and callous criminals (1). McDonald (2) states that the absence of a motive, premeditation, planning, attempt at concealment, and partial or complete loss of memory for the crime is pathognomic for a seizureless epileptic. Thompson (3) states "some sexual psychopaths who engaged in extremely bizarre and socially unacceptable behavior had prominent theta activity in the EEG." Finally, Jonas (1) concludes: "The guises under which epileptic equivalents masquerade as psychopathic syndromes are many."

If one accepts the tantalizing hypothesis that many criminals of all ages are actually ictally or subictally afflicted, then they could be included in the general term of minimal brain damage or minimal brain dysfunctions (i.e., MBD), a term universally used to describe a whole host of emotional disturbances. Also, it should be just as logical to include geriatrics suffering from arteriosclerotic brain disease and simple senile degeneration in the wastebasket term of brain dysfunction and/or ictal and subictal states. Certainly, one can see a parallelism in many of the symptoms in all of the above-mentioned categories.

I would like now to briefly discuss the actions of several major classes of psychotropic agents on the epileptic equivalents with a twofold goal: (1) the obvious goal of therapy and management and (2) the responses of the symptoms to the psychotropic drugs as an aid to differential diagnosis in the absence of confirmatory EEG and neurologic signs—as a test of the scheme presented in this paper and so beautifully elaborated in Jonas's book (1). In order to keep within the time allotted for this discussion, I will only discuss a few of the classes of psychotropic agents—this does not mean that these are the only classes of agents of significance to our discussion.

## THE AMPHETAMINES

In 1937, Bradley (4) introduced the use of Benzedrine Sulfate (20 mg/day) in the treatment of children who since infancy had been irritable, hyperactive, and aggressive, with a short attention span, and whose behavior and mood varied unexplainably from time to time. Bradley referred to this as the "organic reaction type" of behavior. Phenobarbital, on the other hand, was shown to be of doubtful value. Bradley also used Benzedrine Sulfate parenterally as an emergency sedative in these hyperactive children. Cutts and Jasper (5) in 1939 noted clinical improvement with Benzedrine Sulfate (20 mg/day) in 7 of 12 children (aged 7–10) who were asocial, hyperactive, impulsive, and destructive. Phenobarbital aggravated the symptoms in 9 of the 12 children, while producing no change in 3. Lindsley and Henry (6) in 1942 noted marked improvement in 13 behavior problem children treated with Benzedrine Sulfate (i.e., lessening of hyperactivity, impulsiveness, destructiveness, aggressiveness, distractibility, seclusiveness, sex play, stealing, lying, etc.). Phenobarbital, given after Benzedrine improved the behavior of the children, caused an exacerbation of the symptoms. Laufer and Denhoff (7) in 1959 stated:

> In our experience amphetamine is a specific for the treatment of the hyperkinetic syndrome. A favorable response to amphetamine is supportive evidence for a diagnosis of the hyperkinetic syndrome. Phenobarbital or other barbiturates are ineffective on the hyperkinetic syndrome. Instead the great majority of children with this syndrome react adversely to such medication. They often become more irritable, unmanageable, and active. This reaction is so marked as almost to provide a specific diagnostic test in itself.

Leon Eisenberg and Keith Conners (8) reporting the results of many studies conclude that stimulants such as dextroamphetamine (Dexedrine) 10 mg/day and methylphenidate (Ritalin) 30 mg/day are useful in controlling hyperkinetic and aggressive behavior disorders in children and adolescents and that phenobarbital can be considerably worse than placebo. Thus, children with hyperkinesis or the organic brain syndrome respond paradoxically to the amphetamines and the barbiturates. Further work is needed to determine whether normal children show this paradoxical effect. This paradoxical effect to the stimulants, however, is found also in certain adults. Hill (9) in 1947 found that amphetamines improved the behavior of psychopaths. He described his subjects as "aggressive" and "bad-tempered." After taking Benzedrine, the subjects' personalities are described as "more integrated" and having a "more mature expression of the primary appetitive drives." J. J. Shovron (10) in 1947 treated three adult psychopaths with Benzedrine. He reported that the patient's aggression lessened as a result of the drug. In 1959, Tong (11) treated psychopaths whom he described as "affectionless schizoid" with amphetamine. Also, it has been the clinical impression of our group that many geriatric patients suffering from arteriosclerotic brain disease and simple cerebral degeneration also show a paradoxical effect to the stimulants, such as the amphetamines and Ritalin. In addition, Parkinson patients may also show this paradoxical effect to the stimulants.

It is tempting to postulate that the symptoms of hyperkinesis in children, of psychopathy in adults, and of irritability and hostility in the agitated geriatric patient are the results of ictal or subictal events and are epileptic equivalents. Thus, one could postulate a decreased threshold of excitation in the affected areas of the brain. That this may be so is indicated by the work of Laufer and Denhoff (7) who demonstrated that children with the hyperkinetic syndrome demonstrate a low threshold for photometrazol activation of the EEG by the technique of Gastaut. They further demonstrated that Dexedrine resulted in a significant raising of the threshold value toward that characteristic of their comparison group. It would be interesting to see if such is the case with adult psychopaths and geriatrics with cerebral degeneration. These authors also postulate that the hyperkinetic syndrome in children may result from injury to or dysfunction of the diencephalon in early life, thus interfering with the normal cortical-diencephalic interplay. These workers, as well as Bradley (4), suggest that the amphetamines raise synaptic resistance in the diencephalon. It is of interest in this connection to mention that animal data suggest that the amphetamines have anticonvulsant properties. Thus, we may state at this time that the amphetamines and methylphenidate are worthy of further trial in the treatment of juvenile delinquents and adult criminals.

In summary, the amphetamines have been shown to be effective in the treatment of MBD in children (4) and in the treatment of aggressive psychopaths (9, 10). The reasons for this may be as follows: (a) the amphetamines have been shown to possess anticonvulsant properties; (b) the amphetamines are sympathomimetic agents; therefore they are anticholinergic in action. Thus, presumably, they could act as polysynaptic inhibitors in those areas of the CNS where transmission is cholinergic. That this could possibly be a mechanism of action of the amphetamines is strengthened by the observations of many investigators that the antihistamines, such as Benadryl, have been found effective in the treatment of MBD or hyperkinesis in children (7). The antihistamines are powerful anticholinergic agents and thus could be expected to inhibit polysynaptic transmission where acetylcholine is the neurotransmitter. The phenothiazines are also very powerful anticholinergic agents. However, their usefulness may be counteracted by their ability to become epileptogenic and also to produce iatrogenic Parkinsonism, with an impairment of the extrapyramidal motor system. It is of interest to mention here that both the amphetamines and the antihistamines have a beneficial effect on Parkinsonism. Hornykiewicz (12) has shown that in Parkinsonism there are lesions in the basal ganglia and substantia nigra, the only areas of the brain known to contain significant amounts of dopamine. Could one consider the paradoxical effects of the sympathomimetic amphetamines in Parkinson patients as replacement of dopamine, in organic behavior syndrome in children and in psychopaths as replacement of norepinephrine and epinephrine in the hypothalamus? It is of interest in this connection that Laufer and Denhoff (7) postulate that the hyperkinetic syndrome in children may result from injury to or dysfunction of the diencephalon in early life, thus interfering with the normal cortical-diencephalic interplay.

## THE ANTICONVULSANTS

Many investigators have found the anticonvulsants, especially diphenylhydantoin (DPH), to be effective in varying degrees in most, if not all, of the ictal and subictal states or epileptic equivalents. Jonas (1) believes that a positive response to DPH might serve as a basis for diagnosing symptoms as being associated with ictal or subictal events. As stated above, the symptoms associated with ictal or subictal events are so widespread that diagnosis is most often very difficult indeed.

The literature on the use of DPH in the treatment of the ictal and subictal events or epileptic equivalents is extremely voluminous and is discussed in depth in Jonas's book (1). Therefore, I shall confine my remarks here to the use of DPH in the treatment of explosive behavior anomalies in both adults and children.

Diphenylhydantoin has been widely used in the therapy of grand mal and psychomotor epilepsy since 1938. In addition to the control of seizures, DPH was reported to produce improvement in behavior, well-being, cooperation, alertness, general attitude, irritability, temperament, and personality of many of the epileptic patients. Recently William J. Turner (13) has reported on the use of Dilantin in the treatment of nonepileptic neurotics. Dr. Turner states: "Diphenylhydantoin is an effective agent in the relief of symptoms in a variety of neurotic disturbances. It is particularly effective in relief of neurotic depression and impotent rage, especially in persons with obsessive or passive-dependent personalities."

McCullagh and Ingram (14) studied a series of patients from their private practice who suffered from migraine-type headaches and emotional disturbances characterized by paroxysmal outbursts of hostility or temper tantrums. The patients ranged from 5 to 48 years of age and included both males and females. Many of the patients were found to have cerebral dysrhythmias, and in some cases a familial tendency for such dysrhythmias was also observed. In one male subject, the outbursts occurred only after the ingestion of alcohol. The EEG, obtained when the patient did not have any alcohol to drink, was well within the normal limits. All of the cases reported were treated successfully with DPH, 100 mg b.i.d. together with 25 mg Thorazine per day. Jonas (1) cites many references of investigators who demonstrated a frequent incidence of abnormal EEG's in nonepileptic prison inmates, motiveless murderers, and juvenile delinquents. He further states:

> Many individuals charged with automotive manslaughter, robbery, and murder claim that they were under the influence of alcohol at the time of their crimes and that they had no recollection of them. The alcohol seems to have activated seizures of a latent focus in the temporal lobe followed by altered consciousness, fugue states, abnormal rages, automatism and destructive behavior.

In 402 such cases, Marinacci (15) found evidence of temporal lobe seizures, following the ingestion of alcohol, in 18 patients. Hill and Pond (16) reported a high incidence of abnormal EEG's in persons who committed motiveless murders and who were not under the influence of alcohol at the times the crimes were committed.

During the past 30 years, behavior disorders in children have been extensively studied. The concept of minimal brain damage, delayed cerebral maturation, or hyperkinesis encompasses a heterogeneous group of children with a great variety of neurological and/or behavioral disorders. Much work seems to indicate that many of the behavioral symptoms in children may be common to many disorders, regardless of their etiology. Whether there is a known organic etiology or not, one may assume that in some way the child's behavior is the result of a cerebral dysfunction. The absence of a recognizable neurologic deficit or of an abnormal EEG does not rule out cerebral dysfunction. It only means that methods are not yet available to detect many, if not most, cases of abnormal brain function and chemistry. A list of symptoms commonly seen in children with minimal brain damage or hyperkinesis includes the following:

1. overactivity from an early age, often in infancy
2. impulsive and uninhibited behavior
3. emotional lability with fluctuation of moods
4. short attention span with easy distractibility and poor concentration
5. unpredictable performance with behavior variability
6. inability to delay gratification
7. explosiveness and irritability related to low frustration tolerance
8. exaggerated response to external stimuli
9. specific learning disabilities and erratic school performance

These symptoms are most frequently seen in children below 12 years of age. They may disappear at any age from 8 to 18. Many investigators have reported a high incidence of abnormal EEG tracings in nonepileptic emotionally disturbed children and adolescents, especially the 14 and 6 per sec positive spike patterns. However, in most instances the changes observed in the EEG's are nonspecific and hence do not by themselves aid in making a diagnosis. Thus, many unrecognized brain disorders, with or without detectable abnormal EEG's, may be the cause of behavior problems both in children and in adults.

Lindsley and Henry (6) in 1942 noted marked improvement in 13 behavior problem children (i.e., hyperactivity, impulsiveness, destructiveness, aggressiveness, distractibility, seclusiveness, sex play, stealing, lying, etc.) treated either with Benzedrine Sulfate or DPH. Phenobarbital was ineffective.

Brown and Solomon (17) found in a training school setting that 3 out of

7 boys showed definite improvement on DPH as seen by a reduction in hyperactivity, inattention, less excitability, fewer flare-ups of temper, and more efficient work patterns. Zimmerman (18) gave DPH to a group of 200 children having severe behavior disorders. Improvement was seen in 70 percent of the cases. Less excitability, less severe and less frequent temper tantrums, less hyperactivity and distractibility, fewer fears, etc., were some of the behavior changes reported. Putnam and Hood (19) found DPH useful in the treatment of 24 juvenile delinquents ranging in age from 6 to 14 years of age, with fire-setting patterns, disruptive behavior, and sexual problems. Chao, Sexton, and Davis (20), Pincus and Glaser (21), Baldwin and Kenny (22), Oberst (23), Rossi (24), Itil, Rizzo and Shapiro (25), Tec (26), Campbell (27) and Resnick (28) have also demonstrated the beneficial effects of DPH on emotionally disturbed children (MBD) and juvenile delinquents. Resnick (28) also demonstrated the beneficial effects of DPH in both mood and affect in selected, adult, male prison inmates. Mark, Sweet, Ervin, Solomon, and Geschmind (29) studied patients with focal brain lesions whose symptoms included: unrestrained and senseless brutality, pathological intoxication, sexual assault, and multiple traffic accidents. The authors have studied over 100 patients suffering from this "dyscontrol syndrome." Fifteen of these patients had had surgical implantation of the medial temporal lobe with electrodes. The frequent expression of aggressive or assaultive behavior in the interictal period was a most disabling symptom. DPH was found of value in certain of these cases.

From the literature we find ample evidence for the beneficial effects of DPH and other anticonvulsants in neurotics, psychotics, psychopaths (30), and emotionally disturbed children. In some cases, the etiology is known or inferred to be cerebral injury related to trauma or encephalitis, cerebral maldevelopment, delayed cerebral maturation, intense emotional stress, sensory deprivation, cultural deprivation, and the like. In most cases, the etiology cannot be determined nor inferred. In some cases, there are abnormal EEG patterns; in just as many cases, there are no discernible abnormal EEG patterns. Thus DPH seems to affect many heterogeneous groups of patients. However, if these groups of patients are closely examined, one finds commonality with respect to certain behavioral characteristics. These are explosiveness, low frustration tolerance, irritability, impulsive behavior, compulsive behavior, aggressive behavior, erratic behavior, inability to delay gratification, mood swings, short attention span, undirected activity, and the like. Perhaps we may postulate that the presence of one or more anatomical or chemical lesions in the brain, from whatever cause, may disorganize the physiology of the remaining intact brain and thus result in a disorganization of synchrony in the firing of the neurones. This may lead to a decreased threshold of excitation with almost continuous firing of the neurones or it may lead to a spiking pattern of activity resulting in convulsive seizures. Concomitantly, there may result continuous abnormal behavioral changes or abrupt abnormal behavioral changes. That this may be so, in part at least, is indicated by the work of Laufer and Denhoff (7), who demonstrated that children with the hyperkinetic syndrome demonstrate a low threshold for photometrazol activation of the EEG by the technique of Gastaut. Laufer et al. also postulate that the hyperkinetic syndrome in children may result from injury to or dysfunction of the diencephalon in early life, thus interfering with the normal cortical-diencephalic interplay.

Since 1938, DPH has been shown to be one of the most effective drugs for the treatment of major motor epilepsy, psychomotor or temporal lobe epilepsy, and nonconvulsive epileptic equivalents. DPH has also been shown to be effective in the treatment of cerebral dysrhythmias, without clinical evidence of seizures. DPH has now been demonstrated to be effective in the treatment of behavioral and emotional symptoms concomitant with a wide variety of cerebral dysfunctions. The effectiveness of DPH may be due to its ability to decrease the excitability of hyperexcitable cells, in this case, nerve cells. This may result in the re-establishment of normal patterns of brain activity.

Experiments have shown that the aggressive pattern of behavior occurs in almost every case when the hypothalamic area of the brain is damaged. After studying cases of verified lesions of the hypothalamic area, Alpers (31) concluded that the aggressive behavior of his patients had markedly increased. In addition, "obvious antisocial tendencies and partial or complete loss of insight occurred." Fulton and Ingraham (32) made surgical incisions injuring the hypothalamic region of healthy, friendly cats. Immediately after the operation, the cats' behavior changed from playfulness to violent, impulsive sham rage. Patting their backs produced snarling aggressiveness. A similar experiment with dogs, involving removal of the entire thalamic area, brought about a condition of chronic anger (33). Disease, as well as injury, can cause an increase in antisocial behavior. In 1942, after analyzing a great many postencephalitic children, Laruetta Bender concluded that the disease increased aggressiveness and decreased the patients' anxiety concerning his uninhibited behavior (34). Thus, the similarity between the behavior of brain-damaged patients and the sociopath or psychopath may indicate similar cerebral dysfunctions.

Perhaps a biochemical similarity may also be shown to exist. In 1937, Bradley (4) demonstrated the usefulness of the amphetamines in the treatment of the organic behavior syndrome in children. This was considered by many to be a paradoxical effect of the amphetamines. Hill (9) and Shovron (10) reported beneficial, albeit temporary, effects of the amphetamines on aggressive, bad-tempered psychopaths. This could also be considered as a paradoxical effect of the amphetamines. The amphetamines also produce a paradoxical effect in Parkinson patients. It is of great interest to the author that in all areas where the paradoxical effects of amphetamines have been observed, DPH also produces beneficial effects.

## BENZODIAZEPINES

### Chlordiazepoxide (Librium) and Diazepam (Valium)

The benzodiazepine compounds are of interest in this discussion because they are prescribed very extensively for the treatment of the following conditions: tension and anxiety states; somatic complaints which are concomitants of emotional factors; psychoneurotic states manifested by tension, anxiety, apprehension, fatigue, depressive symptoms, or agitation; acute agitation, tremor, delirium tremens, and hallucinosis due to acute alcohol withdrawal; adjunctively in skeletal muscle spasm due to reflex spasm to local pathology; spasticity caused by upper motor neuron disorders; athetosis; stiff-man syndrome; convulsive disorders; and the like.

These conditions are similar to those that are now being treated very extensively with DPH. There appear to be great similarities in the actions of Librium and Valium on the one hand and DPH on the other—both clinically and on an animal level. Schallek and Kuehn (35) investigated the effects of Librium on the limbic system, which is also referred to as the visceral brain or the rhinencephalon. The limbic system is thought to play a fundamental role in "mood" and "affect." The limbic system is composed of the septum, amygdala, and hippocampus. Following electrical stimulation of component parts of the limbic system in decamethonium-immobilized cats, Librium (10 mg/kg i.v.) inhibited EEG after discharge. Specifically, Librium reduced the duration of after-discharge in the septum and hippocampus and reduced the amplitude of discharge in the amygdala. In freely moving cats with electrodes permanently implanted in the brain, Librium in low doses slowed electrical activity at statistically significant levels only in the hippocampus, amygdala, and septum. The cortex was noticeably affected only at higher doses. In addition, naturally vicious laboratory monkeys consistently show aggressive behavior toward their handlers. On Valium, they become quite tame, yet remain alert and coordinated (36). Kalina (37) has reported excellent success with the use of diazepam (Valium) for the control of the destructive rampages of psychotic criminals. To complete the analogy between DPH and the benzodiazephines (Librium, Valium, Serax), many reports have appeared indicating the effectiveness of parenteral diazepam (Valium) in the treatment of status epilepticus. Surely, more work is indicated on the use of the benzodiazephines in juvenile delinquents and prisoners.

## PHENOTHIAZINES

Eisenberg and Conners (8) report that "stimulants such as dextroamphetamine and methylphenidate are useful in controlling hyperkinetic (and aggressive) behavior disorders in children and adolescents; that phenothiazines such as prochlorperazine and perphenazine may be no better than placebo; and that phenobarbital can be considerably worse." Jonas (38) has reported that the phenothiazine tranquilizers are contraindicated in the treatment of epileptic equivalents (e.g., the ictal or subictal neuroses). He further states that "the administration of tranquilizers to an irritable and impulsive youngster who suffers from epileptic equivalents will only intensify his symptoms." He concludes that the major phenothiazine tranquilizers are contraindicated in cases of cerebral dysrhythmia and in suspected cases of epilepsy, both in children and adults. Furthermore, the phenothiazines may actually precipitate or aggravate an epileptic state or an ictal or subictal neurosis. There is ample evidence in the literature to indicate that phenothiazines are of little value or contraindicated in the treatment of MBD in children, of ictal and subictal states in children and adults, and of chronic brain syndrome in geriatric patients. These findings seem to be quite paradoxical when one considers that the phenothiazines are very powerful anticholinergic, antihistaminic, and antiserotoninergic agents. The sympathomimetic amines (e.g., the amphetamines) and the antihistamines (e.g., Benadryl) are also anticholinergic and antihistaminic and yet are beneficial in the treatment of the conditions discussed in this paper. A possible explanation of this paradox would seem to be that the major phenothiazines are epileptogenic, that is, they lower the threshold of excitation and may precipitate or aggravate an epileptic state. Hankoff (39) reported that 6 patients in a group of 56 developed epileptic seizures following promazine treatment. Fabish (40) administered chlorpromazine to epileptics and observed an increase in paroxysmal and hypersynchronous activity in the EEG's. Ingvar and Soderberg (41) produced spindles and slow waves in cats following chlorpromazine, i.v. Since we have assumed that rages, tantrums, acting out, character problems, and all of the epileptic equivalents represent "seizureless epilepsies," certainly agents with "epileptogenic" properties would be contraindicated. On the other hand, a phenothiazine tranquilizer which in clinically effective dosages is usually *not* epileptogenic would be beneficial in the treatment of the conditions discussed in this paper. As is well known by clinicians, thioridazine (Mellaril) is such a phenothiazine tranquilizer—effective in children, adults and geriatric patients.

Kamm and Mandel (42) administered thioridazine to 42 epileptics with severe ictal manifestations, who had responded poorly to other phenothiazines. He reports that "favorable effect was obtained in 37 patients, 19 exhibiting marked to moderate improvement. The absence of any increase in seizures constitutes a significant advantage in using thioridazine for the treatment of behavior disorders associated with, or related to, epilepsy."

Another possible explanation for the paradoxical effects of the phenothiazines in the treatment of the ictal and subictal symptoms would seem to be that the phenothiazines can produce extrapyramidal complications. It is of interest in this connection that the incidence of extrapyramidal complications produced by thioridazine is extremely low.

It would seem that drugs capable of raising the threshold of excitation of neurones of the CNS would be of use in the treatment of the aggressive, explosive behavioral anomalies. This, of course, is the mechanism of action of Dilantin. It is well known that the monoamine oxidase inhibitors (i.e., the psychic energizers) also raise the seizure threshold. Thus, more work with this class of agents is indicated. In addition, drugs that are anticholinergic, antihistaminic, and antiserotoninergic, but are not epileptogenic, would also be of use in treating the ictal and subictal states. The tricyclic antidepressants, such as imipramine (Tofranil) would be examples of this. Tofranil has been found to be especially useful for the treatment of enuresis in children with emotional problems.

Another drug that possesses anticholinergic, antihistaminic, and antiserotoninergic properties and is not epileptogenic is hydroxyzine (Atarax, Vistaril). Hydroxyzine has been found useful in the treatment of the ictal and subictal manifestations, such as tension, anxiety, psychomotor agitation, psychosomatic complaints, behavior problems in children, and the like. Thus, more information on the effects of this drug in aggressive, explosive anomalies is indicated.

## BARBITURATES

As mentioned above, Cutts and Jasper (5) reported that phenobarbital aggravated the symptoms in 9 of 12 children who were asocial, hyperactive, impulsive, and destructive. Lindsley and Henry (6) reported that phenobarbital, given after benzedrine improved the behavior of emotionally disturbed children, caused an exacerbation of the symptoms. Leon Eisenberg (8) concludes that phenobarbital is considerably worse than placebo in controlling hyperkinetic and aggressive behavior disorders in children and adolescents. It has been the experience of the author that phenobarbital may be contraindicated in the treatment of geriatrics with chronic brain syndrome or simple senile degeneration. The adverse effects of phenobarbital in the treatment of aggressive, explosive behavioral anomalies must surely rank as the most "paradoxical" of all the reactions discussed here. Since phenobarbital is an excellent anticonvulsant, one would expect this drug to produce beneficial effects in the aggressive, explosive anomalies, as well as in the ictal and subictal symptomatology. A possible explanation might be the concept, held by many investigators, that places the primary site of action of the barbiturates at the diencephalic rather than the cortical level. We have already mentioned that Laufer and Denhoff (7) postulate that the hyperkinetic syndrome in children may result from injury to or dysfunction of the diencephalon in early life, thus interfering with the normal cortical-diencephalic interplay. Should the barbiturates depress the diencephalon more than the cortex, then the normal cortical-diencephalic interplay would be interfered with, thus actually producing a cerebral dysrhythmia with concomitant behavioral manifestations. Certainly much more work is indicated in this area.

## REFERENCES


1. Jonas, A. D.: *Ictal and Subictal Neurosis, Diagnosis and Treatment.* Charles C Thomas, Springfield, Ill., 1965.
2. McDonald, J. M.: *Psychiatry and the Criminal.* Charles C Thomas, Springfield, Ill., 1958.
3. Thompson, G. N.: Relationship of sexual psychopathy to psychomotor epilepsy and its variants. *J. Nerv. Ment. Dis.* **121** : 374, 1955.
4. Bradley, C.: The behavior of children receiving benzedrine. *Am. J. Psychiat.* **94**: 577, 1937.
5. Cutts, K. K., and Jasper, H. H.: Effect of benzedrine sulfate and phenobarbital on behavior problems of children with abnormal EEG. *Arch. Neural. Psychiat.* **41**: 1138, 1939.
6. Lindsley, D. B., and Henry, C. E.: The effect of drugs on behavior and the electroencephalograms of children with behavior disorders. *Psychosomat. Med.* **4**: 140, 1942.
7. Laufer, M. W., and Denhoff, E.: Hyperkinetic behavior syndrome in children. *J. Pediatrics* **50**: 463, 1957.
8. Eisenberg, L., and Conners, C. K.: Behavioral manifestations of cerebral damage in childhood, *Brain Damage in Children,* H. G. Birch, ed. The Williams and Wilkins Co., 1964.
9. Hill, D.: Amphetamine in psychopathic states. *Brit. J. Addiction.* **44**: 50, 1947.
10. Shovron, J. J.: Benzedrine in psychopathy and behavior disorders. *Brit. J. Addiction.* **44**: 58, 1947.
11. Tong, J.: *Stress Reactivity in Relation to Delinquent and Psychopathic*

*Behavior*, 1959. Cited by Craft, M., *in* Psychopathic personalities: A review of diagnosis, etiology, prognosis and treatment. *Brit. J. Criminol.* **1**, 3, 1961.
12. HORNYKIEWICZ, O. The occurrence of dopamine (3-hydroxytyramine) in the central nervous system: Its relationship to Parkinsonism. *German Med. Monthly*. 7: 344, 1962.
13. TURNER, W. J.: The usefulness of diphenylhydantoin in treatment of non-epileptic emotional disorders. *Intern. J. Neuropsychiat.* **3**: Suppl. 2, 58, 1967.
14. MCCULLAGH, W. H. and INGRAM, W., JR.: Headaches and hot tempers. *Dis. Nerv. Sys.* 17 (9): 279, 1956.
15. MARINACCI, A. A.: Special type of temporal lobe seizure following ingestion of alcohol. *Bull. Los Angeles Neurol. Soc.* **28**: 241, 1963.
16. HILL, D., and POND, D. A.: Reflections on 100 capital cases submitted to EEG. *J. Ment. Sci.* **98**: 23, 1952.
17. BROWN, W. T., and SOLOMON, C. I.: Delinquency and the electroencephalograph. *Am. J. Psychiatry* **98**: 499, 1942.
18. ZIMMERMAN, F. T.: Explosive behavior anomalies in children on an epileptic basis. *N.Y. State J. Med.* **56**: 2537, 1956.
19. PUTNAM, T. J., and HOOD, O. E.: Project Illinois: A study of therapy in juvenile behavior problems. *Western Med.*, July 1964, 231.
20. CHAO, D., SEXTON, J. A., and DAVIS, S. D.: Convulsive equivalent syndrome of childhood. *J. Pediatrics* **64**: 499, 1964.
21. PINCUS, J. H. and GLASER, G. H.: The syndrome of minimal brain damage in childhood. *New England J. Med.* **275**: 27, 1966.
22. BALDWIN, R., and KENNY, T. J.: Learning disabilities *in Learning Disabilities*, J. Hellmuth, ed., vol. 2, 313, 1966.
23. OBERST, B. B.: Preventive care of infants and children. *The Lancet* **86**: 331, 1966.
24. ROSSI, A. O.: Psychoneurologically impaired child. *N.Y. State J. Med.* **67**: 902, 1967.
25. ITIL, T. M., RIZZO, A. E., and SHAPIRO, D. M.: Study of behavior and EEG correlation during treatment of disturbed children. *Dis. Nerv. Sys.* **28**: 731, 1967.
26. TEC, L.: Efficacy of diphenylhydantoin in childhood psychiatric disorders. *Am. J. Psychiatry* **124**: 156, 1968.
27. CAMPBELL, E. W., JR., and YOUNG, J. D., JR.: Enuresis and its relationship to electroencephalographic disturbances. *J. Urol.* **96**: 947, 1966.
28. RESNICK, O.: The psychoactive properties of diphenylhydantoin: Experiences with prisoners and juvenile delinquents. *Intern. J. Neuropsychiat.* **3**: (2) 530, 1967.
29. Personal communication.
30. SILVERMAN, D.: The electroencephalograph and therapy of criminal psychopaths. *J. Crimin. Psychopathol.* **5**(3): 439, 1944.
31. ALPERS, B.: Hypothalamic destruction. *Psychosom. Med.* **2**: 286, 1944.
32. FULTON, J. F., and INGRAHAM, F. D.: Emotional disturbances following experimental lesions of the base of the brain. *J. Physiol.* **90**: 353, 1929.
33. EAST, W. N.: Psychopathic personality and crime. *J. Ment. Sci.* **91**: 426, 1945.
34. BENDER, L.: Postencephalitic behavior disorders in childhood, *in* Neal, Josephine B.: *Encephalitis*. Grune & Stratton, New York, 1942.
35. SCHALLEK, R. W., and KUEHN, A.: Effects of psychotropic drugs on limbic system of cat. *Proc. Soc. Exptl. Biol. Med.* **105**: 115, 1960.
36. RANDALL, L. O., SCHALLEK, W., HEISE, G. A., KEITH, E. F., and BAGDON,

R. E.: The psychosedative properties of methaminodiazepoxide. *J.P. E.T.* 120: 963, 1960.
37. Kalina, R. K.: Use of diazepam in the violent psychotic patient: A preliminary report. *Colorado GP* 4: 11, 1962.
38. Jonas, A.: The emergence of epileptic equivalents in the era of tranquilizers. *Intern. J. Neuropsychiat.* 3: 40, 1967.
39. Hankoff, I. D.: Convulsions complicating ataractic therapy. *N.Y. State J. Med.* 57: 2967, 1957.
40. Fabish, W.: The effect of chlorpromazine on the EEG of epileptics. *J. Neurol. Neurosurg. and Psychiat.* 20: 185, 1957.
41. Ingvar, D. H., and Soderberg, U.: Effects of chlorpromazine on cerebral circulation and EEG in cats. *Arch. Neurol. Psychiat.* 78: 254, 1957.
42. Kamm, I., and Mandel, A.: Thioridazine in the treatment of behavior disorders in epileptics. *Dis. Nerv. System* 28: 46, 1967.

# 15

## *The Effectiveness of a New Drug, Mesoridazine, and Chlorpromazine with Behavior Problems in Children*

THOMAS J. KENNY, DAVOOD BADIE, RUTH W. BALDWIN

Increased attention has been focused on behavior problems in the school age population. The recent interest in minimal brain damage has brought in an intensified effort to determine pharmacological agents capable of modifying aberrant behavior and thus enabling the child to stay in school. The phenothiazines have been reported as one of the most effective of the tranquilizing agents when used with this group of children (3–8). Chlorpromazine (Thorazine) and thioridazine (Mellaril) seem to be the two most frequently examined drugs in the phenothiazine family.

An earlier experience with thioridazine showed it was safe and effective with this group of children (1). Mesoridazine (TPS-23)[1] is a new side chain derivative of thioridazine which has been reported three times as potent (9, 11). A clinical trial of mesoridazine produced significant change in a group of children with behavior problems, including those who were retarded, brain-damaged, and epileptic (2). The success of the clinical trial led to a fuller evaluation of the

From the *Journal of Nervous and Mental Disease*, Vol. 147, No. 3, 1968, pp. 316–321.


[1] Supplied as Serentil by Sandoz Pharmaceuticals, Hanover, N. J.

effectiveness of this new agent. The present study is a comparison of mesoridazine and chlorpromazine designed to evaluate: (a) the relative value of the drugs; (b) the specific target symptoms affected by the drugs, stressing change in the normal behavioral environment (home and school); and (c) a means of controlling the placebo effect usually encountered in drug studies of this type.

## METHOD

### Subjects

The study group consisted of 21 children referred to the Clinic for the Exceptional Child, University of Maryland Hospital, because they showed serious behavior problems in school and at home. The group ranged in age from 7 to 14 years and included 19 boys and 2 girls. In all cases, the behavior problem had sufficient magnitude and duration to make the child a poor risk for continuing in school. Behavior in the home and neighborhood was equally bad.

To be eligible for the study, the children had to be in school, with intelligence above the mentally retarded level, and be capable of outpatient follow-up. Four children included in the study were subsequently dropped for nonparticipation, leaving a total of 17 (15 boys and 2 girls) who formed the trial group.

### Clinical Evaluation and Ratings

Upon referral to the Clinic for the Exceptional Child, each child was given the usual evaluation for new patients. This consisted of an interview with the child and a parent, a thorough history, a physical and neurological examination, and an electroencephalogram. The majority of the subjects, 14, were diagnosed as having minimal brain damage, but this diagnosis was not essential for the child's inclusion in the study. The child's behavior was the major criterion.

At the time of the initial evaluation, the physician made a rating of the child's behavior by using the Behavior Rating Scale from the Clinic for the Exceptional Child (Figure 1). This rating served as a base line score for each subject. This and all subsequent ratings were a composite of an interview with the parent and the child, plus the physician's observation of the child during the interview. To minimize rater variability, one physician served as rater for the total group. To encourage objectivity, the rating scale was removed from the child's chart as it was filled out and replaced by a blank scale to be filled out at the time of the next follow-up visit. This completed stage 1 of the study (Figure 2), after which each subject was started on a pink placebo, Parke-Davis no. 2 capsule (stage 2). The child and parent returned to the clinic in 1 month for a follow-up visit. If at this time the parent's report showed that the child had shown no response to the placebo, the child advanced to stage 3 of the study. If there was a positive response to this placebo, the child was continued in stage 2 until the parent reported dissatisfaction. In no case was it necessary to extend the period in stage 2 beyond 1 month.

## Drug Schedule and Dosage

Stage 3 of the study was a double blind cross over study comparing mesoridazine (TSP-23), chlorpromazine (Thorazine), and a second placebo. All of these were in tablet form to make their difference from the pretreatment placebo obvious. The parents were told that the subjects would be given different medicines during the study and that the tablets could look the same but be different. They were instructed to ignore the size and color of the tablets and attend only to the child's behavior. The physician rating the child never saw the medication issued. Mesoridazine and chlorpromazine were assumed to have equal potency so that the physician following the child, using the dosage levels recommended by the manufacturer, simply prescribed the dosage appropriate for the child's age, size, and condition. Dosages ranged from 30 to 100 mg per day, with the average at 50 mg per day. When the dosage was selected, the chief investigator then supplied the appropriate compound according to a predetermined drug schedule. To control for any possible additive or sequential drug effect, the order of drug presentation was counterbalanced and assignment to the drug order was made at random.

The children were seen at monthly intervals during stage 3, and the Behavior Rating Scale was scored on each visit. Laboratory studies were completed at the beginning of the study and at monthly intervals throughout the study. These included white blood count, hemoglobin, differential, serum glutamic-oxaloacetic transaminase, urea nitrogen, and urinalysis. Funduscopic studies were completed on the same schedule. Electrocardiograms were made randomly for some of the subjects.

## RESULTS

The mean score on the Behavior Rating Scale was computed for each treatment stage (Table 1), and the scores were compared by using an analysis of variance technique. The results are presented in Table 3. There was a significant change noted during the treatment stage with a resulting drug effect exceeding statistical significance at the .01 level ($F = 5.39$—obtain $F = 49.00$). A breakdown of the drug effect indicates that mesoridazine produced a change significant beyond the .01 level ($F = 7.57$—obtained $F = 40.47$). Chlorpromazine failed to produce a change that reached statistical significance ($F = 7.57$—obtained $F = 0.40$).

Individual items on the Behavior Rating Scale were repeatedly analyzed to determine the specific effectiveness of each agent on target symptoms.

Table 2 presents the results of the analysis using the nonparametric Signs Test (12) to ascertain the significance. It will be noted that mesoridazine produced a change on all nine items when compared to the base line rating, while chlorpromazine showed positive change on seven of nine items and placebo produced no change. When compared to the placebo score, mesoridazine still registered change on all nine items, while chlorpromazine produced a change on five items. In a

**Figure 1** Behavior rating scale

University of Maryland

School of Medicine

Department of Pediatrics — Clinic for the Exceptional Child

BEHAVIOR RATING SCALE

Child's name____________________ Date________________

Instructions to rater: Please read instructions carefully. Rate the child by selecting the most appropriate statement on the scale. Try to rate every item, but only one rating per trait.

A. Hyperactivity-Constantly active, unproductive, restless; may be destructive.

| | | | | |
|---|---|---|---|---|
| No problem; calm | Better than average | Average | Overactive; disturbs others | Constant activity; difficult to contain in class |

B. Irritability-Easily angered; subject to temper tantrums; impatient.

| | | | | |
|---|---|---|---|---|
| Not easily provoked, generally pleasant | Better than average control | Average; can be upset; sometimes picks or is picked on | Frequently upset; flies off easily | Frequent tantrums; needs own way; very impatient |

C. Aggressiveness-Attempts to dominate others; fights; may hit, pinch, shove, or bite.

| | | | | |
|---|---|---|---|---|
| Well controlled; avoids fighting | Does not choose to aggress | Average; will fight if provoked | Frequently resorts to aggression | Very aggressive; no control |

D. Emotional Excitability and Control

| | | | | |
|---|---|---|---|---|
| Accepts change or excitement without upset | Better than average control of emotions | Average control; can be excited | Easily excited; below average control | Emotionally volatile; very poor control |

E. Social Adjustment

| | | | | |
|---|---|---|---|---|
| Well adjusted; a leader | Better than average adjustment | Average | Below average adjustment; does not interact easily | Poor adjustment; few friends |

F. Conformity-Conforms or reacts according to taught or accepted standards.

| | | | | |
|---|---|---|---|---|
| Very good | Better than average | Average | Poor | Very poor |

G. Planfulness-Able to develop and use plans; can work independently.

| | | | | |
|---|---|---|---|---|
| Well organized | Better than average planning | Average planfulness | Below average; needs direction | Very poor; accomplishes little without supervision |

**Figure 1** (continued)

H. Attention Span–Ability to attend to one subject and maintain interest.

| | | | | |
|---|---|---|---|---|
| Good attention; able to sustain interest | Better than average attention; usually attentive | Average | Below average; sustains interest briefly | Poor attention span |

I. Distractibility–Attention easily drawn to objects or individuals moving.

| | | | | |
|---|---|---|---|---|
| Not easily distracted; controls attention | Distracted infrequently | Average | Easily distracted | Always distracted |

REMARKS:

**Figure 2** Stages in drug study

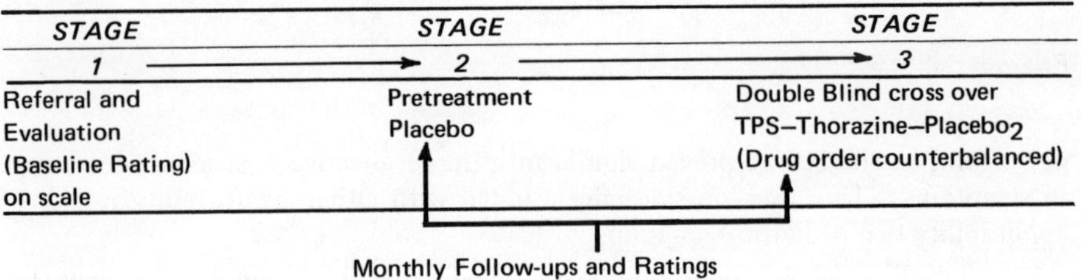


direct comparison of the two active compounds, mesoridazine produced significantly greater change than chlorpromazine on five items (reducing hyperactivity, aggressiveness, irritability, and distractibility).

All laboratory studies, funduscopic examinations, and electrocardiograms were within normal limits. No side effects were encountered under any drug condition.

## DISCUSSION

The present study provides meaningful information in three areas. (a) It evaluates the relative and specific effectiveness of two phenothiazines in modifying behavior in a preadolescent population. (b) The study proves a reasonable means to measure pertinent behavior change, that is, target symptoms in an outpatient population. (c) The design of the study effectively controlled the placebo effect, thus allowing for a more meaningful comparison of the active agents.

As was to be expected from the reports in the literature, chlorpromazine proved an active agent capable of ameliorating extreme behavior. However, the

**TABLE 1. Scores on Rating Scale**

| *Subject* | *Base* | *Placebo (A)* | *Mesoridazine (B)* | *Chlorpromazine (C)* | *Dosage (mg)* | *Drug Order* |
|---|---|---|---|---|---|---|
| 1 | 18 | 21 | 29 | 29 | 50 | BCA |
| 2 | 14 | 12 | 30 | 14 | 50 | BCA |
| 3 | 21 | 23 | 26 | 27 | 50 | BCA |
| 4 | 19 | 15 | 28 | 20 | 40 | BCA |
| 5 | 16 | 22 | 30 | 20 | 50 | BAC |
| 6 | 17 | 19 | 18 | 30 | 75 | BAC |
| 7 | 18 | 17 | 28 | 20 | 100 | CBA |
| 8 | 20 | 25 | 30 | 28 | 30 | CBA |
| 9 | 17 | 10 | 20 | 20 | 75 | CBA |
| 10 | 16 | 16 | 20 | 18 | 30 | CBA |
| 11 | 19 | 20 | 30 | 30 | 30 | ABC |
| 12 | 20 | 20 | 19 | 26 | 50 | ABC |
| 13 | 19 | 20 | 26 | 26 | 50 | ACB |
| 14 | 21 | 18 | 30 | 19 | 50 | ACB |
| 15 | 20 | 22 | 29 | 24 | 50 | ACB |
| 16 | 20 | 18 | 20 | 20 | 50 | CAB |
| 17 | 17 | 20 | 30 | 20 | 50 | CAB |
| | $\bar{x}$ = 18.47 | $\bar{x}$ = 18.71 | $\bar{x}$ = 26.06 | $\bar{x}$ = 23.06 | $\bar{x}$ = 52 | |
| | $\bar{u}$ = 1.73 | $\bar{u}$ = 3.60 | $\bar{u}$ = 4.35 | $\bar{u}$ = 4.35 | | |

Behavior Rating Scale range = 10 to 50.

new agent, mesoridazine, proved significantly more effective over a broader range of symptoms. There were no side effects noted with either agent, indicating their applicability to a pediatric age group.

The plan to use parent interview and physician's rating on the Behavior Rating Scale proved to be a realistic means for assessing change in the child's behavior in the everyday setting rather than in an artificial, sheltered environment

**TABLE 2. Comparison by Item on Behavior Rating Scale**

| | *Comparison with Base Line Rating* | | | *Comparison with Placebo Rating* | | *Between Drugs* | |
|---|---|---|---|---|---|---|---|
| *Item* | *TPS* | *Thorazine* | *Placebo* | *TPS* | *Thorazine* | *TPS* | *Thorazine* |
| 1. Hyperactivity | + | + | 0 | + | + | + | 0 |
| 2. Irritability | + | 0 | 0 | + | + | + | 0 |
| 3. Aggressiveness | + | + | 0 | + | 0 | + | 0 |
| 4. Emotional excitability | + | 0 | 0 | + | + | + | 0 |
| 5. Social adjustment | + | + | 0 | + | + | 0 | 0 |
| 6. Conformity | + | + | 0 | + | + | 0 | 0 |
| 7. Planfulness | + | + | 0 | + | 0 | 0 | 0 |
| 8. Attention span | + | + | 0 | + | 0 | 0 | 0 |
| 9. Distractibility | + | + | 0 | + | 0 | + | 0 |

*N* = 17. + = statistically significant change over comparison rating. 0 = no significant change.

**TABLE 3. Analysis of Variance of Behavior Ratings**

| *Source of Variance* | | *SS* | | *df* | *MS* | *F* |
|---|---|---|---|---|---|---|
| Between subjects | | 477 | | 16 | | |
| Within subjects | | 934 | | 34 | | |
| Drugs | 692 | | 3 | | 346 | 49* |
| Residual | 242 | | 32 | | 7 | |
| Total | | 1411 | | 50 | | |

$F_{.99}$ ($df$ = 30, 2) 5.39

Between drugs—TPS $F = \frac{SS_{e1}}{MS_{res.}} = \frac{283.33}{7} = 40.47^{*}$

($F$ = .99 = 7.56)

Thorazine $F = \frac{SS_{e2}}{MS_{res.}} = \frac{2.83}{7} = .40$

($F$ = .99 = 7.56)

| | |
|---|---|
| Pretreatment rating | $\bar{x} = 19$ |
| Placebo rating | $\bar{x} = 19$ |
| Thorazine rating | $\bar{x} = 23$ |
| TPS rating | $\bar{x} = 26$ |

such as an institution. The children in the study group were in an outpatient situation throughout the study and regularly attended a public school program. That they stayed in school was in a large part the result of the effectiveness of the drugs; even more important, the school officials provided a practical check for any questionable behavior report. Several teachers reported problems within 1 to 2 days after a child was put in the placebo cycle of the study, which would indicate a rather intent observation of behavior throughout the study.

Zrull (14) and Eisenberg (10) have mentioned in separate papers the problem of placebo effect in evaluating tranquilizing agents. The use of the pretreatment placebo in this study effectively controlled this problem. A comparison of pretreatment ratings and placebo ratings showed equivalent means, and a *t* test of difference (13) revealed no significant change between the two conditions. A coefficient of correlation of .511 was obtained between these two sets of scores.

An examination of the individual response to treatment showed that three subjects failed to benefit from either mesoridazine or chlorpromazine. Each of these cases had special complications. In one case, the parents were at the clinic against their wishes and felt that the authorities were harassing them because of their religion (Black Muslim). Their cooperation with the clinic was poor, and it is very questionable whether or not the boy received his medication. The school teacher reported that the boy told her he was not taking his medication. In another case, the family situation was so chaotic that any judgment of change would be less than reliable. The mother was so unstable she was finally referred for psychiatric treatment herself. In the third case, the family was inadequate to the extent that all cooperation was erratic and difficult.

## SUMMARY

Seventeen preadolescent children with severe behavior problems participated in a double blind evaluation of two phenothiazines, mesoridazine, a new sulfoxy derivative of thioridazine, and chlorpromazine. Results were evaluated by means of a Behavior Rating Scale. An analysis of variance indicated that mesoridazine was a significantly effective agent, producing positive change in all items on the rating scale. Chlorpromazine was more effective than placebo but less effective than this new agent. A special pretreatment placebo stage improved the discrimination of drug effect in the double blind section of the study. Laboratory work done at monthly intervals was negative, and no side effects were noted during the study. Mesoridazine was especially effective in reducing hyperactivity, aggressiveness, irritability, and distractibility.

## REFERENCES

1. Baldwin, R., and Kenny, T. Thioridazine in the management of organic behavior disturbances in children. *Curr. Ther. Res.*, 8: 373–377, 1966.
2. Baldwin, R., Kenny, T., and Badie, D. A new drug for behavior problems in children: A preliminary report. *Curr. Ther. Res.*, 9: 457–461, 1967.
3. Eveloff, H. Psychopharmacologic agents in child psychiatry. *Arch. Gen. Psychiat.*, **14**: 472–481, 1966.
4. Fish, B. Drug therapy in child psychiatry: Pharmacologic aspects. *Compr. Psychiat.*, **1**: 212–227, 1960.
5. Freed, H., and Frignito, M. Tranquilizers in child psychiatry: Current status on drugs, particularly phenothiazine. *Penn Psychiat. Quart.*, **1**: 39–48, 1961.
6. Garfield, S. L., Helper, M. M., Wilcott, R. C., and Muffly, R. Effect of chlorpromazine on behavior of emotionally disturbed children. *J. Nerv. Ment. Dis.*, **135**: 147–154, 1962.
7. Gatski, R. L. Chlorpromazine in the treatment of emotionally maladjusted children. *J. A. M. A.*, **157**: 1298–1300, 1955.
8. Grant, G. R. Psychopharmacology in childhood emotional and mental disorders. *J. Pediat.*, **61**: 626–637, 1962.
9. Mena, A., Grayson, H., and Cohen, S. A. study of thioridazine and its side chain derivative, mesoridazine, in chronic male hospitalized psychiatric patients. *J. New Drugs*, 6: 345–348, 1966.
10. Molling, P., Lockner, H., Sauls, R., and Eisenberg, L. Committed delinquent boys: The impact of perphenazine and of placebo. *Arch. Gen. Psychiat.*, 7: 70–76, 1962.
11. Prusmack, J., Hollister, L., Overall, J., and Shelton, J. Mesoridazine (TPS-23), a new anti-psychotic drug. *J. New Drugs*, 6: 182–188, 1966.
12. Siegel, S. *Non-Parametric Statistics*. McGraw-Hill, New York, 1956.
13. Winer, B. J. *Statistical Principles in Experimental Design*. McGraw-Hill, New York, 1962.
14. Zrull, J. P. Critique. *Amer. J. Psychiat.*, **120**: 464, 1964.

# 16

# *The Effects of Methylphenidate (Ritalin) on the Motor Skills and Behavior of Children with Learning Problems**

ROBERT M. KNIGHTS and GEORGE G. HINTON

This study investigates the effects of a 6-week trial of methylphenidate on the performance and behavior of children who have learning difficulties at school. Forty children were included in the double blind design with placebo control. The children were assessed medically and psychologically and rated by their parents and teachers prior to taking the drug or placebo and just before terminating the 6-week period. The principal findings were significant differences in heart rate, diastolic blood pressure, weight loss, motor coordination, and Wechsler Intelligence Scale for Children (WISC) performance abilities. In addition both the parents and teachers rated the methylphenidate group as less distractible and more attentive. Other physical measures and electroencephalographic (EEG) results were not significant. The psychological test data are interpreted to indicate that methylphenidate is associated with improved attention span and this is the basis for the better motor coordination and performance skills. Attempts to relate the magnitude of drug response to medical history, psychological test scores or patterns of behavior were unsuccessful.

Several papers have reviewed the use of drugs in the treatment of children with learning and behavioral difficulties who are classified under the heading minimal brain dysfunction (6, 9, 19). In general, stimulant drugs have been found helpful in the treatment of children who are hyperactive or have behavior problems. The drugs tend to quiet or inhibit their behavior. Methylphenidate (Ritalin) is a stimulant which has been reported to be the most effective with the fewest side effects on the basis of both clinical impressions (14–16) and partially controlled studies (18, 25).

Two controlled studies using a double blind design with placebo control have found methylphenidate more effective than the placebo in groups of retarded and institutionalized children. Eisenberg (6) reported an investigation done with retarded pediatric outpatients who were referred for hyperkinesis and poor school behavior. These children were rated by mothers and school teachers as improving significantly during the methylphenidate period in a cross-over design. The second controlled study by Conners and Eisenberg (3, 4) was conducted with homeless and disturbed institutionalized children. None were diagnosed as brain-damaged, defective, or overtly psychotic. The children were rated by their cottage parents or

From the *Journal of Nervous and Mental Disease,* Vol. 148, No. 6, 1969, pp. 643–653.

* This study was supported by a grant from CIBA Co. Ltd., Dorval, Quebec, and Grant 53 of the Ontario Mental Health Foundation.

child care workers on a symptom check list and learning tasks administered before and after the drug administration. The results indicate, in general, a significant improvement in the methylphenidate group over the placebo group on the symptom ratings and learning tasks.

Several authors (3–6, 15) have suggested that methylphenidate has a positive effect on some types of motor performance and improves attention span. The present study investigates the effect of methylphenidate on several motor performance tasks in an attempt to determine the type of motor ability affected by the drug. In addition, teacher and parent ratings are used to assess its clinical effects on a group of outpatient children with learning problems.

## METHOD

### Subjects

The study includes 40 children referred to a pediatrician (the second author) within a 24-month period prior to the drug study. These children represent 40 consecutive patients with a diagnosis of minimal brain dysfunction. They were included in the study on the basis of the following criteria: IQ above 80, chronological age 8 or above; no obvious brain lesions; and the child had taken an extensive psychological test battery (13). All of the children had been referred to the pediatrician for evaluation of school problems. Table 1 lists the chief presenting complaint of the 40 children. Many of the children had a secondary complaint such as mild behavioral or emotional difficulty, but only the chief complaint is listed in this table.

The children ranged in age from 8 to 15, with a mean age of 10.5 years and a standard deviation of 1.6 years. The mean WISC full scale IQ, on the first testing, was 108.1 with a range of 80 to 134 and a standard deviation of 11.9. There were 35 boys and 5 girls in the sample.

### General Design and Measures

Each child's history had been obtained and a medical and neurological exam had been conducted by the pediatrician, prior to the beginning of the present study. When the child returned to participate in the study, he was reexamined medically and neurologically and the psychological tests were administered. In addition, the child's parent and his teacher completed the rating scales. The child was then placed on medication for approximately 6 weeks. Just prior to the time when the medication was discontinued, the same medical, psychological, and

**TABLE 1. Chief Presenting Complaint of the 40 Children**

| *Chief Complaint* | *No. of Children* |
|---|---|
| Hyperactive, poor attention span, distractible | 17 |
| Reading, spelling, arithmetic problems | 12 |
| Generally slow progress, failure | 7 |
| Clumsy, poor coordination | 4 |

rating procedures were repeated. Several of the children had been on stimulants prior to the beginning of this study.

The medication was coded and administered on a double blind basis for approximately 6 weeks. This resulted in a random assignment of 20 children on methylphenidate and 20 children on placebo. The code was not broken until the study was complete. The mean number of days on the medication was 46 and duration ranged from 33 to 62 days.

The parents were instructed to follow a standardized increase in dosage up to 40 mg/day. For the first 2 days the child was given 20 mg in the morning, for the next 2 days 20 mg in the morning and 10 mg at noon, and for the remaining days 20 mg in the morning and 20 mg at noon. Each parent was asked to telephone at the end of the first 5 days to report on the child's progress. All except one parent cooperated in this plan and administered 40 mg of methylphenidate per day, or its equivalent in placebo.

### *Measures*

Table 2 lists the pediatric, behavioral and psychological assessment used prior to and at the conclusion of the 6-week medication period. Only the pediatric procedures which could be statistically analyzed are listed in the table. The findings from the neurological exam were not frequent enough to analyze statistically.

The rating scales used were the Peterson-Quay scale (21) and the Werry-Weiss-Peters activity scale (24). The Peterson-Quay lists 66 behaviors of children related to conduct and personality disorders. The Werry-Weiss-Peters activity scale includes 31 behaviors related to behavior during meals, watching television, doing homework, playing, behavior away from home except school, and behavior at school. On both of these scales the rater checks one of three categories for each behavior—"none," "moderate," or "severe"—indicating the intensity of the symptom. The parents completed both scales and the teachers only the Peterson-Quay.

The psychological tests included a WISC, three tests of motor coordination, (maze, holes, and pegboard) and the Bender Gestalt scored by the Koppitz

**TABLE 2. Measures Used before and at the End of Six Weeks on Medication**

Pediatric
1. Height, weight, blood pressure, heart rate
2. Urine pH
3. EEG

Behavior ratings
1. Parents
   a. Peterson-Quay behavior rating
   b. Werry-Weiss-Peters activity scale
2. Teachers
   a. Peterson-Quay behavior rating

Psychological tests
1. Wechsler Intelligence Scale for Children
2. Maze test of steadiness during movement
3. Holes test of steadiness while resting
4. Pegboard test of fine motor speed and coordination
5. Bender Gestalt

(17) system. A detailed description and normative data on the maze, holes, and pegboard tests are available (12).

The maze test is a measure of steadiness during motion, in which the child moves a stylus through a maze, twice with each hand. Three scores are obtained for each hand—the number of contacts with the edge, the duration of contact, and the speed of completion. The holes test is a measure of steadiness while resting, in which the child tries to hold a stylus, for 10 seconds, in the center of a series of progressively smaller holes, without touching the edge. Two scores are obtained for each hand—the number and duration of contacts with the edge. The pegboard test is a measure of fine motor manipulation and speed, in which keyhole-shaped pegs are inserted in similarly shaped holes, as rapidly as possible. The two scores obtained for each hand are speed (total time) and errors (number of pegs dropped).

In addition to the tests administered before and at the conclusion of the 6-week medication period, a more extensive test battery described by Knights and Watson (13) had been administered to the children within 18 months prior to the beginning of the study. These tests included the category, formboard, tapping, trails, aphasia screening, speech perception and target from the Reitan (22) battery and four other tests: auditory closure (11), sentence memory (1), oral fluency (23) and wide range achievement (10). This entire test battery was administered to each child at the conclusion of the 6-week medication period. The mean time between the initial testing and the beginning of the drug study was 5½ months.

## RESULTS

The medication of three children was discontinued during the study. The mother of one child decided not to participate after 3 days. Two other children, who had been on a stimulant prior to the beginning of the study, drew the placebo on the double blind procedure and the parents felt compelled to stop the medication after 2 weeks because of deterioration in school work and aggressive behavior at home. There were three other parents who wished to stop the medication but were encouraged to continue for at least 30 days, and the data from these children was included in the analyses. These three children had also drawn placebo and had been on stimulants prior to the present study.

In order to compare the predrug performance of the children randomly assigned to the Ritalin and placebo groups, *t* tests were computed on the CA (chronological age), IQ, and initial test scores. None of these results was significant. The predrug and final test data are analyzed in an analysis of variance design in which the drug group (Ritalin and placebo) is a between group comparison and the hand (right and left) and test (first and second) variables are within group comparisons. The handedness variable is not included in the analysis of the WISC or Bender Gestalt.

Table 3 presents a summary of the results of the analyses of variance on the psychological tests for the first and second testings. In reviewing the table, each vertical column will be discussed separately. All of the tests showed a non-

**TABLE 3. Analyses of Various Results for the Pre- and Final Testings for the Two Drug Groups**

| | *Main Effects* | | | *Interactions* | | | |
|---|---|---|---|---|---|---|---|
| *Variable* | *Drug* | *Hand* | *Test* | *Drug by Hand* | *Hand by Test* | *Drug by Test* | *Triple Interaction* |
| WISC | | | | | | | |
| Verbal IQ | NS | | NS | | | NS | |
| Performance IQ | NS | | <.05 | | | <.05 | |
| Full scale IQ | NS | | <.05 | | | NS | |
| Maze | | | | | | | |
| Counter | NS | <.001 | <.01 | NS | NS | NS | NS |
| Duration | NS | <.001 | NS | <.05 | NS | <.05 | NS |
| Speed | NS | <.01 | <.05 | NS | <.01 | NS | NS |
| Holes | | | | | | | |
| Counter | NS | NS | NS | NS | NS | NS | NS |
| Duration | NS | <.001 | NS | NS | NS | <.05 | <.05 |
| Pegboard | | | | | | | |
| Time | NS | <.001 | <.01 | <.01 | NS | NS | NS |
| Errors | NS | NS | NS | NS | NS | NS | NS |
| Bender Gestalt | NS | | NS | | | NS | |

significant main effect of drug. This indicates that over the two testings no differences in scores were found between the Ritalin and placebo groups. This is an important finding since it establishes that there were no differences in the initial performances of the children later assigned to the Ritalin and placebo groups. The significant main effect of hand on the maze, holes, and pegboard indicates that the dominant hand performance was superior to the nondominant. The significant main effect of test shows that there is an improved performance on the second testing over the first, due to practice effects. There are three double interactions and one triple interaction presented in Table 3. The drug-by-hand interaction indicates that the difference in performance of the dominant versus nondominant hand was greater for the placebo group than for the Ritalin group collapsed over both testings. The significant hand-by-testing interaction on the maze speed score is due to the greater increase in speed with the nondominant hand, compared to the dominant, on the second testing, both for the Ritalin and placebo groups.

The most important interaction for this study is the drug-by-testing interaction. This was significant for the performance IQ and the duration scores of the maze and holes tests. The improvement in performance IQ over the two testings was significant for the children taking Ritalin. They increased a mean of 11.4 IQ points while the placebo group increased a nonsignificant 4.0 IQ points on performance. Examination of the subtest scores indicates that this was due to the relatively greater improvement in coding, picture completion, and block design, in that order of magnitude. On the WISC the mean verbal IQ increase was 5.3 IQ points for the Ritalin group and 4.2 points for the placebo. This difference was not significant.

On the maze and holes tests the children on Ritalin showed a greater improvement in terms of a shorter duration of contact between the stylus and the edge of the channel or hole than did the placebo group. This indicates a faster correction or recovery when the edge of the maze or holes tests was touched. The one significant triple interaction on the holes duration score indicates that over the two testings the improvement of the nondominant hand relative to the dominant was greater in the Ritalin group than a similar change in the placebo group.

### Seven-Month Interval

Two-way analyses of variance were computed on the test scores obtained 5½ months prior to the beginning of the study and the scores obtained at the conclusion of the study. This was a time interval of approximately 7 months. Although a majority of the test scores showed a significant improvement due to practice and maturation effects, only one test score revealed a significant differential effect related to the use of Ritalin over placebo. In general these results indicate that over this extended 7-month period the 6-week treatment with Ritalin or placebo had no differential effect. This finding is not unexpected since during the time prior to the study some of the children in both groups had been under treatment of various kinds including tutoring in special skills, counseling with teachers and parents, and drug therapy. The remaining "Results" and the "Discussion" deal only with the 6-week treatment period.

### Parent and Teacher Ratings

In general, the children in both drug and placebo groups were rated as showing an improvement in their behavior. The teachers and parents knew the children were involved in the study of a drug which was considered helpful in modifying the behavior of their children, and this positive attitude probably contributed to the overall improvement.

On the Peterson-Quay scale, the teachers of the children on Ritalin rated 88 percent as improved, and the teachers of the children on placebo rated 67 percent as improved. The parents' rating was similar in direction but lower in magnitude with 73 percent of the Ritalin and 54 percent of the placebo children rated as improving. Neither of these differences was significant at the 5 percent level.

On the Werry-Weiss-Peters scale the parents of the children on Ritalin rated 71 percent as improved, while for the placebo group 37 percent were considered to improve. This difference was significant ($\chi^2 = 2.42$; $df = 1$; $p < .05$).

Table 4 presents the statistical analyses of the rating scale data as completed by the teachers and parents at the beginning and end of the medication period. A total score was obtained from each rating scale by combining the three subcategories which indicated the severity of symptom. The difference score shown in the table was calculated by subtracting the total of the second rating from the total of the first rating. The *t* test comparisons are between the Ritalin and placebo difference scores. Nine parents did not answer every item on the Peterson-Quay and the size of the groups in Table 4 is reduced.

In general the difference score analysis shows the Ritalin group as improv-

**TABLE 4. Mean Difference Scores Showing Improvement in Behavior as Rated by Teachers and Parents**

| | *Drug* | *N* | *Mean Difference* | *t* | *p* |
|---|---|---|---|---|---|
| Teachers | | | | | |
| Peterson-Quay scale | Ritalin | 17 | 13.3 | 1.44 | <.20 |
| | Placebo | 17 | 7.1 | | |
| Parents | | | | | |
| Peterson-Quay scale | Ritalin | 12 | 9.9 | 1.49 | <.20 |
| | Placebo | 13 | 1.5 | | |
| Werry-Weiss-Peters scale | Ritalin | 17 | 6.2 | 2.45 | <.05 |
| | Placebo | 16 | −1.1 | | |

ing more than the placebo group on both scales. Only the difference score on the Werry-Weiss-Peters scale reached significance at the 5 percent level of probability.

A more detailed examination was made of each of the items of both the Peterson-Quay and Werry-Weiss-Peters scales in order to determine whether ratings on particular symptoms had changed significantly. *t* tests were computed on the symptom change scores between the initial and final treatment ratings for the Ritalin and placebo groups. Table 5 presents the symptoms which showed a significant reduction or increase in mean change scores, and they are listed from top to bottom in order of magnitude of significance level. In general the symptoms showing a greater reduction in the Ritalin group, over the placebo, have to do with distractibility and activity level.

## Side Effects and Physical Findings

At the end of the first week of treatment the parents phoned to report on the progress of their children. The number of side effects mentioned were: 12 with appetite loss; 11 with increased restlessness; 4 with stomach and neck aches; 3 with sleeping difficulty, and 2 who were more irritable. Inspection of the frequency of these side effects revealed a significantly greater occurrence of appetite loss in the Ritalin group over the placebo group ($\chi^2 = 11.9$; $df = 1$; $p < .05$). No other group comparisons were significant.

**TABLE 5. Symptoms Rated as Showing a Significant Change in the Ritalin Group over and above That of the Placebo Group**

| *Teachers and Parents: Peterson-Quay* | *Parents: Werry-Weiss-Peters* |
|---|---|
| ***Reduced*** | |
| 1. Laziness | 1. Restlessness while shopping |
| 2. Distractibility | 2. Wiggling during homework |
| 3. Restlessness | 3. Periods at quiet play |
| 4. Disobedience | |
| 5. Fluctuating performance | |
| ***Increased*** | |
| 1. Stomach aches | 1. Fiddles with things at meals |
| 2. Aloofness | |

**TABLE 6. Physical Exam Data for the Ritalin and Placebo Groups before and at the End of the 6-Week Treatment**

| | *Drug* | *Predrug* | *Final* | *Difference* | *t* | *p* |
|---|---|---|---|---|---|---|
| Height (in) | Ritalin | 58.2 | 58.4 | 0.2 | | |
| | Placebo | 57.0 | 57.3 | 0.3 | | |
| Weight (lb) | Ritalin | 79.8 | 78.3 | −1.5 | 1.92 | <.10 |
| | Placebo | 74.6 | 75.0 | 0.4 | | |
| Blood pressure | | | | | | |
| Systolic | Ritalin | 117.2 | 118.8 | 1.6 | | |
| | Placebo | 113.5 | 114.5 | 1.0 | | |
| Diastolic | Ritalin | 73.4 | 75.3 | 1.9 | 1.72 | <.10 |
| | Placebo | 74.0 | 71.3 | −2.7 | | |
| Heart rate | Ritalin | 78.3 | 93.9 | 15.6 | 3.41 | <.01 |
| | Placebo | 81.1 | 82.0 | 0.9 | | |
| Urine pH | Ritalin | 5.8 | 6.2 | 0.4 | | |
| | Placebo | 6.0 | 6.2 | 0.2 | | |

Table 6 shows the mean data for selected items from the physical examination done before and after 6 weeks on medication. *t* tests of the difference scores were computed and show a significant weight loss, a significant change in diastolic blood pressure, and a significant heart rate increase in the Ritalin group relative to the placebo group.

## EEG Findings

Thirty-nine of the 40 patients had an electroencephalogram. One patient from a broken home made several appointments but eventually refused to cooperate in the study. Records were made with a 16-channel Grass or 8-channel Schwartzer. Sixteen scalp electrodes and two reference electrodes on the ear were used with the Gibbs system of electrode placement. Both monopolar and bipolar records were made. The EEG recordings were made in the morning and no attempt was made to get sleep records because special emphasis was placed on the presence of muscle artifact. Only 2 children slept during recording.

The records were interpreted after the study by the electroencephalographer, who knew neither the identity nor drug status of the patient. Six children had single records only, leaving 33 who were studied both on and off the drug. Two of the 6 who refused further study had spike and wave abnormalities, and another had excessive posterior slow.

Twenty-two or 66 percent of the children had normal resting records without medication. There were slight increases in slow or irregular rhythms in 6 of these, but since the records were considered "within normal limits" they are included as normal. This frequency of abnormal EEG records is similar to the 41 percent reported by Paine (20) in his study of children with minimal cerebral dysfunction. Using a more rigorous definition of normality would have given 16 children (48 percent) unequivocally pristine records, similar to other studies in children with learning disabilities (2, 20).

Table 7 presents the number of children with normal and abnormal EEG records taken when the child was not on medication and then during the drug study.

**TABLE 7. Frequency of Normal and Abnormal EEG Records off and on Medication**

| No Medication | | | On Medication: Ritalin | On Medication: Placebo |
|---|---|---|---|---|
| Normal | 22 | Normal | 10 | 10 |
| | | Abnormal | 1 | 1 |
| Abnormal | 11 | Normal | 2 | 1 |
| | | Abnormal | 2 | 6 |
| Total | 33 | | 15 | 18 |

The abnormalities seen in the 11 resting records were all minor, consisting of 6 with increased slow activity, 3 with a generally irregular background, and 2 with some posterior quadrant sharp. Two of those with increased slow activity showed abnormal bursts on placebo, and 1 of these children had a history of seizures. Of the 22 children with normal control records 2 were abnormal while the child was on medication, and of the 11 abnormal control records, 3 were considered normal when the child was on medication.

One of the most interesting observations regarding the electroencephalogram was related to the presence of excessive muscle artifact, usually regarded as a nuisance by technician and electroencephalographer alike. No data could be found on the amount of muscle artifact in children, and so a control group was selected from patients having EEG's for any reason other than learning difficulties.

An activity index was created by counting the number of distinct muscle bursts in each record, dividing by the number of EEG pages and multiplying by 10. The activity index, therefore, represents the number of distinct muscle movements in 10 pages or 100 sec of recording. Table 8 presents the EEG activity index for two control groups and the children included in this study, both off and on medication. The most remarkable characteristic of the children with learning problems is the increased amount of muscle movement seen in the waking record of the electroencephalogram. The difference in the activity index between the children with learning problems while off medication and the control children was highly significant ($p < .001$). When the children were on medication, there were no significant differences in activity index between the two drug groups. Similarly, the differences in activity index between the controls and the

**TABLE 8. EEG Activity Index**

| | *N* | *Mean* | *Standard Deviation* |
|---|---|---|---|
| | *No medication* | | |
| Controls, age 7-12 | 20 | 0.59 | 0.45 |
| Controls, age 12-18 | 20 | 0.55 | 0.32 |
| Learning problems | 33 | 3.12 | 2.25 |
| | *On medication* | | |
| Learning problems | | | |
| Ritalin | 15 | 1.57 | 1.82 |
| Placebo | 18 | 1.55 | 1.20 |

drug groups were not significant although the mean scores of the drug groups were twice as high. The reduction in activity index for the children in the study is assumed to be related to the children becoming familiar with the variety of special procedures they experienced.

## DISCUSSION

In general, the children taking methylphenidate showed a greater improvement than the placebo group on both the test results and behavior ratings. On the tests this change was revealed in performance skills, rather than in verbal abilities. A detailed examination of the performance results suggests that the ability to pay attention, rather than motor speed or motor control, was influenced by the methylphenidate. For example, on the maze and holes tests the counter score, which measures the number of contacts between the stylus and edge of the channel or hole and is interpreted as a measure of motor control, was not different between the two drug groups, while the duration score was. This duration score is a measure of the length of time the stylus touches the edge, and the more rapid recovery or removal of the stylus by the Ritalin group suggests that attention to the task was influenced, rather than motor control. Examination of the significant results of the WISC subtests provides the basis for a similar conclusion. The coding and block design subtests require good motor coordination as well as other abilities, but the picture completion test, which also showed a significant Ritalin effect, requires primarily sustained attention and visual and oral skills. The most appropriate explanation of the pattern of test results is that the child's ability to attend was improved, and this permitted more accurate motor control.

In a study of Ritalin and reserpine using reaction time tasks, Zimmerman and Burgemeister (25) reported greater improvement in the Ritalin group. Comparing their results with the present study, an improvement in reaction time is consistent with the improved motor steadiness scores, but it may be that the improvement in reaction time was the result of an increased ability to attend to the task.

In another study of the effects of a stimulant on children's test performance, Epstein, Lasagna, Conners, and Rodriguez (7) administered dextroamphetamine (Dexedrine) to pediatric outpatients. They used the same holes test of static motor steadiness and found a significant improvement in the counter score but did not report the duration score. Epstein et al. interpreted the improvement in fine motor coordination as an increased determination to perform, and the results of the present study are consistent with this conclusion.

Several studies (3–5, 7), which have used the Porteus maze test to measure the effect of a stimulant drug, are relevant to the discussion. The Porteus maze test (not included in the present study) requires both sustained attention and fine motor control. It has two scores—a test quotient which assesses planning, judgment, and attention and a qualitative score which assesses motor control. Each study found the drug group (Ritalin, Benzedrine, or Dexedrine) performed significantly better than the placebo group in terms of test quotients, while the qualitative scores were not significantly different. This finding suggests that the stimulant affected attention abilities more than motor control skills.

In a direct attempt to assess the effects of amphetamine on children's ability to pay attention, Conners and Rothschild (5) administered reaction time and vigilance tasks, among other tests, to a group of children with learning disorders. Their sample of children appears to be very similar to the group used in the present study. On these tasks the children on amphetamine performed more accurately and less impulsively than the children on placebo. The authors concluded that attention is substantially improved and said that they "view the effects as consisting of both a greater general alertness or excitation and a greater degree of selective inhibition" (p. 204).

The results of the behavior rating scales completed by both parents and teachers are consistent with the interpretation that methylphenidate is associated with increased ability to attend, although there apparently was not a reduction in rated activity level. Several studies of Ritalin have reported a reduction in hyperactivity (3, 15) in the sense that the child is less restless or distractible, rather than a reduction in the level of motor activity. Eisenberg (6) has noted this distinction between activity level and activity which is inappropriate to a particular situation. The present result on the rating scales and motor tests are consistent with the interpretation that the children on Ritalin were just as active as those on the placebo, but their ability to inhibit distracting influences was enhanced.

An interesting finding by Millichap and Boldrey (18) corroborates this suggestion. They measured the activity level of four children with an actometer and found a significant *increase* in motor activity in the Ritalin group over the placebo, but also reported teacher and parent impressions of "improvements in attention span and motor coordination, more adequate responses, less impulsivity and an increase of useful productivity" (p. 471). The fact that they found an increase in activity level as well as improved attention is generally consistent with the results of the studies discussed and is not contradictory if it is assumed that the ability to pay attention is relatively independent of motor activity.

In general, there is a strong placebo effect in the study. This is apparently due to the fact that both the teachers and parents knew the child was on a drug and considered this a positive treatment. Improvement in the placebo group, according to the parents and teachers, varied from 37 to 67 percent of the children, depending on the rating scale used. This placebo effect is considerably higher than that reported in other drug studies, which typically are reported at approximately 33 percent (8). This positive attitude toward the effects of drug treatment in the children tends to make it more difficult for improved behavior to appear as a function of the drug treatment. There is good evidence, however, that the children on Ritalin were rated as improving more. This is shown by the significant changes in symptom ratings which were done by the parents and teachers without knowledge of the actual medication the child was on. The fact that both the teachers and parents rated the Ritalin group as improving more, and agreed on the type of symptom change, is an impressive finding. Conners and Rothschild (5) reported similar results on parent and teacher ratings.

Some of the side effects of methylphenidate found in this study have been previously reported. Conners and Eisenberg (3), in their controlled study, reported significant decrease in appetite and increases in stomach aches and nail biting. Other clinical studies (15, 18) reported minimal side effects of appetite loss, headaches, abdominal pain, and insomnia, none of which were severe enough to warrant discontinuing the medication. In this study no child was withdrawn because of side effects. The three who did stop taking medication were withdrawn because they were on placebo and became behavior problems.

The medical history, neurological examination findings, and the pattern of psychological test results were all extensively examined in order to determine whether any differences existed between the children who showed either a positive or negative drug or placebo response. No relationships were established between the symptoms, history or test results, and the type of drug response.

A second method of examination of the data to determine if the drug was more effective with a specific subgroup of children was based on separation of both groups into those with and without brain damage. That is, children with physical findings or histories of probable brain damage were compared with those children who had very little evidence for organic brain impairment. Comparisons of the medical data, behavior ratings, and test scores of these groups revealed no differences.

This result is consistent with the observations of Millichap and Boldrey (18), who reported no differences in the Ritalin treatment of organic and nonorganic groups.

The results of this study do not preclude the suggestion that Ritalin is more effective for certain children than others, as evidenced by the fact that there was a dramatic improvement in some children. With this small and heterogeneous group of children, however, no characteristics were identified which would permit predictions about which children would respond to drug or placebo treatment. It is suggested that both the drug and the attitude of the child and his parents toward drug therapy must be evaluated before this type of prediction may be made.

In conclusion, the double blind administration of methylphenidate for 6 weeks to a group of children referred for learning disabilities was associated with greater improvement in motor control and behavior ratings, as compared with a placebo control group. The improved motor control was interpreted to be secondary to a greater ability to pay attention. There was a strong placebo effect, but both the parents and teachers rated the children on methylphenidate as being less distractible and more attentive than the control placebo. In general the results indicate that the prediction of drug effectiveness for an individual child will require a more detailed study of both etiology and family attitude.

## REFERENCES

1. Benton, A. L. *Sentence Memory Test*. Department of Neurology, University Hospital, Iowa City, Iowa, 1965.
2. Capute, A. J., Niedermeyer, E. F. L., and Richardson, F. The electroencephalogram in children with minimal cerebral dysfunction. *Pediatrics*, 41: 1104–1114, 1968.
3. Conners, C. K., and Eisenberg, L. The effects of methylphenidate on symp-

tomatology and learning in disturbed children. *Amer. J. Psychiat.*, **120**: 458–464, 1963.

4. Conners, C. K., Eisenberg, L., and Sharpe, L. Effects of methlyphenidate (Ritalin) on paired-associate learning and Porteus Maze performance in emotionally disturbed children. *J. Consult. Psychol.*, **28**: 14–22, 1964.
5. Conners, C. K., and Rothschild, G. H. Drugs and learning in children. In Hellmuth, J., ed. *Learning Disorders*, vol. 3, pp. 193–218. Special Child Publications, Seattle, 1968.
6. Eisenberg, L. The management of the hyperkinetic child. *Develop. Med. Child Neurol.*, 8: 593–598, 1966.
7. Epstein, L. C., Lasagna, L., Conners, C. K., and Rodriguez, A. Correlation of dextroamphetamine excretion and drug response in hyperkinetic children. *J. Nerv. Ment. Dis.*, **146**: 136–146, 1968.
8. Freed, H. *The Chemistry and Therapy of Behavior Disorders in Children.* Charles C Thomas, Springfield, Ill., 1962.
9. Freeman, R. D. Drug effects on learning in children—a selective review of the past thirty years. *J. Special Educ.*, **1**: 17–37, 1966.
10. Jastak, J. F., Bijou, S. W., and Jastak, S. R. *Wide Range Achievement Test.* Guidance Association, Wilmington, Del., 1965.
11. Kass, C. E. Auditory closure test. In Olson, J. J. and Olson, J. L. *Validity Studies on the Illinois Test of Psycholinguistic Abilities.* Photo Press Inc., Madison, Wisc., 1964.
12. Knights, R. M., and Moule, A. D. Normative data on the motor steadiness battery for children. *Percept. Motor Skills*, **26**: 643–650, 1968.
13. Knights, R. M., and Watson, P. The use of computer test profiles in neuropsychological assessment. *J. Learning Dis.*, **1**: 696–710, 1968.
14. Knobel, M. Diagnosis and treatment of psychiatric problems in children. *J. Neuropsychiat.*, **3**: 82–91, 1959.
15. Knobel, M. Psychopharmacology for the hyperkinetic child. *Arch. Gen. Psychiat.*, **6**: 198–202, 1962.
16. Knobel, M., Wolman, M. B., and Mason, E. Hyperkinesis and organicity in children. *Arch. Gen. Psychiat.*, **1**: 310–321, 1959.
17. Koppitz, E. M. *The Bender Gestalt Test for Young Children.* Grune & Stratton, New York, 1964.
18. Millichap, J. G., and Boldrey, E. E. Studies in hyperkinetic behavior: II. Laboratory and clinical evaluations of drug treatments. *Neurology*, **17**: 467–471, 1967.
19. Millichap, J. G., and Fowler, G. W. Treatment of "minimal brain dysfunction" syndromes. *Pediat. Clin. N. Amer.*, **14**: 767–777, 1967.
20. Paine, R. S., Werry, J. S., and Quay, H. C. A study of minimal cerebral dysfunction. *Develop. Med. Child Neurol.*, **10**: 505–520, 1968.
21. Peterson, D. R. Behavior problems of middle childhood. *J. Consult. Psychol.*, **25**: 205–209, 1961.
22. Reitan, R. M. A research program on the psychological effects of brain lesions in human beings. In Ellis, N., ed. *International Review of Mental Retardation*, pp. 153–218. Academic Press, New York, 1966.
23. Strong, R. T. Verbal Fluency Test. 2804 Townes Lane, Austin, Tex.
24. Werry, J. S. Developmental hyperactivity. *Pediat. Clin. N. Amer.*, **15**: 581–599, 1968.
25. Zimmerman, F. T., and Burgemeister, B. B. Action of methylphenidylacetate (Ritalin) and reserpine in behavior disorders in children and adults. *Amer. J. Psychiat.*, **115**: 323–328, 1958.

## 17

# *Diagnosis and Treatment of Drug Dependence of the Barbiturate Type*

ABRAHAM WIKLER

According to the definitions proposed by the World Health Organization (18):

> Drug dependence of the barbiturate type is described as a state arising from repeated administration of a barbiturate, or an agent with barbiturate-like effect, on a continuous basis, generally in amounts exceeding therapeutic dose levels. Its characteristics include: 1) a strong desire or need to continue taking the drug; the need can be satisfied by the drug taken initially or by another with barbiturate-like properties; 2) a tendency to increase the dose, partly owing to the development of tolerance; 3) a psychic dependence on the effects of the drug related to subjective and individual appreciation of those effects; and 4) a physical dependence on the effects of the drug requiring its presence for maintenance of homeostasis and resulting in a definite, characteristic, and self-limited abstinence syndrome when the drug is withdrawn.

Although patients who display any or all of the first three characteristics are also in need of medical and psychiatric attention, the development of the fourth characteristic, physical dependence, may be fraught with danger to life and therefore demands immediate and skillful treatment. This article will therefore begin with a discussion of the diagnosis and treatment of physical dependence on drugs of the barbiturate type.

## PHYSICAL DEPENDENCE ON BARBITURATES

Understanding of the clinical course and predictable outcome of chronic barbiturate intoxication was greatly advanced by the experimental studies of Isbell and associates (14), Wikler and associates (17), Fraser and associates (8, 10), and Belleville and Fraser (2). Using former narcotic addicts without psychosis, epilepsy, or other central nervous system disease as subjects (all volunteered for the research), these investigators demonstrated that tolerance, though only partial, does develop to the effects of barbiturates on the central nervous system; and that abrupt withdrawal of secobarbital, amobarbital, or pentobarbital after prolonged (one or more months) continuous intoxication results in a characteristic abstinence syndrome. The severity of the latter is at least in part directly related to the daily dose level attained before drug withdrawal.

From the *American Journal of Psychiatry,* Vol. 125, 1968, pp. 758–765. 

Table 1 summarizes the essential features of the "full-blown" barbiturate abstinence syndrome as it develops on abrupt withdrawal of the so-called short-acting barbiturates following chronic intoxication at daily dose levels of 0.8 to 2.2 gm. For convenience in discussion the clinical phenomena may be classified as "minor" (apprehension, muscular weakness, tremors, postural faintness, anorexia, and twitches) and "major" (seizures, psychosis).

As indicated in the table, the minor abstinence phenomena are observable within 24 hours after administration of the last dose of barbiturates and continue beyond the appearance of the major abstinence phenomena which, if they develop, emerge between the second and eighth days.

Among the minor abstinence phenomena, postural faintness (orthostatic hypotension) is of particular value in differentiating the developing barbiturate abstinence syndrome from ordinary anxiety states, but often the differential diagnosis is difficult to make at this stage. The presence of coarse, rhythmic intention tremors in the upper extremities is also a useful but less specific sign

**TABLE 1. The Barbiturate Abstinence Syndrome**
**(After abrupt withdrawal of secobarbital or pentobarbital following chronic intoxication at dose levels of 0.8 to 2.2 gm per day orally, for 6 weeks or more)**

| *Clinical Phenomenon* | *Incidence* | *Time of Onset* | *Duration* | *Remarks* |
|---|---|---|---|---|
| Apprehension | 100% | 1st day | 3-14 days | Vague uneasiness, or fear of impending catastrophe. |
| Muscular weakness | 100% | 1st day | 3-14 days | Evident on mildest exertion. |
| Tremors | 100% | 1st day | 3-14 days | Coarse, rhythmic, nonpatterned, evident during voluntary movement, subside at rest. |
| Postural faintness | 100% | 1st day | 3-14 days | Evident on sitting or standing suddenly. Associated with marked fall in systolic and diastolic blood pressure, and pronounced tachycardia. |
| Anorexia | 100% | 1st day | 3-14 days | Usually associated with repeated vomiting. |
| Twitches | 100% | 1st day | 3-? days | Myoclonic muscular contractions; or spasmodic jerking of one or more extremities. Sometimes bizarre patterned movements. |
| Seizures | 80% | 2nd-3rd day | 8 days | Up to a total of 4 grand mal episodes, with loss of consciousness and postconvulsive stupor. |
| Psychoses | 60% | 3rd-8th day | 3-14 days | Usually resemble "delirium tremens"; occasionally resemble schizophrenic or Korsakoff syndromes; or acute panic states may occur. |

Note: These data are based on a series of 19 cases of experimental addiction to barbiturates. Four developed seizures without subsequent psychosis; one exhibited delirium without antecedent seizures. Three escaped both seizures and delirium.

of barbiturate abstinence. Other minor abstinence phenomena include insomnia, profuse sweating, and tendon hyperreflexia. Even if overt major abstinence phenomena do not develop, paroxysmal discharges may be found in the electroencephalogram after the second day of abstinence in a majority of the patients abruptly withdrawn from such dose levels (5, 17).

When major abstinence phenomena do appear, the seizures are invariably of the clonic-tonic grand mal type clinically indistinguishable from those of idiopathic grand mal epilepsy. It is curious that in the experimental studies on which this discussion is based, no subject had more than four seizures, and the interseizure electroencephalograms were characterized by recurrent 4 per second spike-wave discharges. Also of interest is that none of the subjects having seizures could recall any aura.

The psychoses that develop as major barbiturate abstinence phenomena are more variable. In severe cases the psychosis is indistinguishable from that of alcoholic delirium tremens (also a withdrawal phenomenon) with disorientation, agitation, delusions, and hallucinations (usually visual, sometimes also auditory). Rising core temperature is an ominous sign prognosticating a fatal outcome if not combated vigorously (9). Milder cases may be characterized by hallucinations with relatively clear sensorium, a Korsakoff-like syndrome, or by extreme anxiety.

The data in Table 2, also obtained in experimental studies on former narcotic addicts who volunteered for research, show the relationships between daily dose level and duration of intoxication on the one hand, and the incidence of major and minor abstinence phenomena following abrupt withdrawal of barbiturates on the other. It will be noted that of 20 subjects who were withdrawn from daily barbiturate dose levels of 0.4 gm or less, none developed major, and only one developed significant minor, abstinence phenomena. On the other hand, of 23 subjects withdrawn from 0.6 to 0.8 gm daily, three had convulsions, one displayed hallucinations, and 14 showed significant degrees of minor abstinence phenomena.

**TABLE 2. Summary of Data on Relationship of Dosage of Secobarbital or Pentobarbital to Intensity of Physical Dependence**

| *Patients* | | | | | *No. of Patients Having Symptoms* | | |
|---|---|---|---|---|---|---|---|
| | *No. Receiving* | | | | | | |
| *Total No.* | *Secobarbital* | *Pentobarbital* | *Daily Dose of Barbiturate, Gm.* | *Days of Intoxication in Hospital* | *Convulsions* | *Delirium* | *Minor Symptoms of Significant Degree* |
| 18 | 16 | 2 | 0.9-2.2 | 32-144 | 14 | 12 | 18 |
| 5 | 5 | | 0.8 | 42-57 | 1 | 0 | 5 |
| 18 | 18 | | 0.6 | 35-57 | 2 | 0 | 9 |
| 18 | 10 | 8 | 0.4 | 90 | 0 | 0 | 1 |
| 2 | 1 | 1 | 0.2 | 365 | 0 | 0 | 0 |

Reprinted from J.A.M.A., Vol. 166, 1958, pp. 126-129, by permission of the editor; see Ref. 10.

It may be inferred therefore that chronic intoxication with barbiturates at daily dose levels of 0.6 to 0.8 gm for periods of 35 to 57 days is sufficient to produce a clinically significant degree of physical dependence. The data in Table 2 also indicate that higher daily dose levels of barbiturates induce stronger physical dependence. Thus all of 18 subjects withdrawn from 0.8 to 2.2 gm daily had minor abstinence phenomena, 14 had convulsions, and 12 had delirium (some subjects had both).

Although there is a direct relationship between daily intoxication dosage and severity of barbiturate abstinence phenomena, more information is needed about the relationships that may exist between duration of chronic barbiturate intoxication per se (daily dose level held constant) and the severity of abstinence phenomena.

Initial treatment of patients chronically intoxicated with barbiturates is directed toward withdrawal of the drug in such a manner as to prevent the appearance of the major abstinence phenomena altogether and to minimize the severity of minor abstinence phenomena. To this end the procedure developed by Isbell (13) has proven to be safe, simple, and reliable. Essentially it consists of stabilization of the patient on a so-called short-acting barbiturate (e.g., pentobarbital) at doses (0.2–0.4 gm, orally if possible, intramuscularly if necessary) at four- to six-hour intervals, regulated in such a manner that no abstinence phenomena and a minimal degree of barbiturate-type signs of intoxication are observed.

After two to three days of such stabilization the barbiturate is withdrawn *slowly* at a rate not exceeding 0.1 gm a day regardless of the daily stabilization dose level. If more than the mildest minor abstinence phenomena appear, the reduction schedule is suspended until these signs and symptoms subside, after which it is resumed at the same rate or a slower rate, e.g., 0.05 gm daily, if orthostatic hypotension, marked tremulousness, and/or persistent insomnia develop.

In clinical practice, initiation of this stabilization and reduction procedure will depend of course on the status of the patient on admission. Should the patient be grossly intoxicated or comatose on arrival, no barbiturates are given until these effects have receded completely, but if there is a clear history of chronic barbiturate intoxication or if this is strongly suspected on other grounds, one should not wait until severe minor or any major withdrawal phenomena are observed before instituting the "stabilization" procedure.

In doubtful cases a test dose of 0.2 gm of pentobarbital may be given after all signs of intoxication have disappeared, and if no signs of barbiturate effect (positive Romberg sign, gait ataxia, finger to nose incoordination, nystagmus, slurred speech, drowsiness) are observed one hour later, the same dose may be prescribed every six hours around the clock. During the next 24 hours the patient should be observed for signs of abstinence just *before* each dose and again for signs of barbiturate intoxication one hour *after* each dose.

If during this period clear abstinence phenomena and no signs of barbiturate intoxication are observed, the dose and/or the frequency of administration should be increased and then manipulated upwards or downwards until optimal stabilization is achieved. Often optimal stabilization takes more than 24 hours, but in no case should systematic reduction of daily dosage be initiated before the patient is stabilized.

On the other hand, if the patient reacts to the initial test dose of 0.2 gm of pentobarbital with gross signs of barbiturate intoxication, the diagnosis of physical dependence on barbiturates should be questioned. To be safe it is usually advisable to continue the "assay" at reduced dosage—e.g., 0.1 gm of pentobarbital every six hours with the same observations before and after each dose as already described. If during the next 24 hours no abstinence phenomena are observed and especially if the patient shows signs of increasing barbiturate intoxication, the diagnosis of physical dependence may be rejected and barbiturates may be discontinued altogether.

This testing and stabilization procedure may also be applied to patients who on admission display minor abstinence phenomena. In the case of patients who have already had one or more seizures, the initial dose of pentobarbital should be somewhat larger (0.3 to 0.4 gm) and the stabilization procedure should be accelerated beginning with 0.2 gm of pentobarbital every four hours, and dosage and frequency manipulated thereafter as indicated.

The presence of delirium on admission calls for a somewhat different approach. This condition is not easily reversible in the sense that the stabilization state can be readily achieved. Rather, the aim should be to sedate the patient heavily so that agitation, insomnia, and above all hyperpyrexia are suppressed. To accomplish this, pentobarbital may have to be given intramuscularly or intravenously in whatever amounts may be found necessary for three to five days, after which the degree of sedation may be lightened gradually and slow reduction carried out as in stabilized patients.

Because of its longer duration of action, sodium phenobarbital may be preferable to pentobarbital. Indeed, the Danish workers (16) have used the very long acting barbiturate, barbital (Veronal) with excellent results in the treatment of alcoholic delirium tremens since 1909; probably this venerable agent would be equally effective in the management of barbiturate withdrawal delirium. However, the very long duration of action of barbital may be a disadvantage to physicians who have had little experience with it.

In addition to specific therapy as described, it is of course necessary to ensure that patients displaying barbiturate abstinence phenomena, and especially delirium, are protected from injury. They should be provided with very low beds or mattresses on the floor and should receive adequate fluids and electrolytes, calories, vitamins, and, when indicated, antibiotics.

While theoretically such drugs as paraldehyde or chloral hydrate should readily substitute for pentobarbital in specific therapy, there appears to be no valid reason for employing certain other agents that have been advocated from time to time. Thus neither diphenylhydantoin (Dilantin) nor chlorpromazine (Thorazine) prevents barbiturate withdrawal seizures in the dog (4, 6), and systematic studies on the effectiveness of meprobamate (Miltown, Equanil) or chlordiazepoxide (Librium) in the management of the barbiturate abstinence syndrome have not yet been made.

## DEPENDENCE ON NONBARBITURATE SEDATIVES AND MINOR TRANQUILIZERS

To date, systematic experimental studies on the physical dependence-producing properties of nonbarbiturate sedatives and minor tranquilizers in man have been reported only for meprobamate (11) and chlordiazepoxide (12). However, individual case reports, reviewed by Essig (3), indicate that barbiturate-type abstinence phenomena, both of the minor and major kind, can supervene when not only these agents but also glutethimide (Doriden), ethinamate (Valmid), ethchlorvynol (Placidyl), or methyprylon (Noludar) are withdrawn abruptly after periods of chronic intoxication at high daily dose levels of these drugs.

All of these agents are central nervous system depressants, and the abstinence phenomena that develop after their abrupt withdrawal under the conditions stated closely resemble the barbiturate abstinence syndrome. It may thus be inferred that to a considerable extent at least, there are common neurochemical mechanisms that underlie physical dependence on barbiturates, nonbarbiturate sedatives, and minor tranquilizers. If so, then barbiturates should substitute readily for nonbarbiturate sedatives and minor tranquilizers both in assaying the degree of tolerance and physical dependence that may have developed in patients chronically intoxicated on the latter two categories of drugs and in the clinical management of drug withdrawal.

This principle was applied by Bakewell and Wikler (1) in a study on the incidence of nonnarcotic addiction in a Southern university hospital psychiatric ward, using pentobarbital exclusively as the drug of substitution in the same manner as already described for the diagnosis and treatment of physical dependence on barbiturates. Inasmuch as the earlier studies of Fraser and associates (10) had indicated that the critical daily intoxication dose level for development of physical dependence on barbiturates is 0.6 to 0.8 gm, Bakewell and Wikler (1) adopted as a criterion for classifying patients as physically dependent on nonbarbiturate sedatives and/or minor tranquilizers the ability of the patient to tolerate (i.e., become stabilized on) 0.8 gm of pentobarbital or more daily.

On the basis of this criterion, they found that nine of 132 consecutive patients (6.8 percent) admitted to the psychiatric ward over a 14-month period were physically dependent on nonnarcotic central nervous system depressants including glutethimide, meprobamate, chlordiazepoxide, diazepam, paraldehyde, and barbiturates, alone or in various combinations (Table 3).

It is of interest that Ewing and Bakewell (7) concluded from a chart study that in 7.6 percent of 1,686 patients admitted to another Southern university hospital psychiatric ward over a three-year period, the diagnosis of drug dependence was made either on admission or during hospitalization. In their series, however, the drugs implicated included not only barbiturates, nonbarbiturate sedatives, and minor tranquilizers, but also bromides, amphetamines, alcohol, and narcotics.

Theoretically the testing, stabilization, and slow reduction procedures could be carried out with the nonbarbiturate sedative or minor tranquilizing

**TABLE 3. Case Summaries**

| Patient No. | Sex | Age (Years) | Drugs of Abuse: Agent | Drugs of Abuse: Estimated Average Daily Intake (mg) | Daily Pentobarbital Stabilization-Dose Level (Oral, mg.) |
|---|---|---|---|---|---|
| 1 | M | 36 | Glutethimide | 2,500 | 800 |
| 2 | F | 59 | Glutethimide | 5,000 | 1,200 |
| 3 | F | 44 | Glutethmide | 2,000 | 900 |
| 4 | M | 60 | Glutethmide | 4,000 | 1,200 |
| 5 | F | 49 | Glutethmide | 1,000 | 800 |
| | | | Meprobamate | 4,000 | |
| 6 | F | 60 | Glutethimide | ? | 800 |
| | | | Chlordiazepoxide | 100? | |
| 7 | F | 53 | Amphetamine-amobarbital (elixir) | ? | 800 |
| | | | Pentobarbital (elixir) | ? | |
| | | | Aprobarbital (elixir) | ? | |
| 8 | M | 61 | Secobarbital | ? | 1,000 |
| | | | Pentobarbital | ? | |
| | | | Butabarbital | ? | |
| | | | Phenobarbital | ? | |
| | | | Propantheline and phenobarbital | ? | |
| | | | Diazepam | ? | |
| 9 | M | 29 | Paraldehyde | ? | 800 |

Reprinted from J.A.M.A., Vol. 196, 1966, page 711, by permission of the editor; see Ref. 1.

drug on which the patient had become physically dependent rather than with pentobarbital. But since far less is known about the duration of action of the drugs in the former classes, the pentobarbital substitution method is preferable, at least at the present time.

However, differences in duration of action between pentobarbital on the one hand and certain of the nonbarbiturate sedatives and minor tranquilizers on the other may require some modifications of the stabilization and slow reduction procedures described when pentobarbital is substituted for drugs in the other two categories. Thus, patients physically dependent on glutethimide or chlordiazepoxide may seem to be well stabilized on a given daily dose of pentobarbital, only to have convulsions a day or two later while still stabilized, or after a modest reduction of pentobarbital dosage has been made. In the cases of primary physical dependence on glutethimide or chlordiazepoxide, therefore, it might be well to delay initiation of pentobarbital reduction for a few days after initial stabilization.

## PSYCHOTHERAPY AND REHABILITATION

As the series studied by Bakewell and Wikler (1) and Ewing and Bakewell (7) consisted of patients admitted to psychiatric wards, it is not surprising that all of those judged to be dependent on drugs were also found to have antecedent emotional and/or characterological disorders, presumably rendering them addiction prone. However, it is remarkable that 93.2 percent of the patients in the first series and 92.4 percent in the second were *not* drug-dependent.

Whether or not the drug-dependent and the non-drug-dependent populations differed significantly in respect to particular kinds of emotional and/or characterological disorder cannot be decided on the basis of available data. However, it would seem reasonable to suppose that such disorders do play a role—if not a sufficient one—in the genesis of drug abuse. In any case, the existence of emotional and/or characterological disorder calls for treatment of these conditions by whatever means may be indicated.

Generally, psychotherapy of other than the supportive type will be more effective after drug withdrawal has been accomplished. Indeed, "painless" drug withdrawal may facilitate development of a favorable psychotherapeutic relationship between physician and patient. It has also been the author's impression that ignorance on the part of the patient, his relatives, and sometimes his physician of the dangers involved in escalation of dosage and/or frequency of administration of central nervous system depressant drugs has contributed to the development of physical dependence. Appropriate education is certainly indicated in such cases.

A difficult question to answer is the extent to which barbiturates, nonbarbiturate sedatives, and minor tranquilizers may be used in the treatment of addiction-prone patients, especially if they had become physically dependent on such drugs on one or more occasions in the past. Generally, these drugs should be avoided or, if used at all, they should be prescribed in therapeutic doses and for only short periods of time with rigid limitation of prescription refills.

In some cases daytime reduction of anxiety may be achieved with small doses of chlorpromazine, or with imipramine or amitriptyline if depression is a prominent symptom. According to Overall and associates (15), thioridazine possesses not only tranquilizing but also antidepressant properties, and therefore this phenothiazine derivative may be effective in some cases. Persistence of anxiety and/or depression, however, poses a challenge to the psychiatrist's skills which is not met by resorting to the unregulated use of drugs with physical dependence-producing properties, such as barbiturates, nonbarbiturate sedatives, and minor tranquilizers.

## SUMMARY

An abstinence syndrome characterized in its complete form by the appearance of tremulousness, anxiety, insomnia, diaphoresis, postural hypotension, tendon hyperreflexia, convulsions, delirium, and hyperpyrexia can ensue when barbiturates, nonbarbiturate sedatives, or minor tranquilizers are withdrawn abruptly following prolonged periods of intoxication at daily dose levels that exceed therapeutically recommended amounts. Regardless of the drug category involved, withdrawal of these agents may be accomplished safely by initial stabilization on pentobarbital alone in amounts and at intervals that suppress abstinence phenomena throughout the day and night and produce mild signs of barbiturate intoxication. This should be followed by gradual reduction in pentobarbital dosage at a rate not exceeding 0.1 gm daily.

If delirium has already developed when the patient is first seen, the immediate aim of treatment is not stabilization but heavy sedation with pentobarbital or phenobarbital, sufficient to suppress agitation, insomnia, and hyperpyrexia. Such heavy sedation is maintained for three to five days with appropriate supportive medical and nursing care, after which the degree of sedation is lightened gradually and slow reduction of the barbiturate is carried out as in the stabilized patient.

Psychotherapy and other treatment of psychiatric disorders associated with drug dependence of the barbiturate type is of course indicated, with due regard for the dangers involved in treating addiction-prone individuals with drugs that are capable of producing physical dependence.

## REFERENCES


1. Bakewell, W. E., Jr., and Wikler, A.: Symposium: Nonnarcotic Addiction—Incidence in a University Hospital Psychiatric Ward, *J.A.M.A.* **196**: 710–713, 1966.
2. Belleville, R. E., and Fraser, H. F.: Tolerance to Some Effects of Barbiturates, *J. Pharmacol. Exp. Ther.* **120**: 469–474, 1957.
3. Essig, C. F.: Addiction to Nonbarbiturate Sedative and Tranquilizing Drugs, *Clin. Pharmacol. Ther.* **5**: 334–343, 1964.
4. Essig, C. F., and Carter, W. W.: Failure of Diphenylhydantoin to Prevent Barbiturate Withdrawal Convulsions in Dogs, *Neurology* **12**: 481–484, 1962.
5. Essig, C. F., and Fraser, H. F.: Electroencephalographic Changes in Man During Use and Withdrawal of Barbiturates in Moderate Dosage, *Electroenceph. Clin. Neurophysiol.* **10**: 649–656, 1958.
6. Essig, C. F., and Fraser, H. F.: Failure of Chlorpromazine to Prevent Barbiturate-Withdrawal Convulsions, *Clin. Pharmacol. Ther.* **7**: 466–469, 1966.
7. Ewing, J. A., and Bakewell, W. E., Jr.: Diagnosis and Management of Depressant Drug Dependence, *Amer. J. Psychiat.* **123**: 909–917, 1967.
8. Fraser, H. F., Isbell, H., Eisenman, A. J., Wikler, A., and Pescor, F. T.: Chronic Barbiturate Intoxication: Further Studies, *Arch. Intern. Med.* **94**: 34–41, 1954.
9. Fraser, H. F., Shaver, M. R., Maxwell, E. S., and Isbell, H.: Death Due to Withdrawal of Barbiturates: Report of a Case, *Ann. Intern. Med.* **38**: 1319–1325, 1953.
10. Fraser, H. F., Wikler, A., Essig, C. F., and Isbell, H.: Degree of Physical Dependence Induced by Secobarbital or Pentobarbital, *J.A.M.A.* **166**: 126–129, 1958.
11. Haizlip, T. M., and Ewing, J. A.: Meprobamate Habituation: A Controlled Clinical Study, *New Eng. J. Med.* **258**: 1181–1186, 1958.
12. Hollister, L. E., Motzenbecker, F. P., and Degan, R. O.: Withdrawal Reactions from Chlordiazepoxide (Librium), *Psychopharmacologia* **2**: 63–68, 1961.

13. ISBELL, H.: Manifestations and Treatment of Addiction to Narcotic Drugs and Barbiturates, *Med. Clin. N. Amer.* 34: 425–438, 1950.
14. ISBELL, H., ALTSCHUL, S., KORNETSKY, C. H., EISENMAN, A. J., FLANARY, H. G., and FRASER, H. F.: Chronic Barbiturate Intoxication: An Experimental Study, *Arch. Neurol. Psychiat.* 64: 1–28, 1950.
15. OVERALL, J. E., HOLLISTER, L. E., MEYER, F., KIMBELL, I., JR., and SHELTÔN, J.: Imipramine and Thioridazine in Depressed and Schizophrenic Patients—Are There Specific Antidepressant Drugs? *J.A.M.A.* 189: 605–608, 1964.
16. SØRENSON, B. F.: Delirium Tremens and Its Treatment, *Danish Med. Bull.* 6: 261–263, 1959.
17. WIKLER, A., FRASER, H. F., ISBELL, H., and PESCOR, F. T.: Electroencephalograms During Cycles of Addiction to Barbiturates in Man, *Electroenceph. Clin. Neurophysiol.* 7: 1–13, 1955.
18. WORLD HEALTH ORGANIZATION EXPERT COMMITTEE ON ADDICTION-PRODUCING DRUGS: Thirteenth Report. WHO Technical Report Series no. 273, Geneva, 1964.

# 18

## *Experimental Effects of Amphetamine: A Review*

SHERWOOD O. COLE

The present review is designed to demonstrate some of the important experimental effects of amphetamine on behavior. Although different amphetamine compounds differ in the degree of their effect, the direction of their action appears to be the same. Of the amphetamine compounds most widely used in experimental studies (d-amphetamine sulfate, amphetamine sulfate, and methamphetamine), d-amphetamine sulfate appears to be the most active and to differ from the other compounds in its greater strength as a CNS stimulant. No attempt is made here to distinguish differences in effect due to the type of amphetamine compound employed unless such information helps to clarify contradictory findings on the drug's action. Since amphetamine is similar in structure to the catecholamines (epinephrine and norepinephrine), it mimics many of their central effects, including the arousal of systems in conflict with cholinergic inhibitors. For a discussion of the relationship of amphetamine to the catecholamines and the importance of this relationship to the central activating functions of the drug, see Carlton (1963).

Although the present review does not attempt to exhaust all the material related to the experimental effects of amphetamine, an attempt has been made to select studies which are representative of the general action of the drug as well as studies which indicate the limitations of such action. With these guidelines in mind, the effects of amphetamine are discussed in terms of the depressant and facilitating action of the drug.

## DEPRESSANT ACTION

### Effect on Food Consumption

Ersner (1940) demonstrated the clinical effectiveness of amphetamine in producing a decrease in food consumption and loss of weight in a large number of human subjects. Other studies (Knapp, 1952; Lesses & Myerson, 1938; Nathanson, 1937) have demonstrated a similar anorexic effect of the drug with chronic administration, although other effects were also observed. Using male albino rats, Siegal and Sterling (1959) found a depressant action of amphetamine on food consumption even when the strength of the feeding response had been varied by experimental feeding techniques. The decrease in food consumption following amphetamine injections is apparently due to a sensation of satiety or subdued appetite (Goetzl & Stone, 1948). This anorexic effect varies with the amount of concomitant food deprivation (Cole, 1963, 1965) and apparently interacts with other experimental conditions, such as electric shock (Teitelbaum & Derks, 1958).

Since amphetamine has been observed to depress food consumption in the absence of peripheral bodily changes (Nathanson, 1937) and following surgical interruption of gastric hunger contractions (Harris, Ivy, & Searle, 1947), this anorexic effect appears to be mediated primarily by CNS sites. The changes in amphetamine anorexia following lesioning of the CNS further indicate the importance of central sites to the drug's effects on food consumption.

### Exaggerated and Attenuated Effects Following Brain Lesions

Harris, Ivy, and Searle (1947) observed that human subjects with frontal lobotomies were less susceptible to the anorexic effect of amphetamine than were normal subjects. These findings were supported by Andersson and Larsson (1957), who used dogs as subjects, although the depressant effect on food consumption was not consistent in all instances following prefrontal lobotomies.

In response to the findings of Brobeck, Larsson, and Reyes (1956) which suggested that amphetamine depresses eating by "mimicking" the inhibitory activity of the ventromedial (VM) hypothalamus, several investigators have studied the effect of the drug in combination with VM lesions. Although the findings of Brobeck, Larsson, and Reyes suggested that the depressant action of amphetamine on eating would be less or eliminated following lesioning of the VM region, Epstein (1959) and Reynolds (1959) found the effect to be exaggerated following such lesions. However, Sharp, Neilson, and Porter (1962), using cats, found support for the "mimicking hypothesis" since the effect of amphetamine was attenuated following VM lesioning. Although the discrepancy in these findings was pointed out by Meyer and Meyer (1963), no attempt has been made to explain this apparent contradiction. A closer examination of the studies suggests that a species difference (rats versus cats) and a difference in experimental procedure might have been partially responsible.

More recent studies suggest that the role of CNS sites in the mediation of amphetamine anorexia is much more complex than was suggested by the findings of Brobeck et al. (1956). Cole and Hudspeth (1964) and Cole (1966b) reported that anterior hypothalamic (AH) lesions exaggerate the depressant effect of amphetamine on eating, and Carlisle (1964) found that lateral hypothalamic (LH) lesions attenuate such an effect. Apparently, a large portion of the hypothalamus is involved in the mediation of amphetamine anorexia as well as more specific systems of restraint and facilitation. The evidence suggests that VM and AH sites constitute a retarding system on amphetamine action which is interrupted by lesioning these areas (Cole, 1966b; Cole & Hudspeth, 1964; Epstein, 1959; Reynolds, 1959) thereby giving rise to an exaggerated drug effect, and that inhibition of the LH "facilitatory eating center" might be the specific central action mediating the effect of the drug (Carlisle, 1964).

Apparently, areas of the brainstem are also involved in executing the central mediation of amphetamine anorexia since Carlisle and Reynolds (1961) observed an exaggerated effect of the drug following lesions of the area postrema.

### Effect on Food-Motivated Behavior

Hearst (1961) and Poschel (1963) demonstrated the effectiveness of amphetamine in depressing the lever-pressing performance of rats to get food. Other studies have also demonstrated a depression of response rates following amphetamine administration under fixed-ratio (FR) schedules of food reinforcement in pigeons (Davis, 1965) and in rats (Kelleher, Fry, Deegan, & Cook, 1961; Owen, 1960). Although the depressant effect of amphetamine under FR schedules of food reinforcement is quite consistent, Brown (1965) found that rats subjected to daily dosages of 3.0 mg/kg of d-amphetamine develop a tolerance to the action of the drug. In addition to the depressing effect of amphetamine on lever-pressing performance, Carlson, Doyle, and Bidder (1965) found the drug effective in producing a decrement in food-motivated runway performance. Apparently, amphetamine allowed the interference of irrelevant responses during the runway performance. The depressant action of amphetamine on food-motivated performance is, apparently, a reflection of the anorexic properties of the drug.

Several other studies clearly demonstrate the limitations of the depressant effect of amphetamine on food-motivated performance. Kelleher and Cook (1959) found that amphetamine increased rather than decreased response rate under the experimental conditions of differential reinforcement of low rates (DRL), and Kelleher et al. (1961) found similar results with certain variable- and fixed-interval schedules of reinforcement. Ferster, Appel, and Hiss (1962) observed that amphetamine increased response rate under FR schedule when such a schedule was further complicated by an experimental pre–time-out condition. Apparently, the depressant action on food-motivated performance breaks down under complex schedules of reinforcement, where greater discrimination is required by the subject, or under conditions where reinforcement is contingent upon certain time characteristics rather than performance characteristics. A similar breakdown in a complex discriminatory task of a different type has been observed in the monkey following amphetamine administration (Thurmond, 1965).

## FACILITATING ACTION

### Effect on Intellectual and Motor Performance

Talland and Quarton (1965) measured the effect of methamphetamine on several types of human motor performance, using students as subjects. Methamphetamine speeded performance in simple repetitive motor tasks but apparently did not have any significant effect on a manual reaction-time task. Lovingood (1964) and Nash (1962) also reported an amphetamine enhancement of performance on a wide range of motor and intellectual tasks. A similar facilitating effect of the drug has been observed by Plotnikoff, Reinke, and Fitzloff (1962) on the motor performance of mice in a rotating-rod task, although the amount of facilitation clearly interacted with the speed of the "rotarod." Since Kiernan (1965) demonstrated that amphetamine produced more responses for the onset of a dim light only when subjects had had previous experience in a Skinner box without light onset, the effect of the drug on motor performance appears to depend upon previous experience and possibly other conditions under which it is administered.

Other studies have thrown considerable light on the possible mode of amphetamine facilitation of motor and intellectual tasks. Since amphetamine does not significantly affect reaction time (Costello, 1964) and has even been observed to decrease the extent of motor movement in a lever-response task (Rachman, 1961), the drug does not facilitate such performance by merely augmenting the level of motor activity. Apparently, the drug facilitates the monitoring of cues in such tasks without actually increasing the response time. Studies in which amphetamine has been observed to decrease cognitive fluctuation (Anderson & Zingle, 1961) and to facilitate the physiological correlates of alertness (Hauty, Payne, & Bauer, 1957) strongly support a cue-monitoring mode of facilitation in motor and intellectual tasks.

Although an increased alertness or improved discrimination is the apparent mode of amphetamine facilitation in these tasks, such an effect only partially compensates for other important conditions related to alertness, such as amount of sleep. Kornetsky, Mirsky, Kessler, and Dorff (1959) found that with 44 and 68 hours of sleep loss, amphetamine was able to bring the performance of only those tasks least impaired by the sleep deprivation up to the non-sleep-deprived level. Those measures of performance most affected by sleep loss were still far below the non-sleep-loss level after administration of the drug. Thus, as is true with the effect of amphetamine on other variables, the effect on motor and intellectual tasks depends upon the state of the organism at the time of administration as well as the nature of the task. A more extensive review of the enhancing effects of amphetamine on human performance has been given by Weiss and Laties (1962).

Studies have also indicated the facilitating effect of amphetamine on self-stimulation performance in infrahuman subjects. Using an apparatus where rats could turn stimulation on by pressing one bar and turn it off by pressing a second bar, Miller (1957, 1958) reported that methamphetamine significantly increased the speed with which the stimulus was turned on and reduced the speed with which it was turned off. Poschel and Ninteman (1966) trained rats to press a lever for rewarding electrical stimulation of the lateral-posterior hypothalamus and demonstrated the effectiveness of small dosages of methamphetamine in producing a recovery of such behavior when it had been suppressed by alphamethyl-tyrosine. Since Olds (1962) reported that amphetamine sensitizes self-stimulation sites in the AH, the potentiating effect of the drug on self-stimulation performance is apparently due to a lowering of the threshold for the central rewarding effects of such stimulation.

Meyer, Horel, and Meyer (1963) also demonstrated that amphetamine is able to produce a recovery of the visual and tactile placing response in the cat for the duration of the drug when such a response has been eliminated by extensive lesions of the neocortex. Such findings strongly suggest that the drug plays a facilitating role in the expression of "higher order" reflexive patterns in addition to facilitating motor performance resulting from training.

### Effect on Personality and Social Behavior

Cameron, Specht, and Wendt (1965) demonstrated that college students given a normal clinical dosage of amphetamine liked the way the drug made them feel, were more optimistic, friendly, energetic, talkative, decisive, egotistic, keyed up, light headed, and were less drowsy, languid, bored, dissatisfied, depressed, and grouchy than their placebo controls. Smith and Beecher (1964) tested graduate and undergraduate college students in a situation where they had to solve 25 calculus problems and afterward estimate the number of correct solutions. Although the subjects significantly overestimated the number of correctly solved problems after taking placebo, the amount of overestimation was greater with amphetamine. Weitzner (1965) also used amphetamine in combination with low-, middle-, and high-anxiety groups screened with the Taylor Manifest Anxiety (MA) scale. When tested on three types of tasks, high-MA subjects were superior on noncompetitive tasks, and low-MA subjects were superior on competitive tasks as expected. However, amphetamine significantly facilitated performance on all three tasks, indicating that the drug was more successful than MA levels in affecting performance on a wide variety of tasks. The drug appeared to act more as a nonspecific drive factor on performance than did MA level. These general pictures of elation (Cameron et al., 1965), overestimation of one's performance (Smith & Beecher, 1964), and nonspecific drive (Weitzner, 1965) are consistent with the increased need to achieve under amphetamine found by Evans and Smith (1963). The central subjective effects of amphetamine on personality variables appear earlier than the effect of the drug on more objective measures (Frankenhaeuser & Post, 1964) and very well may be basic to the influence of the drug on intellectual and motor performance. As is true with the effect of amphetamine on other aspects of behavior, the effect of the drug on mood and personality appears to depend upon age and the social context (Krugman, Ross, & Lyerly, 1964), as well as other conditions under which it is administered.

Heimstra (1962a) demonstrated that amphetamine significantly increased the social behavior of rats where both the dominant and submissive members of a group were given the drug. Since the dosage (0.5 mg/kg) was not large enough to produce an increase in activity, the increased social behavior cannot be attributed to a general increase in bodily activity and probably reflects the monitoring of social cues. Other studies indicate that the facilitating effect of amphetamine on social behavior is further enhanced by atropine (Rumelhart & Mueller, 1963) and is dependent upon the stimulus conditions of the social context (Heimstra & McDonald, 1962).

### Effect on Bodily Activity

Amphetamine has been observed to increase general activity (Cole, 1963; Hearst & Whalen, 1963; McGaugh, de Baron, & Longo, 1963). Although such a facilitation of bodily activity interacts with varying amounts of food deprivation, the effect appears to be an ordered one when deprivation conditions are collapsed for purposes of data analysis (Cole, 1964). Using a modified activity platform, Cole (1964) found that the mean activity measures for independent groups of male albino rats during a 1-hour test period were 381.75, 826.44, 1589.38, and 1956.13 for the dosage levels of 0.00, 0.50, 1.25, and 2.50 mg/kg, respectively. Yagi (1963) also found that relatively small doses of methamphetamine (3 mg/kg) markedly increased activity measured in an activity wheel. However, with larger doses (6 mg/kg), a striking but temporary decrease in activity was observed. This reversal effect on activity with larger doses is not uncommon and has also been observed with the established hoarding behavior of rats (Zucker & Milner, 1964). Since Davis (1957) found that amphetamine drastically reduced the sterotyped pacing of the already hyperactive animal, the effect of the drug on bodily activity appears to depend upon the activity level of the subject at time of administration as well as other important experimental conditions.[1]

Gunn and Gurd (1940) found that aggregation increased the facilitating effect of amphetamine on the activity of mice, and Hardinge and Peterson (1963) have presented evidence that such an aggregate effect in turn may increase the toxicity of the drug. Although the evidence for social enhancement of the effect of amphetamine on activity is clear, the amount of enhancement appears to vary with social conditions and dosage levels (Heimstra, 1962b).

Contrary to the effect of amphetamine on food-motivated performance, activity measures do not reflect the development of tolerance to the drug (Schuster & Zimmerman, 1961) but reflect a prolonged action of the drug even in the case of a single administration (Ross & Schnitzer, 1963). Although Alexander and Isaac (1965) found that amphetamine significantly decreased the activity of the macaque under different levels of illumination, they suggested that their findings may have been due to the uniqueness of the experimental setup and a

[1] The importance of experimental procedure and type of apparatus employed in the evaluation of the effect of psychotropic drugs on activity has been pointed out by Kinnard and Watzman (1966).

difference in the diurnal activity of the macaque in comparison to the more commonly used rat. Alexander and Isaac pointed out that the decrease in activity produced by amphetamine under varying levels of illumination does not rule out a facilitating effect of the drug on activity when illumination is not concomitantly varied.

## Effect on Peripheral Systems

The facilitating effect of amphetamine on peripheral systems has also been observed. Myerson, Loman, and Dameshek (1936) found an increase in blood pressure following the administration of 40 mg of amphetamine to human subjects, and Beyer (1939) demonstrated the effectiveness of the drug in increasing metabolic activity and blood pressure in humans. Using rats as subjects, Ehrich and Krumbhaar (1937) found that injections of 40–80 mg/kg of amphetamine daily produced an increase in blood constituents, an increase in blood urea, and an initial increase in blood glucose. Such peripheral effects are observed primarily with larger dosages of amphetamine and are relatively independent of the central anorexic action of the drug since amphetamine has been observed to depress eating in the complete absence of any metabolic or cardiovascular changes (Nathanson, 1937).

The amphetamine depression of gastric hunger contractions in the dog found by Sangster, Grossman, and Ivy (1948) might appear to contradict the general facilitatory effect of the drug on peripheral systems. However, it may merely reflect, again, the importance of the state of the organism at the time of administration. Although such a depression of hunger contractions seems to be a logical explanation for the depressant action of the drug on eating, evidence does not support such a position. Harris et al. (1947) demonstrated that amphetamine was effective in reducing food intake in dogs after the action of the drug on the gastrointestinal tract had been interrupted by bilateral vagotomies and bilateral sympathectomies.

Since such peripheral changes as increases in blood pressure, metabolic activity, and blood constituents frequently accompany increases in bodily activity, both appear to reflect the more peripheral sympathomimetic action of amphetamine.

## Effect on Avoidance Conditioning

Krieckhaus (1965) and Krieckhaus, Miller, and Zimmerman (1965) found that amphetamine facilitated the conditioned avoidance response (CAR) in a modified Miller-Mowrer shuttle box. Since the drug reduced freezing, the facilitating effect of the drug was interpreted to be the result of a reduction in freezing behavior produced by CS. Stein (1965) also found a facilitating effect of amphetamine on the CAR in a shuttle box with no barrier dividing the box into compartments. Similar facilitating effects of the drug on the CAR have been found by Hearst and Whalen (1963) and by Carlton and Didamo (1961) where conditioning involved lever pressing in response to a CS in order to avoid shock. The facilitating effect of amphetamine on avoidance conditioning appears to be similar to the effect of septal lesions on active avoidance tasks (Kenyon &

Krieckhaus, 1965) but quite dissimilar to the effect of such lesions on passive avoidance tasks (Fox, Kimble, & Lickey, 1964).

Using chronic administration of methamphetamine (6 mg/kg daily for 35 days), Moriguchi (1963) found that avoidance learning was more difficult for experimental than for control subjects. Although these findings place some important restrictions on the facilitating action of the drug on avoidance conditioning, they are not necessarily inconsistent with such an effect. A larger dosage of methamphetamine is usually required to produce the same effect as smaller dosages of the other amphetamine compounds; however, Moriguchi's procedure probably produced some cumulative effect far in excess of the dosage levels used in the previously mentioned studies. Since a reversal in the facilitating effect of amphetamine on avoidance conditioning has been observed with larger dosages in a bar-pressing situation (Weissman, 1959), an augmented effect due to the cumulative action of the drug may partially explain Moriguchi's (1963) directionally different findings.

Although Powell, Martin, and Kamano (1965) did not find a facilitation of the CAR by amphetamine in the shuttle-box apparatus, some reconciliation of their findings with those of Krieckhaus (1965) and Krieckhaus et al. (1965) has been suggested by Cole (1966a) in terms of the interaction of the drug with the different CS conditions employed and the effect of the drug on bodily activity. Since the amphetamine's action on consummatory behavior has been observed to interact with food-deprivation conditions (Cole, 1965) and with shock conditions (Teitelbaum & Derks, 1958), the effect of amphetamine on avoidance conditioning also may vary with differences in the experimental CAR conditions.[2] Furthermore, the decreased efficiency of lever-pressing avoidance produced by amphetamine when such a condition was further complicated by a time-out period (Owen, 1963) or a mixed schedule of avoidance and extinction (Stone, 1964) suggests, again, that the facilitating effect of the drug breaks down when greater discrimination is required. The similarity of this breakdown in time discrimination under avoidance conditioning to that observed under more complex appetitive-controlled situations has been pointed out by Sidman (1956).

### Effect on Escape Behavior

Barry and Miller (1965) found that methamphetamine not only facilitated avoidance performance in a straight alley but also facilitated escape behavior, and to an even greater degree. Although escape behavior developed more slowly and attained a lower stable overall rate when noise was used as the aversive stimulus instead of the usual shock, a facilitating effect of amphetamine has also been observed under such conditions (Harrison & Abelson, 1959). The facilitating effect of smaller dosages of methamphetamine (0.5–2.0 mg/kg) on escape performance is consistent with the effect of the other amphetamine compounds on such behavior, and suggests even more strongly that the reversal effect of

[2] The importance of seemingly minor procedural differences in producing substantially different effects of drugs on avoidance conditioning has been pointed out by Barry and Buckley (1966).

methamphetamine on avoidance conditioning found by Moriguchi (1963) was the result of an augmented dosage action.

Since amphetamine has shortened the actual latency of response in escape behavior (Mize & Isaac, 1962) and has also increased the actual speed of running to escape shock (Hamilton, 1960), facilitation of such performance appears to involve the peripheral action of the drug on motor systems. This decreased latency and increased running speed may be another expression of the sympathomimetic action of the drug on peripheral systems.

## CONCLUSION

The multitudinous effects of amphetamine are due to the fact that it is one of several psychotropic drugs having both a central and peripheral action on behavior. Although this dual action assures a wide variety of experimental tasks in which the effects of the drug can be studied, at the same time it increases the complexity of predicting the behavior resulting from such effects. For example, amphetamine-induced anorexia is mediated primarily by the central action of the drug; however, such an effect is not completely independent of the effect of the drug on bodily activity which appears to be mediated by sympathomimetic action on the more peripheral motor systems. Changes in activity may determine the amount of time the subject actually spends in contact with the food dish and thus indirectly influence the amount of food consumed. Although the central and peripheral actions of amphetamine might be quite specific, the resulting behavior frequently demonstrates the interactive effect of the actions.

Since sufficient evidence has been presented to clearly indicate the limits of the general depressant and facilitating effects of amphetamine and the dependency of such effects on the experimental conditions, much still remains to be done before the action of the drug can be predicted with any degree of accuracy. In an attempt to provide guidelines for future investigation, the following suggestions are offered.

1. Increased attention should be given to the effects of amphetamine in relation to dosage levels employed. Reversal effects or inconsistent effects are frequently related to larger than normal dosage levels (e.g., Moriguchi, 1963; Yagi, 1963) and may reflect the "spilling over" of the drug's action into other systems.
2. Increased concern is needed for the specific experimental conditions under which the effects of the drug are studied. Contradictory findings already have been noted in studies which employed different experimental stimulus conditions (e.g., Krieckhaus et al., 1965 vs. Powell et al., 1965). If the effect of amphetamine on avoidance conditioning is different in the presence of a tone CS than it is in the presence of a light CS, the importance of this difference in experimental procedure cannot be ignored. Furthermore, if the effect of the drug on avoidance conditioning is interpreted in terms of its influence on the stimulus condition (i.e., CS-induced freezing), such a difference in experimental conditions

becomes crucial indeed. Since similar contradictory findings have also been noted in studies which employed a difference in time-discrimination requirements, the need for clearly specifying the experimental variables in amphetamine studies seems clear if the action of the drug on avoidance conditioning or any other type of performance is to be understood.

## REFERENCES

ALEXANDER, M., & ISAAC, W. Effect of illumination and d-amphetamine on activity of the rhesus macaque. *Psychological Reports*, 1965, **16**, 311–313.

ANDERSON, C. C., & ZINGLE, H. W. Two experimental tests of a hypothesis concerning the determinants of function fluctuation. *British Journal of Psychology*, 1961, **52**, 371–376.

ANDERSSON, B., & LARSSON, S. Water and food intake and the inhibitory effect of amphetamine on drinking and eating before and after prefrontal lobotomy in dogs. *Acta Physiologica Scandinavica*, 1957, **38**, 22–30.

BARRY, H. III, & BUCKLEY, J. P. Drug effects on animal performance and the stress syndrome. *Journal of Pharmaceutical Sciences*, 1966, **55**, 1159–1183.

BARRY, H. III, & MILLER, N. E. Comparison of drug effects on approach, avoidance, and escape motivation. *Journal of Comparative and Physiological Psychology*, 1965, **59**, 18–24.

BEYER, K. H. The effects of benzedrine sulfate on metabolism and the cardiovascular system in man. *Journal of Pharmacology and Experimental Therapeutics*, 1939, **66**, 318–325.

BROBECK, J. R., LARSSON, S., & REYES, E. A study of electrical activity of the hypothalamic feeding mechanism. *Journal of Physiology*, 1956, **132**, 358–364.

BROWN, H. Drug-behavior interaction affecting development of tolerance to d-amphetamine as observed in fixed tolerance ratio behavior of rats. *Psychological Reports*, 1965, **16**, 917–921.

CAMERON, J. S., SPECHT, P. G., & WENDT, G. R. Effects of amphetamine on moods, emotions, and motivations. *Journal of Psychology*, 1965, **61**, 93–121.

CARLISLE, H. J. Differential effects of amphetamine on food and water intake in rats with lateral hypothalamic lesions. *Journal of Comparative and Physiological Psychology*, 1964, **58**, 47–54.

CARLISLE, H. J., & REYNOLDS, R. W. Effect of amphetamine on food intake in rats with brain-stem lesions. *American Journal of Physiology*, 1961, **201**, 965–967.

CARLSON, N. J., DOYLE, G. A., & BIDDER, T. G. The effect of DL-amphetamine and reserpine on runway performance. *Psychopharmacologia*, 1965, **8**, 157–173.

CARLTON, P. L. Cholinergic mechanisms in the control of behavior by the brain. *Psychological Review*, 1963, **70**, 19–39.

CARLTON, P. L., & DIDAMO, P. Augmentation of the behavioral effects of amphetamine by atropine. *Journal of Pharmacology and Experimental Therapeutics*, 1961, **132**, 91–96.

COLE, S. O. Interaction of amphetamine with conditions of food deprivation. *Psychological Reports*, 1963, **13**, 387–390.

Cole, S. O. Hypothalamic regulation of eating behavior and amphetamine-induced anorexia. Unpublished doctoral dissertation, Claremont Graduate School, 1964.

Cole, S. O. Further study of interactive effects of amphetamine and food deprivation. *Psychological Reports*, 1965, **16**, 625–630.

Cole, S. O. Comments on the effect of amphetamine in avoidance conditioning. *Psychological Reports*, 1966, **19**, 41–42. (a)

Cole, S. O. Increased suppression of food intake by amphetamine in rats with anterior hypothalamic lesions. *Journal of Comparative and Physiological Psychology*, 1966, **61**, 302–305. (b)

Cole, S. O., & Hudspeth, W. J. Hypothalamic mediation of amphetamine anorexia. Paper presented at the meeting of the Western Psychological Association, Portland, April 1964.

Costello, C. G. The effects of depressant and stimulant drugs on the relationship between reaction time and stimulus light intensity. *British Journal of Social and Clinical Psychology*, 1964, **3**, 1–5.

Davis, G. D. Effects of central excitant and depressant drugs on locomotor activity in the monkey. *American Journal of Physiology*, 1957, **188**, 619–623.

Davis, J. L. Antagonism of a behavioral effect of d-amphetamine by chlorpromazine in the pigeon. *Journal of the Experimental Analysis of Behavior*, 1965, **8**, 325–327.

Ehrich, W. E., & Krumbhaar, E. B. The effects of large dosages of benzedrine sulfate on the albino rat: Functional and tissue changes. *Annals of Internal Medicine*, 1937, **10**, 1874–1888.

Epstein, A. Suppression of eating and drinking by amphetamine and other drugs in normal and hyperphagic rats. *Journal of Comparative and Physiological Psychology*, 1959, **52**, 37–45.

Ersner, J. S. The treatment of obesity due to dietary indiscretion (overeating) with benzedrine sulfate. *Endocrinology*, 1940, **27**, 776–780.

Evans, W. O., & Smith, R. P. Some effects of morphine and amphetamine on intellectual functions and mood. *USA MRL Rep.*, 1963, No. 598 (Abstract)

Ferster, C. B., Appel, J. B., & Hiss, R. A. The effect of drugs on a fixed-ratio performance suppressed by a pre–time-out stimulus. *Journal of the Experimental Analysis of Behavior*, 1962, **5**, 73–88.

Fox, S. S., Kimble, D. P., & Lickey, M. E. Comparison of caudate nucleus and septal area lesions on two types of avoidance behavior. *Journal of Comparative and Physiological Psychology*, 1964, **58**, 380–386.

Frankenhaeuser, M., & Post, B. Time relations of objective and subjective reactions to d-amphetamine and Pentobarbitone. *Scandinavian Journal of Psychology*, 1964, **5**, 99–107.

Goetzl, F. R., & Stone, F. The influence of amphetamine sulfate upon olfactory acuity and appetite. *Gastroenterology*, 1948, **10**, 708–713.

Gunn, J. A., & Gurd, M. R. The action of some amines related to adrenaline cyclohexylalkylamines. *Journal of Physiology*, 1940, **97**, 453–470.

Hamilton, C. L. Effects of LSD-25 and amphetamine on a running response in the rat. A. M. A. *Archives of General Psychiatry*, 1960, **2**, 114–119.

Hardinge, M. G., & Peterson, D. I. The effects of exercise and limitation of movement on amphetamine toxicity. *Journal of Pharmacology and Experimental Therapeutics*, 1963, **141**, 260–265.

Harris, S. C., Ivy, A. C., & Searle, L. M. The mechanism of amphetamine-induced loss of weight. *JAMA: Journal of the American Medical Association*, 1947, **134**, 1468–1475.

Harrison, J. M., & Abelson, R. M. The maintenance of behavior by the termination and onset of intense noise. *Journal of the Experimental Analysis of Behavior*, 1959, **2**, 23–42.

Hauty, G. T., Payne, R. B., & Bauer, R. O. Physiological costs incurred by dextro-amphetamine. *Journal of Comparative and Physiological Psychology*, 1957, **50**, 647–651.

Hearst, E., Effects of d-amphetamine on behavior reinforced by food and water. *Psychological Reports*, 1961, **8**, 301–309.

Hearst, E., & Whalen, R. E. Facilitating effects of d-amphetamine on discriminated-avoidance performance. *Journal of Comparative and Physiological Psychology*, 1963, **56**, 124–128.

Heimstra, N. W. Effects of amphetamine sulfate (Benzedrine) on the behavior of paired rats in a competitive situation. *Psychological Record*, 1962, **12**, 25–34. (a)

Heimstra, N. W. Social influence on the response to drugs: I. Amphetamine sulfate. *Journal of Psychology*, 1962, **53**, 233–244. (b)

Heimstra, N. W., & McDonald, A. L. Social influence on the response to drugs: IV. Stimulus factors. *Psychological Record*, 1962, **12**, 383–386.

Kelleher, R. T., & Cook, L. Effects of d-amphetamine, meprobamate, phenobarbital, mephenesin, or chlorpromazine on DRL and FR schedules of reinforcement with rats. *Journal of the Experimental Analysis of Behavior*, 1959, **2**, 267.

Kelleher, R. T., Fry, W., Deegan, J., & Cook, L. Effects of meprobamate on operant behavior of rats. *Journal of Pharmacology and Experimental Therapeutics*, 1961, **133**, 271–280.

Kenyon, J., & Krieckhaus, E. E. Enhanced avoidance behavior following septal lesions in the rat as a function of lesion size and spontaneous activity. *Journal of Comparative and Physiological Psychology*, 1965, **59**, 466–468.

Kiernan, C. C. Modification of the effects of amphetamine sulfate by past experience in the hooded rat. *Psychopharmacologia*, 1965, **8**, 23–31.

Kinnard, W. J., & Watzman, N. Techniques utilized in the evaluation of psychotropic drugs on animal activity. *Journal of Pharmaceutical Sciences*, 1966, **55**, 995–1012.

Knapp, P. H. Amphetamine and addiction. *Journal of Nervous and Mental Disease*, 1952, **115**, 406–432.

Kornetsky, C., Mirsky, A. F., Kessler, E. K., & Dorff, J. E. The effects of dextro-amphetamine on behavioral deficits produced by sleep loss in humans. *Journal of Pharmacology and Experimental Therapeutics*, 1959, **127**, 46–50.

Krieckhaus, E. E. Decrements in avoidance behavior following mammillothalamic tractotomy in rats and subsequent recovery with d-amphetamine. *Journal of Comparative and Physiological Psychology*, 1965, **60**, 31–35.

Krieckhaus, E. E., Miller, N. E., & Zimmerman, P. Reduction of freezing behavior and improvement of shock avoidance by d-amphetamine. *Journal of Comparative and Physiological Psychology*, 1965, **60**, 36–40.

Krugman, A. D., Ross, S., & Lyerly, S. B. Drugs and placebos: Effects of instructions upon performance and mood under amphetamine sulfate and chloral hydrate with younger subjects. *Psychological Reports*, 1964, **15**, 925–926.

Lesses, M. F., & Myerson, A. Benzedrine sulfate as an aid in the treatment of obesity. *New England Journal of Medicine*, 1938, **218**, 119–124.

Lovingood, B. W. The effects of dextro-amphetamine sulfate and caffeine on selected psychomotor, strength, and intellectual performance tasks and physiological parameters of young white men exposed to a restricted environment. *Dissertation Abstracts,* 1964, **24,** 3625. (Abstract)

McGaugh, J. L., de Baron, L., & Longo, V. G. Electroencephalographic and behavioral analysis of drug effects on an instrumental reward discrimination in rabbits. *Psychopharmacologia,* 1963, **4,** 126–138.

Meyer, D. R., & Meyer, P. M. Brain functions. *Annual Review of Psychology,* 1963, **14,** 155–174.

Meyer, P. M., Horel, J. A., & Meyer, D. R. Effects of dl-amphetamine upon placing responses in neodecorticate cats. *Journal of Comparative and Physiological Psychology,* 1963, **56,** 402–404.

Miller, N. E. Experiments on motivation. *Science,* 1957, **126,** 1271–1278.

Miller, N. E. Central stimulation and other new approaches to motivation and reward. *American Psychologist,* 1958, **13,** 100–108.

Mize, D., & Isaac, W. Effects of sodium pentobarbital and D-amphetamine on latency of the escape response in the rat. *Psychological Reports,* 1962, **10,** 643–645.

Moriguchi, N. Avoidance learning under the condition of abulia induced by chronic administration of methamphetamine hydrochloride (Philopon). *Annual of Animal Psychology,* 1963, **13,** 49–55.

Myerson, A., Loman, J., & Dameshek, W. Physiologic effects of benzedrine and its relationship to other drugs affecting the autonomic nervous system. *American Journal of the Medical Sciences,* 1936, **192,** 560–574.

Nash, H. Psychological effects of amphetamines and barbituates. *Journal of Nervous and Mental Disease,* 1962, **134,** 203–217.

Nathanson, M. H. The central action of benzedrine. *JAMA: Journal of the American Medical Association,* 1937, **108,** 528–531.

Olds, J. Hypothalamic substrates of reward. *Physiological Review,* 1962, **42,** 554–604.

Owen, J. E., Jr. The influence of dl-, d-, and l-amphetamine and d-methamphetamine on a fixed-ratio schedule. *Journal of the Experimental Analysis of Behavior,* 1960, **3,** 293–310.

Owen, J. E., Jr. Psychopharmacological studies of some 1-(Chlorophenyl)-2-aminopropanes II: Effects on avoidance and discrimination behavior. *Journal of Pharmaceutical Sciences,* 1963, **52,** 684–688.

Plotnikoff, N., Reinke, D., & Fitzloff, J. Effects of stimulants on rotarod performance of mice. *Journal of Pharmaceutical Sciences,* 1962, **51,** 1007–1008.

Poschel, B. P. H. Effects of methamphetamine on hunger and thirst motivated variable-interval performance. *Journal of Comparative and Physiological Psychology,* 1963, **56,** 968–973.

Poschel, B. P. H., & Ninteman, F. W. Hypothalamic self-stimulation: Its suppression by blockade of norepinephrine biosynthesis and reinstatement by methamphetamine. *Life Sciences,* 1966, **5,** 11–16.

Powell, B. J., Martin, L. K., & Kamano, D. K. Failure to find improved shuttlebox avoidance performance using d-amphetamine sulfate. *Psychological Reports,* 1965, **17,** 330.

Rachman, S. Effect of a stimulant drug on extent of motor responses. *Perceptual and Motor Skills,* 1961, **12,** 186.

Reynolds, R. W. The effect of amphetamine on food intake in normal and hypothalamic hyperphagic rats. *Journal of Comparative and Physiological Psychology,* 1959, **52,** 682–684.

Ross, S., & Schnitzer, S. B. Further support for a placebo effect in the rat. *Psychological Reports,* 1963, **13,** 461–462.

RUMELHART, D. E., & MUELLER, M. R. Enhancement of amphetamine sulfate effects by atropine in a social situation. *Psychological Reports*, 1963, **12**, 251–254.

SANGSTER, W., GROSSMAN, M. E., & IVY, A. C. Effects of d-amphetamine on gastric hunger contractions and food intake in the dog. *American Journal of Physiology*, 1948, **153**, 259–263.

SCHUSTER, C. R., & ZIMMERMAN, J. Timing behavior during prolonged treatment with dl-amphetamine. *Journal of the Experimental Analysis of Behavior*, 1961, **4**, 327–330.

SHARP, J. C., NEILSON, H. C., & PORTER, P. B. The effect of amphetamine upon cats with lesions in the ventromedial hypothalamus. *Journal of Comparative and Physiological Psychology*, 1962, **55**, 198–200.

SIDMAN, M. Drug-behavior interaction. *Annals of the New York Academy of Science*, 1956, **65**, 282–302.

SIEGAL, P. S., & STERLING, T. D. The anorexigenic action of dextro-amphetamine sulfate upon feeding responses of differing strength. *Journal of Comparative and Physiological Psychology*, 1959, **52**, 179–182.

SMITH, G. M., & BEECHER, H. K. Drugs and judgement: Effects of amphetamine and secobarbital on self evaluation. *Journal of Psychology*, 1964, **58**, 397–405.

STEIN, L. Facilitation of avoidance behavior by positive brain stimulation. *Journal of Comparative and Physiological Psychology*, 1965, **60**, 9–19.

STONE, G. C. Effects of drugs on nondiscriminated avoidance behavior. 1. Individual differences in dose-response relationships. *Psychopharmacologia*, 1964, **6**, 245–255.

TALLAND, G. A., & QUARTON, G. C. Methamphetamine and pentobarbital effects on human motor performance. *Psychopharmacologia*, 1965, **8**, 241–250.

TEITELBAUM, P., & DERKS, P. The effect of amphetamine on forced drinking in the rat. *Journal of Comparative and Physiological Psychology*, 1958, **51**, 801–810.

THURMOND, J. B. Effects of amphetamine on the monkey's visual threshold. *Psychonomic Science*, 1965, **3**, 115–116.

WEISS, B., & LATIES, V. G. Enhancement of human performance by caffeine and the amphetamines. *Pharmacological Review*, 1962, **14**, 1–36.

WEISSMAN, A. Differential drug effects upon a three-ply multiple schedule of reinforcement. *Journal of the Experimental Analysis of Behavior*, 1959, **2**, 271–287.

WEITZNER, M. Manifest anxiety, amphetamine, and performance. *Journal of Psychology*, 1965, **60**, 71–79.

YAGI, B. Studies in general activity: II. The effect of methamphetamine. *Annual of Animal Psychology*, 1963, **13**, 37–47.

ZUCKER, I., & MILNER, P. The effect of amphetamine on established hoarding in the rat. *Psychonomic Science*, 1964, **1**, 367.

# 19

# *The Characteristics of Dependence in High-Dose Methamphetamine Abuse*

DAVID E. SMITH

The Haight-Ashbury Medical Clinic, a volunteer private nonprofit medical facility, serves as a treatment and referral center for the Haight-Ashbury district of San Francisco. The use of intravenous methamphetamine at high dosage has become the major adolescent drug problem in this diverse community of young drug users. Unfortunately, much of the literature on amphetamine abuse relates to oral low dose patterns and has been of little value to the clinic's physicians.

This paper will define the clinical characteristics of high-dose methamphetamine abuse and will discuss some of the special characteristics of this drug pattern relating to tolerance and dependence.

## POPULATION AT RISK

An excellent discussion of the types of individuals now involved in the Haight-Ashbury subculture can be found in *The World of the Haight-Ashbury Speed Freak* (Smith, R., 1969). This paper is based on research done by the University of California Medical Center's amphetamine research project operating in the Haight-Ashbury Medical Clinic's psychiatry annex. Without question, the drug practices of the Haight-Ashbury population have changed dramatically, with a shift in emphasis from the ritualistic use of psychedelic drugs to the compulsive use of amphetamines. Relatively little research, however, has been done on the psychosocial aspects of the population at risk prior to their entry into the Haight-Ashbury subculture. This question is being investigated at present by Mt. Zion's Haight-Ashbury Research Project under the direction of Steven Pittell.

In general, however, one can describe the original Haight-Ashbury population as eccentric, mystical, nonviolent, and articulate. The mass media's coverage of "the hippies" attracted large numbers of disturbed or sociopathic young people, many of whom were already compulsively involved with drugs. This latter group introduced violence and exploitation into the Haight-Ashbury, and most significantly, changed it from an acid to a speed[1] subculture (Smith, D., 1969a).

To understand the toxicological manifestations of high-dose methamphetamine abuse, one must understand the cyclical nature of this drug pattern. The "speed binge" can be divided into an action phase and a reaction phase.

From *The International Journal of the Addictions,* Vol. 4, No. 3, September 1969, pp. 453–459. 

[1] "Speed" is the street name for methamphetamine hydrochloride.

During the action phase the user injects methamphetamine intravenously from one to ten times a day. With each injection the user experiences a "flash" which he describes as a "full body orgasm." Between injections the user is euphoric, hyperactive, and hyperexcitable. This action phase may last for several days in which the individual does not sleep and rarely eats.

For a variety of reasons this action phase is terminated. The user may stop voluntarily because of fatigue, he may become confused, paranoid, or panic-stricken and stop, or he may simply run out of drug. Whatever the reason for termination, the action phase is followed by the reaction phase in which the user goes rapidly from a hyperexcitable state to one of extreme exhaustion. The speed freak[2] may sleep for 24 to 48 hours and upon awakening is quite hungry and may eat ravenously. Unfortunately, when his food and sleep needs are satisfied the user often enters into a prolonged phase of extreme psychological depression. This depression is often so severe and intolerable that in most cases he starts another speed binge and the cycle is repeated.

The speed freak, because of his poor impulse control, seems unable to wait out his depression unless treatment of a supportive nature is available at this crucial time. Unfortunately, voluntary treatment facilities for compulsive amphetamine users are quite limited, and without therapeutic intervention the speed freak treats his own depression by "going back up."

## METHAMPHETAMINE TOXICITY

A wide variety of medical complaints occur with continued use of intravenous methamphetamine at high doses, including hepatitis, malnutrition, skin abscesses, and other dermatological problems (Smith, 1969b; Smith & Rose, 1968). These medical problems, of course, are aggravated by the poor hygiene and crowded living conditions of the user. The acute psychiatric problems seen with this drug pattern can be divided into four categories: the acute anxiety reaction, the psychotic reaction, the exhaustion reaction, and the withdrawal reaction.

Of these, the amphetamine psychosis characterized by visual hallucinations, auditory hallucinations, and a well-defined paranoid system with ideas of reference represents the most dramatic and difficult management problem.

These paranoid characteristics may become so frightening to the speed freak that he may inject barbiturates or heroin as a form of self-medication. Unfortunately, secondary forms of barbiturate and heroin dependence have resulted from this practice.

Ellinwood (1967) feels that personality is the prime variable in differentiating between a nonpsychotic (anxiety) reaction and a psychotic reaction. He states that the sociopathic personality produces primarily nonpsychotic amphetamine reactions whereas the schizoid personality produces primarily psychotic amphetamine reactions.

[2] "Speed freak" is the street name for the compulsive methamphetamine user.

Our research tends to question this hypothesis. For example the "novice" or inexperienced user, when he first begins injecting methamphetamine, has a high incidence of anxiety reactions. However, if he is in a drug subculture such as Haight-Ashbury, where other more experienced users are available, reassurance helps him suppress this anxiety. Continued use produces an increase in tolerance to the effects of intravenous methamphetamine to the point where the user can increase his dosage. It is this prolonged high dosage that produces the amphetamine psychosis.

Support for this hypothesis of environment and dosage as being the prime determinants of the nature of the adverse amphetamine reaction can be found in a series of diverse studies.

Griffith and others at Vanderbilt Medical School, in an unpublished study, found that normal, nontolerant, human volunteers given progressively larger doses of amphetamine developed a transient paranoid schizophrenic-like reaction.

Further, it is known that group factors, including peer group sanction, play a major role in the individual's learning to use a drug. The many experienced speed users in the Haight-Ashbury often teach the novice how to use speed and how to interpret the anxiety reaction as a pleasant, rather than a frightening, experience (Smith, D., 1969a). For example, such terms as "creative paranoia" and "terminal euphoria" are used to describe certain disturbing psychic experiences. With such group support, the individual is able to increase his dosage until an intolerable paranoid schizophrenic reaction occurs.

## TOLERANCE AND DEPENDENCE

The mechanism of tolerance with chronic methamphetamine use is an unsettled scientific question of considerable interest to those working in the drug abuse field.

Goodman and Gilman (1960) describe severe reactions occurring with 30 mgm, and death has been reported with rapid intravenous injection of 120 mgm. Conversely, regular users of methamphetamine have injected 500 to 1000 mgm at a single dose without serious morbidity (Kramer, 1967). Griffith at Vanderbilt was able to induce an acute paranoid schizophrenic reaction in four normal, healthy males with doses of 40 to 220 mgm over a five-day period, and yet patients seen at the Haight-Ashbury have injected 1000 to 5000 mgm of black market methamphetamine without producing an acute amphetamine psychosis (Smith, D., 1969b).

This wide range of dose-effect relationships is demonstrated in the following three case histories:

*Case 1* A 23-year-old white male was brought to the Haight-Ashbury Medical Clinic by two friends. He was fatigued to the point where he had to be supported and aroused to obtain a response, but upon arousal he became agitated. His friends reported that he was a speed freak and had been on a 12 day run and was shooting one spoon (approximately 1 gram) of speed every 4 hours. It was calculated that he had shot approximately 100 grams of speed during this period of time. Management required nothing other than removing his clothes, which he had not changed during this 12-day period, and allowing him to sleep. He awoke approximately 18 hours later and complained of hunger and depression.

*Case 2* A 17-year-old white female came to the Haight-Ashbury Clinic in an acutely agitated state with marked muscle tremors. Her blood pressure was 180/120 and her pulse was 120. She had a history of intravenous methamphetamine use, shooting up to two spoons per day in the past. However, she had not used the drug in approximately 6 months, as she had been in the Mendocino State Hospital program. While at a party in the Haight-Ashbury she decided to try a small quantity of speed and injected a dime bag (approximately 100 mgm). Soon after the injection she felt she was "over-amped" and came to the Haight-Ashbury Clinic in the above condition. The patient was treated with intramuscular chlorpromazine 0/100 mgm and allowed to rest. In two hours her blood pressure was 120/80 with a pulse of 90. She remained somewhat excited for the rest of the day, but there were no longer term sequelae.

*Case 3* A 19-year-old white male was brought to Orange County Hospital after convulsing. He was unconscious, fasciculating, apneic, and cyanotic. The boy was captured by the police in a parking lot after a short chase. During the chase he ingested the drugs he was carrying. On admission to the hospital his temperature was 104° F and his pulse was 102 and irregular. The patient's temperature went to 108° F and despite vigorous attempts at resuscitation, he died. Autopsy recovered two cellophane packets from his stomach which contained methamphetamine hydrochloride. Further toxicological testing found the urine level of methamphetamine hydrochloride to be 55 mgm percent with a blood level of 2.2 mgm percent; liver contained 13.7 mgm percent and brain contained 30.7 mgm percent. There were no other drug levels picked up. The patient had no old needle marks and by history it appeared that he was not a speed freak (Dunlap, 1968).

Tolerance, then, produces tremendous variability in the human response to methamphetamine, and a lethal dose in a nonuser may be an average psychoactive dose for a regular user. The mechanism of this tolerance is not understood, however, for although many people have the clinical impression that physical tolerance occurs in the chronic methamphetamine user, animal experiments (Kramer, in press) and extensive review of the controlled research literature (Smith, D., 1969a) fail to support such an observation.

The development of psychological tolerance or the ability to withstand and suppress adverse effects because of experience still remain possible explanations for the variation in dose-effect relationships.

Without question, the post-speed binge depression is the major factor in the development of a repetitive and compulsive pattern of methamphetamine abuse. Unlike the heroin addict who continues to inject to prevent physical withdrawal, the speed freak continues to inject to treat his depression.

It has been commonly assumed that true physical dependence does not develop to the amphetamines. High-dose methamphetamine use, however, can produce a moderate degree of physical dependence and classic withdrawal reactions lasting 2 to 4 days have been reported (Smith, D., 1969b).

## SUMMARY

High-dose methamphetamine abuse has become a major drug problem and is associated with a high degree of physical and psychiatric toxicity.

As with any drug pattern, it includes a complex interaction of physical, personality, drug and group factors. However, the relative importance of these variables, particularly in the area of tolerance and dependence, has not yet been established. Further research is needed to provide the medical community with a better understanding of this serious and rapidly growing drug problem. However, this research must be creative and innovative. In addition to the factors described above, one of the most promising areas for further investigation may be basic research approaches to the chemistry of the mind. For example, Mandel (1968) found that high-dose methamphetamine inhibited the neurochemical breakdown of serotonin and facilitated a shunt to Bufotenine, a known hallucinogen. He speculated that this shunting mechanism may be the basis for the prolonged hallucinosis occasionally seen in high-dose amphetamine use. Such basic research emphasizes the need for a broad-based research approach to the amphetamine problem, ranging from neurochemical to sociological considerations.

## REFERENCES


DUNLAP, LAWRENCE B. Orange Country Hospital Pathology Laboratory, personal communication. June 1968.

ELLINWOOD, E. H. Amphetamine psychosis: 1. Description of the individuals and process. *The Journal of Nervous and Mental Disease* 144: 4, 273–283, 1967.

GOODMAN, L. S. & GILMAN, A. (Eds.) *The Pharmacological Basis for Therapeutics*. 2nd Edition. New York: Macmillan, 1960, 532–533.

GRIFFITH, J. D., CAVANAUGH, J., and OATES, J. Schizophrenia psychosis induced by large dose administration of D-amphetamine. Department of Psychiatry, Vanderbilt University School of Medicine (unpublished).

KRAMER, J. C. A Summary of experiments with methamphetamine using Swiss-white mice, publication in progress.

KRAMER, J. C., et al. Amphetamine abuse. *Journal of the American Medical Association* **201**: 305–309, July 31, 1967.

MANDEL, A. J., and SPOONER, C. E. Psychochemical research studies in man. *Science* **162**: 1442–1452, December 27, 1968.

SMITH, D. E. Speed freaks vs. acid heads: conflict between drug subcultures. *Clinical Pediatrics*, 8: 4, 185–188, April 1969a.

SMITH, D. E. High dose methamphetamine abuse in Haight-Ashbury. *Journal of Psychedelic Drugs* 2: 2, 1969b.

SMITH, D. E. Speed kills—high dose methamphetamine abuse. *Los Angeles County Medical Society Bulletin*, June 1968.

SMITH, D. E., and ROSE, A. J. Observations in the Haight-Ashbury Medical Clinic of San Francisco: health problems in a "hippie" subculture. *Clinical Pediatrics*, 7: 6, 313–316, June 1968.

SMITH, R. The world of the Haight-Ashbury speed freak. *Journal of Psychedelic Drugs* 2: 2, 1969.

# 20

# *Speed Freaks versus Acid Heads: Conflict between Drug Subcultures*

DAVID E. SMITH

In the Haight-Ashbury district of San Francisco, methamphetamine abuse has become the major youthful drug problem. The *speed*[1] *freak* has replaced or driven away the *acid*[2] *head,* and as a result the Haight-Ashbury has been converted from an *acid subculture* to a *speed subculture.* The two drug patterns have different causes and consequences, and in effect, are antithetical. Segments of the medical community which tend to group these two drug patterns together increase their own misinformation about drug use and abuse. This paper describes and contrasts some of the basic characteristics of a *speed subculture* vs. those of an *acid subculture.*

## HIGH-DOSE METHAMPHETAMINE ABUSE—THE *SPEED* CYCLE

To understand a speed subculture, one must, of course, understand the *speed freak.*[3] As with any drug taker, the *speed freak* has certain motivations and expectations for his drug use. A comparison with the alcohol user would familiarize the dominant culture with this concept. An alcoholic, for example, may take a martini during the week, setting relaxation as his expectation for this drug experience. On Friday or Saturday, since he does not have to get up the next morning, he may set his expectation as intoxication and take three or four martinis, varying the dose to meet his goal. All drug users have expectations. The physician must understand these motivations for drug use not only in terms of acute treatment but also for chronic treatment which includes intervention into a potentially destructive life-style.

The individual who uses high-dose methamphetamine is after the *flash* or the *rush.* He injects the drug and has a rapid reaction which he describes as a *full-body orgasm.* The methamphetamine-induced excitation and agitation that follows is, to the *speed freak,* a secondary consideration. Individuals often start on oral methamphetamines and develop a desire for the *high,* or the excitation of the oral amphetamines, but for various reasons ranging from group pressure to personality problems they find that intravenous injection of the drug is even more

From *Clinical Pediatrics,* Vol. 2, April 1969, pp. 185–192. Reprinted by permission of author and J. B. Lippincott Company.

[1] *Speed* is the street name for methamphetamine hydrochloride.

[2] *Acid* is the street name for LSD.

[3] *Speed freak* is the name given to the compulsive high-dose methamphetamine user.

desirable. This practice leads eventually to a distinctive and destructive pattern of *speed* use.

Methamphetamine interrupts sleep patterns and suppresses appetite. As he becomes more experienced with speed, the individual goes on a *speed binge* lasting three or four days during which he *shoots up* from one to ten times per day, always going for the peak experience. Throughout this time he neither eats nor sleeps. He stays in a continual state of hyperexcitement until for various reasons (exhaustion and fatigue, abnormal psychologic circumstances that are frightening to him, or inability to obtain the drug) he decides to terminate the *speed binge.*

After the *speed binge* is terminated, the reaction phase of the speed cycle follows. Characteristically, this is the exhaustion syndrome. The individual often lapses into a deep sleep which lasts 24 to 48 hours, depending on the duration of the *speed binge.* Upon awakening he may eat ravenously. Management of the exhaustion syndrome is relatively easy. Treatment consists primarily of supportive care.

After the speed cycle, many amphetamine users do not return to a baseline level of personality function. They remain in a prolonged sub-acute phase, in which profound depression dominates. To escape from this depression the *speed freak* often shoots methamphetamine again, thereby beginning another cycle. The intensity of postspeed depression cannot be overemphasized. To quote a 17-year-old girl: "Without speed I feel so lousy that I'd rather shoot speed and live for one week than live for 40 years without it." In these circumstances a situation of depression rapidly develops in which the patient sees no hope for interruption of this drug-use pattern. The only feasible therapy is to remove him from the drug-using subculture. There is a good institutional program at Mendocino State Hospital, and a self-help outpatient program in San Francisco directed by the Haight-Ashbury Clinic. But as long as the *speed freak* maintains himself in an area where many other individuals also are using the drugs, he has difficulty resisting the temptation to *go back up* again.

## MEDICAL AND PSYCHOLOGIC TOXICITY OF HIGH-DOSE METHAMPHETAMINE ABUSE

We recently described 310 cases of high-dose methamphetamine abuse seen at the Haight-Ashbury Clinic during a three-month period (June to September 1967). (1) Analysis of the reactions showed that approximately 40 percent of the patients came to the clinic with physical complaints, whereas in 60 percent these complaints were psychologic.

Among the physical difficulties were an unusually high incidence of hepatitis and a bewildering array of urticarial reactions, abscesses, respiratory complaints, and acute abdominal complaints. Apparently, acute gastrointestinal distress or abdominal cramps are part of the high-dose methamphetamine syndrome. I will not go into detail about the physical complaints, however, since I prefer to focus here on the psychologic consequences that these individuals develop. These consequences can be divided into five categories: (a) anxiety reaction; (b) amphetamine psychosis; (c) exhaustion syndrome; (d) prolonged depression; (e) prolonged hallucinosis.

The principal psychologic complaint encountered was the simple acute anxiety reaction. The drug taker had overdosed himself and had become acutely anxious, fearful, tremulous; he often had tachycardia and somatic symptoms. Virtually all the methamphetamine used locally is synthesized by black-market laboratories. Its source is not therapeutic diet pills diverted into an illegal market. Therefore, it is difficult to obtain an accurate assessment of dosage. The average therapeutic dose for appetite suppression is 5 to 15 mg, but because of the rapid tolerance which develops, the *speed freak* shoots between 1 and 5 grams per day. The tolerance varies so widely among users, however, that one questions whether these differences in tolerance are physical or psychologic. (1) (2)

For the anxiety reactions long-acting sedatives are enough. However, the acute anxiety reaction is self-limiting, and many times the physician tends to overtreat. Transition from the action to reaction phase can be dramatic, and the consequences of the anxiety reaction can be handled easily with a supportive, nonthreatening environment and the cautious use of sedatives.

Amphetamine psychosis, less common than anxiety reaction, is associated with three diagnostic characteristics: (a) visual hallucinations; (b) auditory hallucinations; and (c) a well-defined system of paranoia including ideas of reference. (3) Paranoia is a characteristic part of the reaction and makes treatment difficult because the individual is concerned about entering a hospital or encountering the police. He feels comfortable only in a street facility and often raises questions concerning the police. As an example, I saw an 18-year-old white boy who had been having an amphetamine psychosis. In his well-defined system of paranoia he felt that the police were after him, and that his roommate and he had come to the medical clinic for help. Except for this system of paranoia and distracting hallucinations, he was remarkably lucid. During our interview a staff volunteer of the clinic, wearing a black leather jacket, crossed in front of the door. The patient jumped up and said, "I knew it! You're part of the plot!" and tried to run out the door. While restraining the boy, I called the volunteer and indicated that this was a member of the clinic staff who happened to wear a black leather jacket. He calmed down immediately. The movement in and out of a paranoia delusional system can be dramatic, and the physician may suddenly become part of that system. If the patient is large or violent, the physician may be in some immediate jeopardy.

With the amphetamine psychosis the major psychochemotherapy consists of antipsychotic drugs of the phenothiazine type. The physician also must give serious consideration to hospitalization if facilities are available, since psychotic symptoms often persist.

In prolonged hallucinosis the high-dose amphetamine user experiences auditory and visual hallucinations which may persist for days or weeks after the acute reaction has passed. A minority of the individuals who have amphetamine psychoses manifest this prolonged reaction; we are not certain whether drug factors or personality factors play the major role in this drug-induced thought disorder. (1–3)

Group factors are a major contributor to amphetamine toxicity in chronic high-dosage methamphetamine use. In a series of animal experiments the $LD_{50}$ of D-amphetamine was 100 mg/kg. when the drug was administered to individually housed white mice. But when the animals were grouped together, with all other environmental conditions constant, the $LD_{50}$ decreased markedly to 25 mg/kg. Aggregation of the animals increased the toxicity of the drug fourfold.

This phenomenon of aggregate amphetamine toxicity follows a polyphasic mortality curve. The mortality was high at the 25 mg/kg. dose and then decreased, so that at 75 mg/kg. the drug was less toxic than at 25 mg. Mortality rose again at 100 mg/kg., where a second $LD_{50}$ appeared. When trying to explain this polyphasic mortality phenomenon we found that at the 25 mg/kg. dose, the animals were hyperexcitable and agitated and the mechanism of death was the killing of one animal by another. As the drug dose was increased the dose was not high enough to cause convulsions (the mechanism of death at 100 mg/kg.), but the animals became so disorganized that they could not mobilize directive attacks at one another. (4)

The Haight-Ashbury area in many ways resembles such a giant mouse cage. The residents are taking high doses of central-nervous-system stimulants and interacting in a violent and often destructive fashion. It has become obvious that taking the drug in a high-density population situation increases its toxicity. The physician must be aware of this phenomenon of aggregate toxicity. Treatment of any central-nervous-system stimulant reaction always should include great emphasis on a quiet, supportive, nonthreatening environment. A caustic statement by a physician or a nurse bursting into the treatment room constitutes poor treatment. Individuals who treat drug reactions always must remain aware of the importance of environmental group factors in treating both amphetamine and LSD reactions.

## THE ACID HEAD

In our clinic population, those individuals who take methamphetamine chronically are approximately the same age as those who take LSD chronically. There are noteworthy differences in personality type and socioeconomic background between the two groups of drug users. Of greater significance, however, is that the chronic LSD user exhibits a pattern of thought and behavior which is the antithesis of that of the chronic methamphetamine user. Rather than seeking a *flash* or a thrill as do the *speed freaks,* the chronic LSD user develops a complex set of motivations for his drug use, involving self-psychoanalytic, pseudoreligious, and creative aspirations.

To understand the chronic effects of LSD, one must understand the psychopharmacologic effects of the drug. (5) The individual under the influence of LSD manifests marked perceptual changes. Primarily, these changes are illusionary phenomena (e.g., objects changing shape and color). Perceptual changes may include synesthesia in which one sensory phenomenon becomes translated into another (e.g., a record player gives off colored vibrations or an individual smells purple). Teenagers are well aware of the phenomenon of synesthesia and have immortalized it in songs such as "Good Vibrations."

Hallucinatory activity, the perception of an object in one's sensory environment without the physical manifestation of that object, is relatively rare with LSD.

One may encounter marked alterations in symbolic associations with sensory input. For example, an individual may see a red light and become enamored with the hue of the light, rather than make the symbolic association that the red light means "stop." One also finds marked alterations in ideational functioning. Individuals who have taken LSD often feel that they have had a universal religious experience in which they have found the answer to life. They develop a rather elaborate philosophical position around this sensory pattern and often, particularly in the young, this is carried into their nondrug state. They do not say "It is just a drug reaction that gave me this subjective or illusionary experience"; they say, "I've found the answer to life!" If LSD is taken in a psychedelic informational environment where other individuals have had the same experience, then the interpretation of psychedelic reality is reinforced. Repeated LSD experiences with friends supporting a positive interpretation of the LSD experience produces some dramatic psychologic changes in the *acid head.* (6) I have described these changes in the chronic LSD user as the *psychedelic syndrome.* (7)

One first characteristic of the psychedelic syndrome is a profound belief in nonviolence. The *acid head's* rejection of physical aggression is so profound that often one sees a change in diet to natural, vegetable foods; his rejection of killing may be so great that he may refuse to eat meat. There may be a deep desire to return to nature, shown by adoption of the dress and customs of such cultures as the American Indians. There is emphasis on *natural foods* or foods raised without chemicals, and *natural ways* such as natural childbirth. Many young hippie girls seek consultation at the Haight-Ashbury for natural childbirth and home delivery, with child-rearing occurring in a tribal or communal setting. Another of the significant characteristics of the individual who uses LSD chronically and develops the *psychedelic syndrome* is a belief in *magic:* mental telepathy, astrology, ESP, mysticism, telekinesia. The *acid head* believes that his mind can communicate and produce changes in his physical environment because his LSD experiences demonstrated this. He develops a life-style based around this belief system. An individual may not come to work at the Haight-Ashbury Clinic, for example, because the "stars are wrong," or he says "It's impossible for me to interact or work with that individual because our signs conflict." Recently, sincere belief that a meteorite was going to hit San Francisco developed and a large number in the community left for Colorado.

## MEDICAL SIGNIFICANCE OF THE PSYCHEDELIC SYNDROME

Individuals with *psychedelic syndrome* tend to group together in communal living situations, and the combination of chronic LSD usage and living in the psychedelic community reinforces his behavior. They undergo a profound psychologic conversion to belief in an unstructured psychedelic religion.

The medical significance of the *psychedelic syndrome* is vague. In Dr.

Kay Blacker's studies (6) at the Langley Porter Neuropsychiatric Institute, no classical evidence of organic brain damage was found in chronic LSD users. With visually-evoked EEG responses there was an increase in the number of low-intensity visual responses. But in another test sensitive to intellectual disorganization or schizophrenia—the auditory two-toned evoked potential—the LSD users showed no abnormality. As Dr. Blacker pointed out, an alteration in one type of psychologic testing which may be characteristic of a schizophrenic process does not imply an alteration in an entirely different type of psychologic testing. His assumption is that the chronic LSD user tends to modulate and organize sensory input in a different and unique fashion. In other words, he views the world differently from the non- or casual LSD user. His subjects had intact and intense interpersonal relationships; they could not, using standard nomenclature, be described as schizophrenic—merely as eccentric. The breakdown in interpersonal relationships occurs between the *hip* and the straight community or between the nonpsychedelic and the individual who is involved in the psychedelic subculture. There is mounting evidence that young people who regularly use LSD and involve themselves in the psychedelic subculture develop profound alterations in psychosocial functioning.

Why do I stress this behavior? It is often said that young people who involve themselves in what can be called the psychedelic movement are going through a "phase" and will become "straight" again. The rationalization is: "These young people are only experimenting like we did when we swallowed goldfish or went to fraternity games, and they will come back." I submit that, at the very least, those young people who are deeply and intensely involved in the hip movement will not be able to re-enter the dominant American culture without significant problems, because of a profound conflict in value systems. Individuals with the *psychedelic syndrome*, committed to nonviolence, will have great conflict in a society like ours where the ethic is violence and competition. So long as they remain in the psychedelic subculture their *psychedelic syndrome*, with its characteristics of nonviolence and magical beliefs, is actually respected. They cannot be called mentally ill by the standards of their community—only by the standards of ours. Treatment is indicated and successful only if for various reasons—monetary, parental, etc.—the individual attempts to *re-enter* the straight society. Becoming *straight* can cause severe psychologic problems, and be a much more difficult process than most adults predict.

## THE SUBCULTURES ARE DIFFERENT

All this helps to explain why the *acid-head* community cannot live with the *speed-freak* community. Because of the violent characteristics of the latter, the hippies have left the Haight-Ashbury district and have moved to the country where they can establish small rural communes which tolerate and reinforce their belief systems. Urban areas such as the Haight-Ashbury can never be a permanent haven for the acid subculture, because in the conflict of *speed freaks* versus *acid heads, speed* always drives out *acid*—as in the broader society the philosophy of violence dominates the higher aspirations of nonviolence, peace and love.

## REFERENCES

1. SMITH, D. E., and FISCHER, C. M.: High-dose methamphetamine abuse in Haight-Ashbury. *J. Psychedelic Drugs*. In press.
2. ———: Physical versus psychological dependence and tolerance in high-dose methamphetamine abuse. *Clinical Toxicology*. In press.
3. ELLINWOOD, E. R.: Amphetamine psychosis I: description of the individual and process. *J. Nerv. Ment. Dis.* 144: 273, 1967.
4. SMITH, D. E., FISCHER, C. M., SCHOENFELD, E., and HINE, C. H.: Behavioral mediators in the polyphasic mortality curve of aggregate amphetamine toxicity. *J. Psychedelic Drugs*. In press.
5. ———: Lysergic acid diethylamide; an historical perspective. *J. Psychedelic Drugs* 1: 1, 1967.
6. BLACKER, K. H., JONES, R. T., STONE, G. C., and PFEFFERBAUM, D.: Chronic users of LSD; the acidheads. Presented at the 1966 American Psychiatric Association. In press.
7. SMITH, D. E.: LSD and the psychedelic syndrome. *Clinical Toxicology*. In press.

# 4
# *Hallucinogens*

Although natural hallucinogens such as peyote, psilocybin ("magic mushrooms"), morning glory seeds, jimsonweed, and others have been used since the dawn of history by man to induce visions, religious experiences, and altered states of consciousness, there has been a sudden increase in their popularity during recent years. Much of this marked rise is due to the chemical synthesization of new hallucinogens, such as DMT, STP, and the much publicized LSD. With these hallucinogenic drugs, whether natural or synthetic, come alteration of sensory perceptions: Colors may appear brighter and more vivid, sound may be intensified, stationary objects may move in various directions, and the faces of people may assume strange expressions or distortions. Some of these chemicals are extremely toxic to human beings and near-fatal doses are sometimes necessary to produce the sought-after hallucinations.

Because of their constant exposure in the mass media, many half-truths and distortions about the hallucinogenic drugs have been propagated. At one time LSD was believed to offer great help to schizophrenics, alcoholics, and other psychologically disturbed individuals. It was not as successful as first hoped, but many of the questions still unanswered will have to remain hidden for more years because of the government ban on human research with this drug. The ban was introduced partially because of the great scare over possible genetic damage from the ingestion of LSD. As noted in the conflicting articles included in this chapter, Alexander et al. (1967), Warkany and Takacs (1968), and Geber (1967), all of which appeared in *Science*, recent research with animals has continued to produce inconsistent results. These studies should be read thoughtfully and interpreted with caution. Often there have been insufficient control groups in these studies. Simply injecting large quantities of a drug into a pregnant animal does not prove conclusively that the drug caused the resulting deformed offspring. Care should be taken in ascribing cause–effect relationships and in generalizing the results to humans.

This chapter also includes the article by Schwarz (1968), who presents a review of the literature dealing with the complications of LSD. The study by Ditman et al. (1968) further attempts to elucidate the dimensions of the LSD experience as compared with Ritalin and Librium. Another hallucinogenic drug that is little known is found in morning glory seeds. In their article, Matheson and Thomas (1969) find that this drug increases the motor activity in chickens. Similar results were also found using rats in a later study (Matheson and Levinson, 1969).

## REFERENCES

Matheson, D. W., and Levinson, D. *Drug motivated behavior: the effect of morning glory seeds on motor activity of chicks and rats.* Paper presented at Western Psychological Association Convention, Vancouver, B.C., Canada, June 1969.

# 21

## *The Complications of LSD: A Review of the Literature**

CONRAD J. SCHWARZ

While some would insist that all the symptoms of lysergic acid diethylamide (LSD) are in fact complications in that they involve an alteration of the mental state from normal, the present paper will restrict itself to a more limited definition. A complication is defined as an unplanned sequel to administration of the drug, having deleterious effects on the mental or physical health of the subject or those around him.

The material will be presented in as strict chronological order as possible, and this will involve some degree of repetition. The review is felt to be extensive, but by no means exhaustive. It has been achieved by following up specific medical references to the complications of LSD and by culling from that portion of the literature which has come to attention in the course of reading about the drug.

In retrospect, the first person to suggest dangers in the use of LSD appears to have been Hofman (1943) (42). After accidentally ingesting some of the drug while manufacturing it in his laboratory, he experienced a variety of peculiar mental phenomena which led him to fear at one point that he was going insane.

Over the next 12 years, about 80 papers were published on the subject of LSD, mainly dealing with animal and biochemical studies. However, even after only limited human experimentation, the first serious warning about the drug was given in 1955 by Elkes, Elkes, and Mayer-Gross (15). Basing their observations on use of the drug with normal volunteers and on reliable reports from colleagues, these authors pointed out that the subject under the influence of LSD could be a danger to himself and others and that early psychotic conditions might be aggravated by it. They also stated that a "delayed and exceptionally severe response may take place and be followed by serious after effects lasting several days" (15, p. 719). They urged that until more was known about the drug its use should be restricted to inpatients and even then only when constant supervision by trained personnel was available.

Cooper (1955) followed this up with a letter to the same journal citing his observations on eight patients. He reported that in the acute phase "sometimes dream-like situations were acted out violently" (11, p. 1078). He described in detail some of the reactions which occurred more than 24 hours after administration of LSD. These included mood swings occurring 2 or 3 days later,

From the *Journal of Nervous and Mental Disease,* Vol. 146, No. 2, February 1968, pp. 174–186. 

* Paper read at the annual meeting of the North Pacific Society of Psychiatry and Neurology, Vancouver, B.C., April 6–8, 1967.

childish regression 1 week later, and preoccupation and absent-mindedness persisting for weeks afterwards. Insomnia was described as "a great difficulty" and it was pointed out that adverse reactions were particularly likely to occur when the individual was relaxing for sleep. He also noted that the reactions could begin again after an apparent return to normal behavior.

The first mention of the dangers of extramedical administration was made by Savage (1956), who referred to a woman who became suicidal after taking the drug informally. He also stated that "the average subject was unable to judge when the effect of the drug had terminated. After he considered himself recovered, he might get a renewed or secondary effect of the drug" (37, p. 38).

Martin (1957), reporting on a series of 50 patients attending a day hospital for LSD treatments, mentioned that two of these had "a violent reaction on their first and second treatments, thus rendering them unsuitable for day-patient treatment" (32, p. 189), but no further details were given.

Savage (1957) was the first to describe a suicide in connection with LSD. This occurred in a schizophrenic girl who had been sick for 10 years and who was being treated with LSD weekly. The treatment apparently "mobilized tremendous rage and resentment against both her parents and myself. At this time, unfortunately, she was allowed to go home on a visit, where she borrowed the family car and threw herself under a train. While LSD mobilized feelings and affects which had been successfully handled by nihilistic delusions, it also mobilized the supreme resistance: suicide" (38, p. 436). In the same paper, Savage described another case of a woman outpatient who required 4 days of hospitalization for depression during her course of LSD treatment, which she subsequently discontinued.

Lewis and Sloane (1958) reported a "catastrophic breakdown of defences with fear of impending ego dissolution" (25, p. 24) in two of their normal volunteer controls who also happened to be psychiatrists. Both of them had moderately severe paranoid reactions which were only partially responsive to intravenous amobarbital. One of them felt out of touch with reality for several days afterwards. The authors also reported the recurrence of LSD experiences for some time after the administration, and they felt that "the severity of some reactions precludes that use of the drug in out-patient work." Rather prophetically, they concluded "the use of such a drug might seem to raise almost as many problems as it solves" (25, p. 30).

Eisner and Cohen (1958) (13) reported that they had also noted a "spontaneous occurrence" of LSD-like phenomena at varying intervals following treatment. In commenting on the danger of suicide, they stated that this appeared to be restricted to the higher dosage levels above 75 gamma and to an unfamiliarity with the drug. In this paper they reported that Stoll, who had been involved in the early investigation of LSD with Hofman, had in a personal communication to them reported two suicides in Europe, one of these occurring in a woman who was given the drug without her knowledge. They also noted that transient depressions could occur after LSD and they themselves had "indirectly observed" one case of "treatment precipitated psychosis." They also described an impairment of coordination, and one of their rules in using this drug was that patients should not drive immediately after the treatment. While they generally felt that the drug was safe in the proper hands, they insisted "It is self-evident that the drug should be administered only under medical supervision."

Klee and Weintraub (1959) described four cases of paranoid reactions lasting a few days in "normal" subjects given LSD. They linked these reactions with the previous personalities and emphasized the need for careful screening and handling of volunteers "since paranoid reactions following LSD may become prolonged" (22, p. 460).

Cohen (1960) (7) received replies from 44 out of 62 LSD researchers whom he questioned about the incidence of complications. He estimated that the replies referred to a total of about 25,000 LSD treatments administered to 5,000 individuals. Combining the replies to the questionnaire with a survey of the literature, Cohen reported the following:

1. Adverse reactions during the LSD treatment included unmanageability, disrobing, accidental self-injury, panic episodes, frightening dissociation, acute hyperactive paranoid state, severe physical complaints, and severe catatonic states.
2. During the immediate post-LSD period, there could be a prolongation of the LSD state, with the persistence of anxiety or visual apparitions for another day or two in wavelike undulations. Short-lived depressions were also described during the immediate post-LSD period.
3. Suicide attempts were reported on five occasions by Sandison (two attempted drownings) and by Gillberti et al. (one [suicide report] each).
4. Completed suicides were also reported in five cases by Savage, Hoff (after two 30 gamma sessions), Janiger, Hartman (after one 50 gamma session), and Stoll. This seems to include only one of the two patients referred to by Stoll in the previous paper by Eisner and Cohen. However, Janiger's patient was not considered to be directly linked to LSD administration, since his death occurred 6 months afterwards and was due to nitrous oxide inhalation, to which the subject had been habituated for many years.
5. Prolonged psychosis was reported in eight cases by Hoch and Malitz, van Rhijn, Hoff, Cameron (who also reported a suicide attempt in the same patient), Janiger and Cohen (all one [suicide report] each), and by Sandison (two). All of these psychoses lasted over 48 hours.
6. One grand mal seizure was reported.

In a table in his article, Cohen gives the *estimated* rates of the major complications associated with LSD, but in a personal communication[1] he has indicated that this table was not related to the cases described in the text but utilized additional suicides and attempts, where details of dosage and circumstances were not given. Using this data, he estimated the rate of completed suicide after LSD was given in medical settings to be 0.4 per 1,000 patients. No suicides or attempts were reported in control volunteers given LSD, but psychotic reactions over 48 hours were estimated to occur in 0.8 per 1,000 control subjects, as opposed to 1.8 per 1,000 in patients.

Chandler and Hartman (1960) reported that "fluctuating feelings of well-being, mild euphoria, depression and anxiety can be uncomfortably pronounced

[1] Cohen, S. Personal communication, 1967.

for several hours to several weeks" (4, p. 289) after LSD sessions. They also reported one suicide in a woman after her first treatment with the drug. She had had a long history of alcoholism and narcotic addiction and had made three previous attempts at suicide. She had had extensive treatment previously, including 50 electroconvulsive therapy sessions, and even prior to taking LSD she confessed to the therapist that she intended to end her life that night anyway. Over the weekend following the LSD treatment, after an argument, her husband walked out of the house, leaving her alone all night. When he returned she was dead from a lethal dose of snail poison. These authors also reported one temporary psychosis lasting about 24 hours.

Ling and Buckman (1960), while insisting that the drug could be safely used on an outpatient basis in selected cases, reported one suicide attempt in a male patient "who discovered while feeling about two years old that his mother was a prostitute" (27, p. 45). They also report that the effects of the drug sometimes recurred during the 2 or 3 days following treatment, but their report is somewhat complicated by the fact that they used methedrine in combination with LSD. They warned that "people under 18 are usually too immature" (27, p. 43) for exposure to this drug.

Bierer and Browne (1960) reported "no accidents, except for one girl who committed suicide, not under the influence of LSD but impulsively in reaction to an unhappy love affair" (3, p. 931). No other details are given of this case. The authors, who were using LSD at times in combination with methedrine in a night hospital setting, felt in fact that they had "successfully supported a number of suicidal patients, including one who was a hopeless drug addict" (3, p. 931). This patient did eventually commit suicide a considerable time after LSD treatment had been discontinued.

By 1960, even the treatment of the complications seemed to be raising the possibility of further problems. Abramson et al. reported that oral chlorpromazine, the most commonly used antidote for LSD, produced in some instances "an apparently enhanced reaction to LSD" (1, p. 307). They reported that this effect was not produced by the parenteral administration of chlorpromazine.

Tenenbaum (1961) (43), reporting on electrocardiogram readings on 10 male character disorder patients who were in LSD group therapy, noted abnormalities consisting of T wave regression and S-T segment depression at times occurring without any increase in the heart rate.

Cohen and Ditman (1962), after referring to the 1960 survey, stated "recently we have encountered an increasing number of untoward events in connection with LSD 25 administration" (8, p. 161). They were now able to report on five individual cases of prolonged psychotic reaction in persons who had taken LSD in nonmedical settings or who had been unskillfully handled in therapy. They also reported some acting out behavior and commented on the illicit trafficking which was occurring in relation to the drug. They then went on to describe a "new but not rare entity" (8, p. 162), which they called multihabituation, referring to the frequent indulgence in a variety of stimulants, narcotics, sedatives, and hallucinogens.

Linton and Langs (1962) (28), using a subjective questionnaire on the day following LSD administration, reported the frequent occurrence of depression sufficiently severe to indicate the need for continued supervision of the subjects.

Malitz et al. (1962) noted "increased motor restlessness, mounting anxiety and brief intensification of visual hallucinations" (31, p. 190) following intravenous administration of chlorpromazine to terminate the LSD experience in experimental subjects.

Elkes (1963) pointed out that "delayed reactions may last for days or even weeks" (14, p. 196) after taking LSD. Such reactions included "changes in mood (predominantly depressive), perceptual distortions, depersonalization, confusional states, phobias, and acting out on ideas of reference."

Grinker (1963) in an editorial expressed some of the growing concern about the illicit use of LSD in the following terms:

> Latent psychotics are disintegrating under the influence of even single doses: long continued LSD experiences are subtly creating a psychopathology. Psychic addiction is being developed. . . . This editorial is a warning to the psychiatric profession that greater morbidity and even mortality is in store for its patients unless controls are developed against the unwise use of LSD-25. . . . The affective release interested many psychiatrists, who administered the drug to themselves and some who became enamored with the mystical hallucinatory state eventually in the "mystique" became disqualified as competent investigators (20, p. 425).

Cohen and Ditman (1963) (9) provided more detailed information about complications they had previously reported. Their cases of prolonged psychotic decompensation included one woman who was ill for 2 years after a single LSD treatment, a man ill for 2 years after 8 treatments, and a man ill for 7 months after 25 treatments. In addition, they reported one case of a 10-year-old boy ill for 1 month after accidentally ingesting a sugar cube coated with LSD, and another case of a man resistant to treatment after 200 to 300 illicit self-administrations. They also gave a case illustration of an 8-month agitated depression in a psychoanalyst who had taken one dose of LSD and a paranoid reaction in a psychologist who had taken three doses. The authors still felt, however, that "when properly employed, LSD is a relatively safe and important research tool," but they warned that "the imprudent, cursory use of LSD and allied drugs is unsafe and the complications that sometimes result retard their proper scientific study" (9, p. 480).

Ling and Buckman (1963) (26) reporting on their 4 years' experience with combined LSD and Ritalin in the treatment of 350 neuotics also felt the drug was safe if carefully used. In their series there was one suicide attempt, three patients were taken out of treatment because of the danger of suicide, and three patients were hospitalized for unspecific complications.

Sandison (1964) pointed out that "one of the principal dangers of treatment lies in the production of a drug-addicted sociopathic individual," but he felt that "this state of affairs can only occur when the treatment is not carefully and conscientiously supervised" (36, p. 35).

Geert-Jörgenson et al. (1964) (18) reported on a 3-year follow-up of 129 patients who had severe character disorders and for whom LSD was considered a "last chance" treatment. They stated that the "complications have been few and it seems absurd to tabulate them" (18, p. 375). However, they described one suicide several hours after administration of LSD and another patient who shot himself 6 months after his final treatment. The latter patient had seemed to be doing very well in the interval and the authors were convinced that his suicide had no immediate connection with the LSD treatment. Four patients who attempted suicide during the course of treatment were mentioned, but the authors felt that only one of these could be considered as a serious suicidal attempt. They stated "It is our impression that these suicidal reactions did not occur at times when the patients had been in states attributable to the LSD after-effects repercussions" (18, p. 376). This series included a case of homicide, which will be described in more detail shortly. The authors also reported "a few patients had brief episodes of after-effects repercussion several months after treatment, either in the form of a revival of the LSD seance or as a groundless fear involving no particular inconvenience" (18, p. 375).

Knudsen (1964) (23) described in detail the case of homicide mentioned above. The patient was a 25-year-old woman who had no family history of mental illness and who appeared to be normally adjusted up until about the age of 20, when she left Denmark to work in Norway as a domestic servant. While there. she apparently became involved with a psychopathic individual who influenced her toward heavy indulgence in drugs, alcohol, and sex. She received several hospitalizations during the next few years and was finally given five LSD treatments at spaced intervals. On the morning after her last treatment she left the hospital and fatally stabbed the psychopath, who had intermittently continued to influence her adversely during the previous 5 years. She had no recollection of the actual stabbing itself, but recalled events before and after. The report of the Medicolegal Council which ruled on her case stated, "It must be assumed that the treatment . . . decisively influenced the faculty of the accused for self-control and control of aggressive impulses" (23, p. 394), and she was committed to a mental hospital for further treatment.

Rosenthal (1964) (35) reported a case of "persistent hallucinoses" following repeated administration of hallucinogenic drugs. This occurred in a 23-year-old married female artist who had been briefly hospitalized at the age of 18 with hysterical seizures. She later had one therapy session with LSD and subsequently went on to administer LSD, mescaline, and psilocybin to herself on about 10 or 12 occasions. She developed increasing anxiety and "lost interest in life, in her marriage and in her work, in which she 'could not hope to approach' the experiences which she had had under the influence of the drugs" (35, p. 240). For 5 months after her last exposure to hallucinogenic drugs she experienced spontaneous hallucinations. She had some control over the pleasant ones, but not over the unpleasant ones, which included "terrifying involuntary illusions of people decomposing in the street in front of her" (35, p. 240). For 5 months after her last exposure and in spite of the fact that she had to be hospitalized for treatment of them, she still considered further use of these drugs. Rosenthal stated, "It is likely that many adverse reactions are unreported. . . .

More cases of this condition will occur because of the current fad of unsupervised consumption of hallucinogenic drugs in repeated doses" (35, p. 243).

Cole and Katz (1964) interpreted the state of the LSD controversy at that time as follows: "Rather than being the subject of careful scientific enquiry, these agents have become invested with an aura of magic offering creativity to the uninspired, 'kicks' to the jaded, emotional warmth to the cold and inhibited, and total personality reconstruction to the alcoholic or the psychotherapy-resistant chronic neurotic" (10, p. 758). They went on to point out that "indiscriminate, unsupervised use is clearly dangerous" and stated that there were "reports of insidious personality changes in individuals who have indulged in repeated self-administration" (10, p. 761). They also expressed concern over the possibility that "investigators who have embarked on serious scientific work in this area may have been subject to the deleterious and seductive effects of these agents" (10, p. 761).

Grinker (1964) in another editorial stated, "From experimental subjects there are increasing numbers of reports indicating that temporary or even permanent harm may be induced despite apparently careful pre-therapeutic screening of latent psychoses and careful precautions during the artificial psychoses." He concluded, "The drugs are indeed dangerous even when used under the best of precautions and conditions" (19, p. 768).

Levine and Ludwig (1964) (24) presented a plea for balanced objectivity in relation to the claims for and warnings against LSD. They stated, "The impression one tends to gain from reading many of the articles concerning LSD use is that the drug is fairly dangerous with rather serious complications, most of a mental nature." However, they feel that "in most of the reported cases no direct cause or relationship was established between LSD therapy and subsequent psychotic deterioration or suicide attempts." They concluded that "It would seem that the incidence statistics better support a statement that the drug is *exceptionally safe* rather than dangerous" (24, p. 318).

Cohen (1964) (5) discussed the increased incidence of complications as a result of the illicit use of LSD. He also considered in some detail the dangers to the therapist who becomes overly enthusiastic about the beneficial effects of the drug. He referred to therapists who have themselves suffered depressions and psychotic breakdowns, or have developed megalomaniacal ideas of grandeur, and he also mentioned one who committed suicide. He suggested that the causes of this "impressive morbidity in view of the relatively small number of American practitioners using the hallucinogens" (5, p. 218) might be related to pre-existing disturbances in personality or to adverse reactions due to self-administration of LSD.

Incidentally, Cohen in his book mentioned that during his 1960 survey of researchers using LSD there was one report of coronary occlusion occurring a few days after LSD. This was regarded as coincidental and it was pointed out that no physical complications had been observed in using the drug on debilitated alcoholics.

Downing (1964) (12) reported on his observations on 29 persons who attended the International Federation for Internal Freedom (IFIF) Psychedelic

Training Center at Zihuatenejo, Mexico, during the last 2 weeks before its enforced closure in June 1963. Despite the claim of Leary, the leader of this group, that there had been no problems in using psychedelic drugs in this type of setting, Downing reported that 1 of the 29 persons required psychiatric hospitalization directly from the Center, and that another was hospitalized for treatment of self-inflicted injuries.

Ludwig and Levine (1965) (30) presented information on the general patterns of hallucinogenic drug abuse obtained from intensive interviews of 27 narcotic drug addict inpatients who were being treated at the U.S. Public Health Service Hospital in Lexington, Kentucky. All of them had used hallucinogenic agents at one time or another. One of these patients became so frightened after his first exposure that he "ran his head into the wall to stop the experience, asked a friend to knock him out (the friend tried to cooperate) and later, on his way to the hospital, experienced homicidal impulses towards the cab-driver" (30, p. 96). The authors obtained undocumented reports of people acting out homosexual impulses or becoming more withdrawn, depressed, and paranoid when under the influence of these drugs. One patient reported that an acquaintance of his "tried to stab himself, since he believed himself to be invincible" (30, p. 96). Another tried to jump out of a window, believing that his body was weightless. There were also reports of people trying to walk on the sea and two of the patients themselves reported near accidents while driving under the influence of the drugs. One of the patients described the difference between heroin and the hallucinogens as follows: "You addict yourself with the hallucinogens, whereas heroin addicts you" (30, p. 95).

Savage and Stolaroff (1965) pointed out that "by far the greatest damage has been caused by the illicit use of the hallucinogens" (39, p. 220). They felt that the complications of these drugs arose from improper use due to (a) inadequate preparation of the subject; (b) improper support to the subject; (c) too frequent use of LSD; (d) improper handling of patients; (e) improper dosage; and (f) over-enthusiastic response.

Frosch et al. (1965) described in detail 12 out of 27 patients admitted to Bellevue Hospital with the complications of LSD during a 4-month period. They categorized the complications as being panic reactions with a good prognosis, usually resulting in discharge in 1 to 3 days, reappearance of symptoms up to 1 year after multiple exposures to the drug, and extended psychosis in long-standing schizophrenics who had taken the drug illicitly. The last two categories had a poor prognosis and all 6 patients in these categories "showed some impairment of performance at the time of our last contact with them" (17, p. 1238). One of their patients jumped out of a window, and they emphasized the danger of bodily injury under the influence of the drug, because a person may believe himself to be invulnerable to harm and take unwarranted risks, as several of the patients with panic reactions did.

Cohen (1966) felt that "complications to the extra-legal use of LSD have increased so rapidly that it is now possible to propose a more complete classification of untoward reactions" (6, p. 182). Case descriptions accompanied most of the categories, which are as follows:

## PSYCHOTIC DISORDERS

1. Accidental LSD intoxication in children characterized by anxiety and visual illusions lasting several weeks.
2. Chronic LSD intoxication with ataxia, slurred speech, and incoordination.
3. Schizophrenic reactions occurring in schizoid individuals or ambulatory schizophrenics.
4. Paranoia with relatively appropriate thought processes, except in the area of megalomaniacal delusions.
5. Acute paranoid states usually occurring during the LSD experience itself and involving danger to the subject or to others around him. One death is reported in a young man who stepped into the traffic and tried to stop it and another death in an individual who drowned. Another man drove through traffic convinced that he could change the red lights by concentrating on them. In another case two men took LSD together; one of them was beaten up by the other, subsequently jumped or was thrown out of a fourth-floor window and suffered multiple injuries.
6. Prolonged or intermittent LSD-like psychoses.
7. Psychotic depressions usually associated with agitation and anxiety.

## NONPSYCHOTIC DISORDERS

1. Chronic anxiety reactions associated with depression, somatic symptoms, difficulty in functioning, and a recurrence of LSD-like symptoms such as time distortion, visual alterations, and body image changes for weeks or months.
2. Acute panic states with a potential to self-injury.
3. Dyssocial behavior, involving a complete loss of previously held values and ideas, loss of motivation to study or work, and indulgence in "pseudo-philosophic jargon."
4. Antisocial behavior, involving obliteration of cultural values of good and bad and society's rules of right and wrong, especially in individuals with a previously attenuated moral code.

## NEUROLOGICAL REACTIONS

1. Convulsions, not observed by Cohen but reported by Sandison (one case) and by Baker (five convulsions in 150 patients).
2. Permanent brain damage. This has not yet been demonstrated, but in a personal communication to Cohen, Adey reported prolonged electroencephalographic changes in cats given large amounts of LSD. Cohen suggested that a number of human beings have ingested massive amounts and some of these may in future show brain damage. He also pointed out that the "purity of the illicit LSD is open to question and nothing is known about the toxicity of possible contaminants" (6).

Cohen concluded that "It must be explicitly stated that some individuals should never take drugs of this category and one's friends are not suitable judges of suitable candidates. Furthermore, a secure environment is essential for the patient or the subject who takes LSD, since he is now vulnerable, hypersuggestible and emotionally labile" (6, p. 186).

Rinkel (1966), who had introduced LSD to the United States in 1949, stated that the "dangers are many times multiplied by their illegitimate use. Persons who have taken LSD obtained on the black market become psychotic often weeks or months after the ingestion of LSD. They are being admitted to hospital in an ever-increasing number" (34, p. 1415). He also pointed out that "the cult aspect of the LSD movement has rendered serious damage to the scientific studying of this group of drugs" (34, p. 1416).

Pos (1966), reporting on 24 patients treated over a 3-year period with a total of 56 LSD sessions, felt that "the events of the LSD-25 sessions could not be predicted on the basis of pre-LSD-25 experience with the patient" (33, p. 341), even though the patient had been in intensive psychotherapy. He reported one questionable suicidal attempt during an LSD session and one attempt by jumping out of a window 6 hours after LSD administration.

The American Psychiatric Association produced a position statement on LSD at the meeting of the Council on June 12, 1966, in which it stated "The indiscriminate consumption of this hazardous drug can and not infrequently does lead to destructive physiological and personality changes" (2, p. 353).

Ungerleider et al. (1966) pointed out that "some preparations claimed to be LSD contain impurities, particularly atropine-like compounds" (45, p. 389). They presented a study of 70 patients attending the emergency room at one of the Los Angeles hospitals during a 7-month period. All were showing complications after having taken illicit LSD. The commonest presenting symptoms were hallucinations (29 percent), anxiety (24 percent), depression (21 percent) and confusion (20 percent). A number had exposed themselves to a variety of hallucinogenic agents, but 40 percent had taken only LSD and 29 percent had taken it only once. A total of 66 percent had taken the drug over 1 week before admission to the hospital. Of these 70 patients, 25 required psychiatric hospitalization and 17 were in the hospital over 1 month. The authors raised a question about chlorpromazine being able to reverse the symptoms and described in detail one case which was resistant to up to 2,000 mg of chlorpromazine daily, together with trifluoperazine. They concluded that their findings seemed to contradict statements implying that the complications of LSD are infrequent.

Fink et al. (1966) (16) estimated that 40 percent of the prolonged reactions reported in the literature had not improved at the time of the reports, some of which extended up to 2 years after exposure. In their own series of 158 administrations to 65 chronic hospitalized psychotics, they reported prolonged reactions lasting up to 3 months in 3 patients (2 percent). These reactions occurred in patients who had a phasic history of a schizo-affective type of illness before LSD. The post-LSD picture was one of exacerbation and exaggeration of previous symptoms, with a superimposed confusional, delirious state. One of these patients made a suicidal attempt and 2 of the cases were unresponsive to high doses of chlorpromazine.

Scher (1966), in an interesting if somewhat anecdotal review of patterns and profiles of addiction and drug abuse in Chicago, pointed out that "the abuser of LSD will, in the course of time, tend to develop paranoid ideas. One of the most frequent paranoid impressions is that everyone around the user except himself is homosexual" (40, p. 547). He also pointed out that the illicit synthesis of LSD may be "dangerous to the manufacturers, who are usually in a semi-stupor from the very process of manufacture" (40, p. 547).

Louria (1966) stated that LSD "must be listed as one of the most dangerous drugs in the pharmacopeia of man" (29, p. 47). He referred to one case of homicide in which a former medical student killed his mother-in-law while under the influence of the drug and had no recollection of his action. He described various types of disturbed behavior in approximately 100 patients admitted to one New York hospital in a 13-month period. He also stated, "There is no doubt that even apparently well-adjusted persons can be thrown into an acute psychosis requiring days or weeks of hospitalization. This is true even in the hands of an experienced physician who carefully selects his patients" (29, p. 49).

Keeler and Reifler (1967) (21) described in detail a case of suicide under the influence of LSD which they felt would not have occurred in this particular individual had he not been in a toxic state. The case was that of a 20-year-old college undergraduate, who disrobed and jumped out of a window to his death while under the influence of self-administered LSD, taken when in the company of several other people who were also taking LSD. The young man had been a part of the LSD subculture for several months, during which he had become preoccupied about the homosexual feelings which were frequently brought out and discussed in the group meetings. He seemed to withdraw somewhat and his academic work deteriorated, with irregular class attendance. However, a few days prior to his death he discussed plans for the immediate and distant future with his friends. He "took LSD in the company of others, was observed to pace in and out of the room in which the others were and, without explanation, while by himself disrobed and took his life" (21, p. 885). The authors concluded, "The circumstances strongly suggest that he would not have died at the time he did if he were not in a state of LSD intoxication" (21, p. 885).

Ungerleider and Fisher (1967) (44) reported on a wide range of complications observed by themselves. These included grand mal seizures in a previously nonepileptic person and persistence of episodic recurrences up to 1 year after ingestion. They described one young man who was prevented from throwing his girl friend off a hotel roof under the delusion that he had to offer a human sacrifice after having taken his first LSD trip. They also commented on researchers, themselves LSD users, who "become so enthusiastic that they even refused to consider psychosis and suicide as bad results" (44, p. 51). They pointed out that the occurrence of either acute or chronic side effects cannot be predicted by psychiatric interviews and psychological testing and stated, "Some of the worst reactions have been in persons, often physicians and other professionals, who appeared stable by every indicator" (44, p. 51). These authors also gave several instances of marked changes in personality and values in relation to current social standards.

Schwarz (1967) (41) reported two cases of paradoxical responses to chlorpromazine after LSD. In one case, intravenous chlorpromazine given to terminate an LSD-25 session precipitated a subjective and objective exacerbation of the

LSD phenomena. This patient showed a milder but similar response to oral chlorpromazine the day after. In the other case, a student who had been experiencing spontaneous recurrences for 3 weeks after taking LSD illicitly reported that oral chlorpromazine given to counteract these seemed to precipitate them again. The author discussed possible psychological and biochemical explanations of this phenomenon and suggested that it raises the suspicion that LSD or some metabolite might be present in the brain some time after ingestion of the drug.

## DISCUSSIONS

It should be emphasized that this review of the complications of LSD covers only the medical literature on the subject. Many other reports of adverse reactions are available in the lay press, particularly in relation to the informal use of the drug.

It should be obvious that the total number of incidents mentioned in this paper cannot be taken to indicate any kind of absolute figures. It can be assumed that additional complicated cases, including fatalities, have occurred but have not been reported in either the medical or lay press. No statistical analysis can be attempted, but some general impressions appear justified from the above review.

1. The acute intoxicated state carries risk of acting out in a manner dangerous to the subject or others.
2. For several days after ingestion of LSD, anxiety, depression, or paranoid thinking can occur even in normal control subjects.
3. Spontaneous recurrences some time after ingestion are often mentioned and appear to constitute a common complication of LSD. These phenomena still require explanation, but the apparent precipitation of a similar recurrence by the administration of another chemical compound (chlorpromazine), if supported by observation, should encourage further investigation of the possibility of a continuing process with a biochemical basis.
4. Prolonged mental illnesses, including persistent anxiety, depression, psychosis, and personality deterioration toward a nonactivist role in society have all been reported.
5. Definite physical effects from LSD have not been proven, but there are several slight indices of suspicion in this area. Prolonged electroencephalogram changes have been reported in cats. Epileptic convulsions have been observed in humans. Mildly significant electrocardiogram changes suggestive of coronary insufficiency have been recorded in the only study which could be found using this test. One coronary occlusion has been reported several days after LSD.

In view of the reported complications which might arise in the use of LSD, steps to prevent these are given frequent emphasis in the literature. The recommendations generally follow the classical lines of (a) careful selection of subjects, (b) attention to the setting, (c) safe dosage, and (d) follow-up of subjects. Taken in isolation, each of these criteria appears to harbor some as yet undefined aspect in relation to this particular drug.

Careful selection of the subjects, including detailed knowledge of their backgrounds, psychological testing, and even psychotherapy interviews, does not appear to guarantee freedom from complications.

Attention to the setting does not seem to eliminate the dangers entirely, and complications are reported in a wide variety of medical, research, and informal situations. The setting, however, would appear to be an important factor in the management of adverse reactions when these do arise.

Dosage criteria are also questionable, since one suicide has been reported after two 30-gamma sessions, and one after one 50-gamma session.

Careful follow-up appears to have loopholes in that spontaneous recurrences have an out-of-the-blue character which makes their prediction almost impossible.

Certainly careful attention to *all* four criteria, i.e. subject, setting, dosage, and after-care, will minimize the risks, but the use of LSD would appear to carry an innate unpredictability which makes it a difficult drug to use even in medical settings. This does not make its medical use unjustifiable, since, in the first place, trained personnel and appropriate facilities are available to deal with complications and, secondly, any medical procedure carries a certain risk of morbidity and even mortality. Thus a suicide rate of 0.4 per 1,000 psychiatric patients given LSD, even though it is four times the average suicide rate in the U.S.A. (46), might not be unexpected, particularly in view of the severity of the cases treated.

Such a figure does, however, assume graver significance when it is realized that a number of severely disturbed people and borderline psychiatric patients find self-medication with LSD attractive. In addition to the rejection of the first criterion of control (careful subject selection), the other three criteria (setting, dosage, and after-care) often receive only ineffectual lip service. Finally, there is often a refusal on the part of the user to acknowledge the unpredictability of his own reaction to a substance which he has never ingested before and of which he has only the scantiest knowledge. There is a blind faith in whatever the LSD pusher says about the reliability of an illicitly manufactured chemical which is offered around in a wide variety of sizes, forms, and colors. It is interesting to note that one of the chief characteristics of the LSD reaction, suggestibility, is obvious in some individuals even before they have purchased the drug.

In conclusion, while the therapeutic value of LSD-25 must remain a subject of debate for the time being, there would appear to be little doubt that the informal use of this drug is dangerous.

## REFERENCES

1. Abramson, H. A., Rolo, A., and Stache, J. Lysergic acid diethylamide (LSD-25) antagonists: Chlorpromazine. *J. Neuropsychiat.*, **1**: 307–310, 1960.
2. American Psychiatric Association. Position Statement on LSD. *Amer. J. Psychiat.*, **123**: 353, 1966.
3. Bierer, J., and Browne, I. W. An experiment with a psychiatric night hospital. *Proc. Roy. Soc. Med.*, **53**: 46–50, 1960.
4. Chandler, A. L., and Hartman, M. A. Lysergic acid diethylamide (LSD-25)

as a facilitating agent in psychotherapy. *Arch. Gen. Psychiat.*, **2**: 286–299, 1960.

5. Cohen, S. *The Beyond Within: The LSD Story*. Atheneum Press, New York, 1964.
6. Cohen, S. A classification of LSD complications. *Psychosomatics*, **7**: 182–186, 1966.
7. Cohen, S. Lysergic acid diethylamide: Side effects and complications. *J. Nerv. Ment. Dis.*, **130**: 30–40, 1960.
8. Cohen, S., and Ditman, K. S. Complications associated with lysergic acid diethylamide (LSD-25). *J.A.M.A.*, **181**: 161–162, 1962.
9. Cohen, S., and Ditman, K. S. Prolonged adverse reactions to lysergic acid diethylamide. *Arch. Gen. Psychiat.*, **8**: 475–480, 1963.
10. Cole, J. O., and Katz, M. M. The psychotomimetic drugs. *J.A.M.A.*, **187**: 758–761, 1964.
11. Cooper, H. A. Hallucinogenic drugs. *Lancet*, **268**: 1078–1079, 1955.
12. Downing, J. J. Zihuatanejo: An experiment in transpersonative living. In Blum, R., ed. *Utopiates: The Use and Users of LSD-25*, pp. 142–177. Atherton Press, New York, 1964.
13. Eisner, B. J., and Cohen, S. Psychotherapy with lysergic acid diethylamide. *J. Nerv. Ment. Dis.*, **127**: 528–539, 1958.
14. Elkes, J. The dysleptics: Note on a no man's land. *Compr. Psychiat.*, **4**: 195–198, 1963.
15. Elkes, C., Elkes, J., and Mayer-Gross, W. Hallucinogenic drugs. *Lancet*, **268**: 719, 1955.
16. Fink, M., Simeon, J., Hawue, W., and Itil, T. Prolonged adverse reactions to LSD in psychotic subjects. *Arch. Gen. Psychiat.*, **15**: 450–454, 1966.
17. Frosch, W. A., Robbins, E. S., and Stern, M. Untoward reactions to lysergic acid diethylamide (LSD) resulting in hospitalization. *New Eng. J. Med.*, **273**: 1235–1239, 1965.
18. Geert-Jörgensen, E., Hertz, M., Knudsen, K., and Kristensen, K. LSD-treatment: Experience gained within a three-year period. *Acta Psychiat. Scand.*, **40**: 373–382, 1964.
19. Grinker, R. R., Bootlegged ecstasy. *J.A.M.A.*, **187**: 768, 1964.
20. Grinker, R. R. Lysergic acid diethylamide. *Arch. Gen. Psychiat.*, **8**: 425, 1963.
21. Keeler, M. H., and Reifler, C. B. Suicide during an LSD reaction. *Amer. J. Psychiat.*, **123**: 884–885, 1967.
22. Klee, G. D., and Weintraub, W. Paranoid reactions following lysergic acid diethylamide (LSD-25). In Bradley, P. B., Demicker, P. and Radauco-Thomas, C., eds. *Neuro-psychopharmacology*, pp. 457–460. Elsevier, Princeton, N. J., 1959.
23. Knudsen, K. Homicide after treatment with lysergic acid diethylamide. *Acta Psychiat. Scand.*, **40** (Suppl. 180): 389–395, 1964.
24. Levine, J., and Ludwig, A. M. The LSD controversy. *Compr. Psychiat.*, **5**: 314–321, 1964.
25. Lewis, D. J., and Sloane, R. B. Therapy with lysergic acid diethylamide. *J. Clin. Exp. Psychopath.*, **9**: 19–31, 1958.
26. Ling, T. M., and Buckman, J. *Lysergic Acid (LSD-25) and Ritalin in the Treatment of Neurosis*. Lombardo Press, London, 1963.
27. Ling, T. M. and Buckman, J. The use of lysergic acid in individual psychotherapy. *Proc. Roy. Soc. Med.*, **53**: 43–45, 1960.
28. Linton, H. B., and Langs, R. J. Subjective reactions to lysergic acid diethyl-

amide (LSD-25) measured by a questionnaire. *Arch. Gen. Psychiat.*, **6**: 352–368, 1962.
29. Louria, D. *Nightmare Drugs.* Pocket Books, New York, 1966.
30. Ludwig, A. M., and Levine, J. Patterns of hallucinogenic drug abuse. *J.A.M.A.*, **191**: 92–96, 1965.
31. Malitz, S., Wilkins, B., and Escover, R. A comparison of drug-induced hallucinations with those seen in spontaneously occurring psychoses. In West, L. J., ed. *Hallucinations*, pp. 187–190. Grune & Stratton, New York, 1962.
32. Martin, A. J. LSD (lysergic acid diethylamide) treatment of chronic psychoneurotic patients under day-hospital conditions. *J. Soc. Psychiat.*, **3**: 188–195, 1957.
33. Pos, R. LSD-25 as an adjunct to long-term psychotherapy. *Canad. Psychiat. Ass. J.*, **11**: 330–342, 1966.
34. Rinkel, M. Psychedelic drugs. *Amer. J. Psychiat.*, **122**: 1415–1416, 1966.
35. Rosenthal, S. H. Persistent hallucinosis following repeated administration of hallucinogenic drugs. *Amer. J. Psychiat.*, **121**: 238–244, 1964.
36. Sandison, R. A. Hallucinogens. *Practitioner*, **192**: 30–36, 1964.
37. Savage, C. The LSD psychosis as a transaction between the psychiatrist and patient. In Cholden, L., ed. *Lysergic Acid Diethylamide and Mescaline in Experimental Psychiatry*, pp. 35–43. Grune & Stratton, New York, 1956.
38. Savage, C. The resolution and subsequent remobilization of resistance by LSD in psychotherapy. *J. Nerv. Ment. Dis.*, **125**: 434–437, 1957.
39. Savage, C., and Stolaroff, M. J. Clarifying the confusion regarding LSD-25. *J. Nerv. Ment. Dis.*, **140**: 218–221, 1965.
40. Scher, J. Patterns and profiles of addiction and drug abuse. *Arch. Gen. Psychiat.*, **15**: 539–551, 1966.
41. Schwarz, C. J. Paradoxical responses to chlorpromazine after LSD. *Psychosomatics*, **8**: 210–211, 1967.
42. Stoll, W. A. LSD-25: A hallucinatory agent of the ergot group. *Swiss Arch. Neurol.*, **60**: 279–323, 1947.
43. Tenenbaum, B. Group therapy with LSD-25. *Dis. Nerv. Syst.*, **22**: 459–462, 1961.
44. Ungerleider, J. T., and Fisher, D. D. The problems of LSD-25 and emotional disorder. *Calif. Med.*, **106**: 49–55, 1967.
45. Ungerleider, J. T., Fisher, D. D., and Fuller, M. The dangers of LSD. *J.A.M.A.*, **197**: 389–392, 1966.
46. United States Public Health Service. *Mortality Trends in U.S.A., 1954–63.* Publication 1000, Series 20, Number 2. U.S. Government Printing Office, Washington, D.C., 1964.

# 22

## *Dimensions of the LSD, Methylphenidate, and Chlordiazepoxide Experiences*

KEITH S. DITMAN, THELMA MOSS,
EDWARD W. FORGY, LEONARD M. ZUNIN,
ROBERT D. LYNCH, WAYNE A. FUNK

A great deal has been written about the importance of "set and setting" in producing the therapeutic LSD experience, whether it be of transcendental, cathartic, or abreactive nature (Abramson, 1967; Ling and Buckman, 1963; Malitz, 1966; Savage, et al., 1964, Schoen, 1964). Much less has been written about the therapeutic methylphenidate (Ritalin) experience (Ling and Buckman, 1963), and almost nothing about chlordiazepoxide (Librium) therapy except as an anti-anxiety agent. It surely can be appreciated that the three drugs have different pharmacological properties: LSD is probably the most famous of the psychedelics; methylphenidate is considered a mild stimulant; and chlordiazepoxide one of the newer long-acting sedatives. Ostensibly these drugs, having markedly different pharmacological properties, should produce different psychological effects even when administered in the same environment.

But in deference to the power of the ubiquitous "placebo effect," the question arises: What would be the effects of these drugs in a double-blind study when neither doctors nor subjects know which drug is being administered, *and* when the subjects are oriented only to expect the LSD experience? In other words, would an intravenous injection of a substance *thought to be LSD* produce an LSD reaction, when the "set and setting" remained identical for all subjects—even though the drug were not the expected LSD but at times methylphenidate or chlordiazepoxide? The answer to this question became an adjunctive part of our controlled study to evaluate LSD as a therapeutic agent in the treatment of alcoholism. There have been several encouraging reports about LSD as an effective drug with alcoholics (Abramson, 1967; Kurlander, et al., 1967; O'Reilly and Funk, 1964; Belden and Hitchen, 1963, but very few studies have been reported with control groups, the most outstanding being by Ables and Eng (1967); and there is no large completed double-blind study to our knowledge.

## METHOD

To determine the response to LSD as distinct from the other two drugs, we treated 99 men, all of whom were at an alcoholism rehabilitation camp in

From a research study, supported by Public Health Service Research Grant No. MH-11272 from the National Institute of Mental Health and the Vista Hill Psychiatric Foundation. Reprinted by permission of the author.

California.* The men who volunteered for treatment were selected after a comprehensive screening procedure, which included psychological testing, psychiatric evaluation, and physical examination to eliminate severe depressives, psychotics, chronic drug users (including any history of LSD usage), mental retardates, and those with hazardous physical disabilities. The qualified volunteers were assigned to one of three drug treatments (200 mg of LSD, 75 mg of methylphenidate, or 75 mg of chlordiazepoxide), on a random basis. Methylphenidate was chosen as one control treatment because it could mimic some of the effects of LSD in this dose range; and chlordiazepoxide as the other because it is a long-acting sedative, and therefore a good contrast for the other two drugs. In addition, all three drugs could be injected intravenously. Neither treatment doctors, volunteer helpers, nor subjects knew which drug was administered, or how many drugs were involved in the study. The administrant physician did not participate in the treatment, but was available for possible emergencies or drug complications which might have necessitated breaking the drug code. (No such emergency occurred.) All subjects were given an orientation talk which made them familiar with the wide variety of experiences they might encounter with LSD. Questions from the subjects as to the administration of drugs other than LSD were handled by describing the many possible effects of LSD. The use of drugs other than LSD was denied by the investigators.

To measure their drug experiences, the subjects were given the DWM Card Sort (Ditman et al., 1968) both *before* the therapy session in order to assess the expectancies of the men regarding the approaching drug session, and again *after* the session to determine what, in fact, the men had experienced on their treatment day. The DWM Card Sort consists of 156 descriptive statements chosen to represent most aspects of the LSD experience. These 156 items are classified into 7 categories:

1. Strong Pleasant Emotions (21 items)
2. Self Understanding (20 items)
3. Religious or Mystical Feelings (14 items)
4. Parapsychological Sensations (10 items)
5. Sensory and Perceptual Alterations (52 items)
6. Strong Unpleasant Emotions (29 items)
7. Evaluation of the Experience (10 items)

Each item was rated by each subject on a 5 point scale, by being placed into one of 5 piles, each pile being rated as follows:

1. Very Much Like the Experience
2. A Little Like the Experience
3. Neither Like nor Unlike the Experience
4. A Little Unlike the Experience
5. Very Much Unlike the Experience

In this paper only the post-treatment data are presented. With these data, using one-way analysis of variance, it was possible to learn if there were statis-

* Viejas Treatment Center, San Diego County Department of Honor Camps, San Diego, California.

**TABLE 1. Number of Significant Differences of *t*-Tests Between Pairs of Drugs**

| *Pairs of Drugs* | *p* <.05 | *p* <.01 | *p* <.001 |
|---|---|---|---|
| LSD vs. M | 52 | 46 | 32 |
| LSD vs. C | 82 | 40 | 35 |
| M vs. C | 42 | 20 | 9 |

tically significant differences between the LSD, methylphenidate, and chlordiazepoxide experiences.

## RESULTS

To our astonishment, the analysis of the variance of the 156 items gave 96 *F*-ratios beyond the .05 level, 69 beyond the .01 level, and 47 beyond the .001 level of significance. Clearly, in this double-blind study where "set and setting" remained constant for all subjects, the placebo effect did not override the specific psychopharmacological effects of the 3 drugs in this population of alcoholics.

By contrasting pairs of the 3 drug groups (via *t*-tests) we find that the 3 drugs are not equally different from each other. LSD differed significantly from the other 2 drugs on considerably more items, particularly where extreme differences (beyond the .001 level) are noted. See Table I above. (In this, and all other tables, *M* is the abbreviation for methylphenidate and C for chlordiazepoxide.)

As might be expected, LSD far outranked the other drugs in the category of Perceptual and Sensory Distortions. This category contains 3 subgroups: Visual, Somatic, and Other Distortions. The means of the LSD group on all 10 Visual Distortion items differed from the other drugs beyond the .01 level of significance—and 9 of the items beyond the .001 level. (See Table 2 below. Please note that in this, and all other tables, means are computed from the

**TABLE 2. Visual Distortions**

| *p* | *Statement* | *Mean Position of the 3 Drugs* | | |
|---|---|---|---|---|
| | | *M* | *LSD* | *C* |
| *P* < .001 | Walls or other objects seemed to be breathing. | 4.70 | 2.63 | 4.52 |
| | The walls and floors moved and flowed. | 4.30 | 2.33 | 4.38 |
| | With my eyes closed I saw multicolor moving designs. | 4.23 | 2.03 | 3.93 |
| | Objects seemed to glow around the edges. | 4.40 | 2.48 | 4.17 |
| | Colors seemed brighter. | 3.50 | 1.95 | 3.28 |
| | I had "X-ray" vision. | 4.70 | 3.48 | 4.46 |
| | Other peoples' faces seemed to become changing masks. | 4.43 | 3.05 | 4.21 |
| | My eyesight seemed blurred. | 3.60 | 2.60 | 3.86 |
| | I saw music. | 4.30 | 2.98 | 4.00 |
| *P* < .01 | I kept seeing things after I'd stopped looking at them. | 4.37 | 3.25 | 3.79 |

**TABLE 3. Somatic Distortions**

| *P* | *Statement* | *Mean Position of the 3 Drugs* | | |
|---|---|---|---|---|
| | | *M* | *LSD* | *C* |
| $P < .001$ | My "I" or "Self" seemed to leave my body. | 4.27 | 2.30 | 4.24 |
| | I felt like I was floating in space. | 3.17 | 1.93 | 4.31 |
| | I felt like I was shaking or trembling. | 2.30 | 2.35 | 4.14 |
| | One side of my body felt different from the other side. | 4.40 | 3.13 | 4.48 |
| | I had peculiar sensations on my skin at times. | 3.53 | 2.50 | 4.17 |
| | I became another object or person and yet remained myself. | 3.86 | 2.53 | 3.96 |
| | My body seemed to change size all on its own. | 4.43 | 3.25 | 4.35 |
| | My body seemed to grow younger or older all on its own. | 4.57 | 3.45 | 4.35 |
| | I felt paralyzed. | 4.33 | 3.53 | 4.59 |
| | I felt unsteady and uneasy. | 2.60 | 2.65 | 3.89 |
| $P < .01$ | This was like a bad (alcohol) hangover. | 3.57 | 3.03 | 4.38 |
| | I had nausea, headache or other physical pain which dominated the experience. | 3.93 | 3.43 | 4.55 |
| | My hands and feet felt light, or like they were not attached to my body. | 3.77 | 2.90 | 3.97 |
| | I felt choked or found it hard to breathe. | 3.77 | 3.25 | 4.41 |

5-point scale ratings, where 1 equals "Very Much Like the Experience" and 5 equals "Very Much Unlike the Experience.")

Turning to the subcategory of Somatic Distortions (21 items), LSD again outranked the other drugs—but not exclusively, as Table 3 illustrates, since occasionally methylphenidate either outranks or challenges LSD, as in the items: *I felt as if I were floating in space; I felt like I was shaking or trembling, etc.*

On the third subcategory (Other Sensory and Perceptual Distortions, consisting of 15 items) 11 statements evoked significantly different drug reactions. Table 4 reveals that again LSD far outranked the other drugs on 6 of these items, such as: *My sense of smell became more acute,* and *Everything seemed too bright, too harsh, too loud.* However, methylphenidate was also predominant in such items as: *My mind was flooded with thoughts; I can remember very clearly everything that happened to me during the experience; My thoughts kept shifting rapidly from one idea to another*—items all characteristic of strong mental activity. Chlordiazepoxide produced significantly less intense mood swings than the other drugs; its only distinction in this category.

Similar to Perceptual and Sensory Distortions is the small (6 items) category, Illusions or Hallucinations. Again we find, not surprisingly, that LSD elicited far more intense reactions than the other drugs on 4 of the 6 statements. See Table 5.

Turning now to another area of experience, Mystical or Religious Sensations (14 items), we find that 6 of these statements show a significant difference at the .01 level or beyond. These are listed in Table 6 and show again that LSD produced far stronger sensations of this nature than the other drugs—which

**TABLE 4. Other Sensory and Perceptual Distortions**

| *P* | *Statement* | *Mean Position of the 3 drugs* | | |
|---|---|---|---|---|
| | | *M* | *LSD* | *C* |
| $P < .001$ | My mind was flooded with thoughts. | 1.37 | 1.98 | 3.46 |
| | My sense of smell became more acute. | 4.27 | 2.75 | 4.10 |
| | I had a craving for food. | 4.53 | 3.60 | 2.55 |
| | I had difficulty talking. | 3.60 | 2.35 | 4.00 |
| | Music affected my mood much more intensely than usual. | 3.60 | 1.90 | 2.83 |
| | My thoughts kept shifting rapidly from one idea to another. | 1.57 | 2.23 | 3.25 |
| | Everything seemed too bright, too harsh, too loud. | 4.20 | 3.25 | 1.55 |
| | I can remember very clearly everything that happened to me during the experience. | 1.23 | 2.15 | 1.55 |
| | I lost interest in what I started to say so that a sentence was left unfinished. | 3.13 | 2.53 | 3.93 |
| $P < .01$ | I had intense swings from "high" to "low." | 3.23 | 3.00 | 4.14 |

**TABLE 5. Illusions or Hallucinations**

| *P* | *Statement* | *Mean Position of the 3 Drugs* | | |
|---|---|---|---|---|
| | | *M* | *LSD* | *C* |
| $P < .001$ | Solid objects changed their shapes and even disappeared. | 4.67 | 2.53 | 4.00 |
| | I heard things that I knew were not real. | 4.53 | 3.10 | 4.14 |
| | My own face in a mirror looked quite different; it even turned into different faces. | 4.40 | 3.25 | 4.28 |
| $P < .01$ | Sounds seemed to affect what I saw. | 4.90 | 4.30 | 4.66 |

surely can be anticipated from the wealth of literature on LSD and the mystical or religious experience. Related to mysticism, perhaps, are Parapsychological Sensations; and in this category of 10 items, 3 attain significance at the .01 level or beyond.

Of considerably greater interest, particularly to LSD psychotherapists who are being denied access to the drug currently, are the following findings: all 7 items which proved statistically significant in the Self-Understanding category (21 items) are statements traditionally considered therapeutic in nature—and 6 of the 7 items demonstrate that the methylphenidate experience ranked higher than the LSD experience. See Table 7.

In this context, it perhaps should be mentioned that another 6 items which could also be classified as therapeutic achieved significance between .05 and .01 probabilities. And again, methylphenidate in four of these statements achieved a higher rating than LSD. See Table 8.

In view of the recent unsupervised and non-medical use of LSD which has resulted in an epidemic of "bad trips" sometimes ending in suicide, psychosis,

**TABLE 6. Mystical or Religious Sensations**

| *P* | *Statement* | *Mean Position of the 3 Drugs* | | |
|---|---|---|---|---|
| | | *M* | *LSD* | *C* |
| *P* < .001 | I felt in contact with wonderful, unknown forces in the Universe. | 4.27 | 2.66 | 4.17 |
| | I saw all the mysteries of the Universe in certain objects. | 4.40 | 3.13 | 4.21 |
| | I had levels of thought I can't express in words. | 2.23 | 1.93 | 3.35 |
| *P* < .01 | Hours went by like seconds or one second seemed to last forever. | 1.87 | 2.17 | 3.00 |
| | I learned what it is like to be really dead. | 4.53 | 3.88 | 4.68 |
| | I felt that we are all one in this Universe. | 3.52 | 2.50 | 3.31 |
| | *Parapsychological Sensations* | | | |
| *P* < .001 | Past, present and future all seemed to be one. | 3.20 | 2.30 | 3.90 |
| | I felt as though I were traveling in time. | 3.57 | 2.65 | 4.14 |
| *P* < .01 | I could make an object turn into something else just by wanting it to. | 3.50 | 2.50 | 3.31 |

**TABLE 7. "Therapeutic" Items (Taken from the Self-Understanding Category)**

| *P* | *Statement* | *Mean Position of the 3 Drugs* | | |
|---|---|---|---|---|
| | | *M* | *LSD* | *C* |
| *P* < .001 | I was especially talkative. | 1.23 | 2.93 | 2.75 |
| | I kept thinking of my problems. | 1.57 | 2.95 | 2.35 |
| | I felt like talking it out. | 1.17 | 2.20 | 1.93 |
| | I had the feeling I had much work to do to set me straight. | 1.33 | 2.33 | 2.45 |
| *P* < .01 | I actually seemed to return to certain moments in my childhood and experience myself there. | 2.60 | 2.95 | 3.93 |
| | Things I remembered threw new light on my problems. | 1.73 | 2.10 | 2.97 |
| | I now have a new feeling regarding my family and marriage. | 2.40 | 2.33 | 3.45 |

and/or acute anxiety attacks, it is of considerable interest that LSD ranked highest in the category of Strong Unpleasant Emotions—particularly in the subcategories of Anxiety and Paranoia. It would be well to point out, too, that while the methylphenidate experience was felt to be therapeutic by the subjects, it also included considerable Anxiety when given intravenously in 75 mm dosages. Table 9 shows that 10 of the 16 Anxiety items were significant beyond the .01 level. LSD generated significantly more anxiety on 15 of these items, while on the remaining 5 items, both LSD and methylphenidate produced considerably more anxiety than chlordiazepoxide. Also, of the 6 items in the Paranoia category,

**TABLE 8. "Therapeutic" Items beyond the .05 Level of Significance**

| *P* | *Statement* | *Mean Position of the 3 Drugs* | | |
|---|---|---|---|---|
| | | *M* | *LSD* | *C* |
| $P < .05$ | I saw myself as I really am, and I did not like what I saw. | 2.50 | 3.18 | 3.72 |
| | This experience had no therapeutic value. | 3.73 | 3.88 | 2.83 |
| | I have been greatly helped by the experience. | 1.57 | 1.85 | 2.38 |
| | My conscience bothered me. | 2.47 | 3.25 | 3.39 |
| | I felt more free. | 1.60 | 2.35 | 2.35 |
| | I felt as if I had been reborn. | 3.30 | 2.70 | 3.69 |

**TABLE 9. Strong Unpleasant Emotions**

| *P* | *Statement* | *Mean Position of the 3 Drugs* | | |
|---|---|---|---|---|
| | | *M* | *LSD* | *C* |
| | A. ANXIETY | | | |
| $P < .001$ | I felt on the fringes of sheer horror. | 4.37 | 3.30 | 4.68 |
| | I became afraid I might die. | 4.67 | 3.58 | 4.72 |
| | I felt anxious or tense. | 2.23 | 2.45 | 3.52 |
| | I felt something dreadful was about to happen. | 4.10 | 3.30 | 4.52 |
| | I tried to fight off what was happening. | 4.33 | 3.25 | 4.38 |
| | I felt confused. | 2.63 | 2.63 | 3.93 |
| $P < .01$ | I felt upset and distraught. | 3.33 | 2.90 | 4.24 |
| | I felt separated from everyone and everything. | 3.70 | 2.63 | 3.66 |
| | I was easily distracted and not able to control my thoughts. | 2.87 | 3.13 | 4.03 |
| | Certain things did frighten me. | 3.27 | 2.70 | 4.10 |
| | B. PARANOIA | | | |
| $P < .001$ | At times I had the sensation of someone spying into my mind. | 4.53 | 3.35 | 4.28 |
| $P < .01$ | I resented what was being done to me. | 4.80 | 4.13 | 4.72 |

LSD contributed significantly more of this negative state on 2 items than either of the other drugs. However, it should be observed that on both of these Paranoia items, the average reaction was definitely toward the "*Unlike* the Experience" rating.

Finally: of the 156 items, only 7 were both uniquely and significantly characteristic of the chlordiazepoxide experience. All of these items were trivial in that they relate to the *absence* of a strong sensation, or are characteristic of the relaxing effects to be expected from this anti-anxiety drug. However, one item reveals the unexpected finding that the chlordiazepoxide group experienced almost as much appreciation of music as did the LSD group, thus: *I felt the beauty and meaning of music as never before.*

## DISCUSSION

There is an ever-increasing variety of consciousness-changing substances appearing in the world today, and these substances produce a wide variety of experiences. Much needed is an instrument which will allow the dimensions of these changes to be explored *without the instrument itself containing the experience.* The 156 item DWM Card Sort used retrospectively has shown itself to be a valuable tool for this vital area of study. In the present instance, the Card Sort clearly differentiated the three drug experiences under observation.

In fact, our findings in certain areas were unexpected, and puzzling. One area is, of course, the therapeutic domain which has been frequently described as part of the LSD experience. In our population the reported therapeutic effects of methylphenidate at least rival—and often surpass—those of LSD. In this context, it should be mentioned that methylphenidate has been used in combination with LSD for psychotherapy with good results by Ling and Buckman (1963). But a strong word of caution: while methylphenidate appears to have the therapeutic properties of ventilation, catharsis, and abreaction (including the re-experiencing of childhood trauma)—it should be stressed that *it has strong addictive properties* which makes it dangerous as a drug for therapy if not used under the strictest medical supervision (Moss and Ditman, 1968).

The second finding. As was to be expected, LSD totally dominated the field in the area of Sensory and Perceptual Distortions (including Hallucinations and Illusions); and for the most part dominated the fields of Religious or Mystical, and Paranormal Sensations. However, occasionally methylphenidate rivaled or surpassed LSD on such items as: *Hours went by like seconds, or one second seemed to last forever*; *I felt like I was floating in space*; *I could make an object turn into something else just by wanting it to*; and *I actually seemed to return to childhood and experienced myself there.* These statements seem to have the flavor of the mystical or paranormal—both of which have become increasingly important areas of experience to the drug (ab)users, who apparently are turning more and more to oral and intravenous injections of stimulants such as the amphetamines (Kihlbom, 1967; Connell, 1967; Marusak, 1967; Moss and Ditman, 1968) in order to obtain a "high" similar to LSD but without the danger of a "bad trip" so common to LSD experience when taken in nonmedical settings. It would seem that the search is on for the "trip," the "high," or the psychedelic experience, but without the famous psychedelic drug, LSD, which has been made illegal in many areas of the world. This search for intoxicants, not yet illegal, has extended to ingredients like Hawaiian wood roses, morning glory seeds, and even the banana peel—presumably because, from their ingestion, mystical and paranormal sensations can be obtained. In addition, methysergide maleate (Sansert), a potent anti-serotin which is used in the treatment of vascular headache, is known to be (ab)used to induce an LSD-like intoxication (Moss and Ditman, 1960). However, almost all these ingredients, like methlyphenidate, can create anxiety when not used in a medical setting (where the anxiety can be explored and analyzed; or if not, can be terminated by the administration of another drug). In fact, the indiscriminate usage of these herbs and drugs can cause severe mental and emotional turmoil often necessitating psychiatric treatment. In a paper by Ditman et al. (1968), such drug users were studied, and it was found that the majority of hospitalized and out-patient subjects had experimented with many such drugs and were classified as "multi-drug" users.

The anti-anxiety drugs, however, seem not to produce these effects. Certainly in the present study it was found that chlordiazepoxide calmed the subjects, without arousing any sensory or perceptual distortions or mystical sensations. Nor did the drug seem to aid in Self-understanding. In fact, its only positive contribution seems to have been to produce relaxation and to create in the subject a deeper appreciation and understanding of music—in this one respect rivaling the LSD experience.

Finally: it should be emphasized that these results were derived from a retrospective Card Sort administered the day after one single 8-hour session, where all subjects (chronic alcoholics) believed they were receiving LSD. Whether the apparently therapeutic methylphenidate and LSD experiences will actually lead to beneficial changes in these men, particularly in relation to their drinking behavior, remains to be seen when the follow-up studies are completed over the next months. And, since the methylphenidate experience was actually reported to be more "therapeutic," we wonder if, in the ensuing follow-up of our subjects, it will prove to be the more valuable drug.

## SUMMARY

Through the retrospective use of the 156 item DWM Card Sort, the experiences from a single intravenous dose of 200 mg of LSD, 75 mg of methylphenidate (Ritalin) and 75 mg of chlordiazepoxide (Librium) were compared in a population of 99 chronic male alcoholics treated in an "LSD setting" in a double-blind study. Surprisingly, 96 of 156 items proved significantly different among the 3 groups. LSD was unique in producing Sensory and Perceptual Distortions (including Hallucinations or Illusions), and Mystical, Religious, or Paranormal Sensations. However, contrary to expectation, LSD did not uniquely produce the traditional "therapeutic" experience, but appeared to be surpassed in that area by methylphenidate. Both drugs also caused some anxiety, while chlordiazepoxide produced relaxation, and enhanced music appreciation.

## REFERENCES

Ables, M., & Eng, E. Group treatment of chronic alcoholics with LSD-25. Read at the 12th Annual Conference of the Veterans Administration, March, 1967.

Abramson, H. A. (Ed.) *The Use of LSD in Psychotherapy and Alcoholism.* Bobbs-Merrill, New York, 1967.

Belden, E., & Hitchen, R. The identification and treatment of an early deprivation syndrome in alcoholics by means of LSD-25. *American Journal of Psychiatry,* **119**: 985–988, 1963.

Connell, P. Personal communication.

DITMAN, K., TIETZ, H., PRINCE, B., FORGY, E., & MOSS, T. Harmful aspects of the LSD Experience. *Journal of Nervous and Mental Disease*, **145**: 464–474, 1968.
KIHLBOM, M. Personal communication.
KURLANDER, A., UNGER, S., SHAFFER, J., & SAVAGE, C. Psychedelic therapy utilizing LSD in the treatment of the alcoholic patient: a preliminary report. *American Journal of Psychiatry*, **123**: 1202–1209, 1967.
LING, T., & BUCKMAN, J. *Lysergic Acid (LSD-25) and Ritalin in the treatment of neurosis*. Lombardo Press, London, 1963.
MALITZ, S. The role of Mescaline and D-lysergic acid in psychiatric treatment. *Diseases of the Nervous System*, **27**: 39–42, 1966.
MARUSAK, C. Personal communication.
MOSS, T., & DITMAN, K. Personal communication.
O'REILLY, P., & FUNK, A. LSD in chronic alcoholism. *Journal of the Canadian Psychiatric Association*, **9**: 250–251, 1964.
SAVAGE, C., HARMAN, W., SAVAGE, ETHEL, & FADIMAN, J. Therapeutic effects of the LSD experience. *Psychological Reports*, **14**: 111–120, 1964.
SCHOEN, S. LSD in psychotherapy. *American Journal of Psychiatry*, **18**: 35–51, 1964.

# 23

## *LSD: Injection Early in Pregnancy Produces Abnormalities in Offspring of Rats*

G. J. ALEXANDER, B. E. MILES,
G. M. GOLD, R. B. ALEXANDER

As part of a continuing investigation of toxic effects of psychotropic drugs (1), we have studied the influence of subcutaneous injections of "psychedelic" doses of lysergic acid diethylamide (LSD) on the course of pregnancy. Here are some preliminary results.

Obtained several years ago (2), the LSD was kept dry in the dark pending solution in saline at 5 μg/ml. Ultraviolet and fluorescence analyses revealed no significant degree of oxidation of the material. Healthy female rats, Wistar strain, 250 g, were mated with selected healthy males weighing 450 g. Pregnant females were divided into matched groups: one group received saline subcutaneously; the other, LSD at 5 μg/kg of body weight. This dosage was selected to correspond in rats to the human hallucinogenic dose which is said to range from 100 to 400 μg pr person—1.7 to 6.7 μg/kg for a person weighing 60 kg (3).

In the first experiment five rates received a single injection of LSD on the

From *Science*, Vol. 157, July 28, 1967, pp. 459–460. 

4th day of pregnancy, with no further treatment (Table 1). Of these, one produced no young; autopsy showed that pregnancy had presumably terminated in abortion; ovaries and uterus were somewhat irregular and enlarged, one horn of the uterus being markedly constricted, with no trace of fetuses. Two rats that received LSD on the 4th day of pregnancy produced abnormal young: six of a litter of 13 were stillborn, as were all nine of the second litter. One rat injected with LSD delivered a litter of eight of which seven appeared normal, one being definitely stunted. The last injected rat delivered a normal litter of 16. Matched controls, given saline, delivered 11, 11, 13, 13, and 16 offspring, all apparently normal and healthy.

In the second experiment one animal that received LSD on the 4th day of gestation did not come to term. The weight curve indicated that pregnancy was interrupted during the 3 days following treatment with LSD. Another treated animal delivered a litter of 14, three of which were stillborn, with one more dying within 24 hours. A third rat delivered a litter of 11 including one stillborn. A fourth animal gave an unusually small litter of four normally appearing offspring. The last one delivered a healthy litter of ten. Again, matched controls produced apparently healthy normal litters averaging 13.

In the third experiment, five animals received similar single injections of LSD late in pregnancy (Table 1). There was no obvious effect on the apparently healthy offspring totaling 51—against 65 for the controls.

**TABLE 1. Effects of Prenatal Treatment of Rats with LSD[a]**

| Rat (No.) | Offspring: In Litter (No.) | Offspring: Nature |
|---|---|---|
| | *Experiment 1* | |
| 2-3-2 (4) | 0 | Fetuses resorbed |
| 2-5-2 (4) | 9 | All stillborn (2 stunted) |
| 2-2-1 (4) | 13 | Six stillborn, remainder normal |
| 2-6-2 (4) | 8 | Seven normal, one small |
| 2-1-2 (4) | 16 | Normal |
| | *Experiment 2* | |
| 1-2-1 (4) | 0 | Presumed abortion |
| 2-6-1 (4) | 14 | Three stillborn, one died within 1 day |
| 2-4-2 (4) | 11 | One stillborn |
| 1-1-1 (4) | 4 | Normal; litter unusually small |
| 2-4-1 (4) | 10 | Normal |
| | *Experiment 3* | |
| 1-3-2 (7) | 10 | Normal |
| 1-4-2 (8) | 11 | Normal |
| 1-2-5 (10) | 13 | Normal |
| 1-1-5 (13) | 9 | Normal |
| 1-1-4 (16) | 8 | Normal |

[a]Each rat had a matched control, which was injected with saline; all controls delivered normal litters of 8 to 17 offspring. The day of gestation on which each rat was treated appears in parentheses.

Gross examination of the young from all experiments revealed some overall stunting of development in the case of three stillborn and one that survived for 6 weeks, but no other abnormalities. Offspring from rats treated with LSD weighed at birth as much on the average as the controls; later some of them grew as well, but others failed to develop at the same rate. For example, average control offspring weighed 64 g at 10 days, while an average offspring of treated rat No. 2-4-1 weighed only 44 g; of treated rat No. 2-4-2, 44 g; and of treated rat No. 2-6-1, 16 g. The stunted offspring of treated rat No. 2-6-2 weighed only 54 g at 36 days, while his apparently healthy littermates weighed 80 to 106 g, averaging 96.5 g.

Our results possibly may be explained by the recent finding of chromosomal abnormalities in cultured cells grown in the presence of LSD (4).

## REFERENCES AND NOTES

1. L. Roizin, M. Lazar, G. Gold, *Federation Proc.* **25**, 253 (1966).
2. From Sandoz Pharmaceutical Co.; FDA permit IND 3632.
3. H. A. Abramson, in *The Use of LSD in Psychotherapy* (Josiah Macy, Jr., Foundation, New York, (1960).
4. M. M. Cohen, M. J. Marinello, N. Back, *Science* **155**, 1417 (1967).
5. Aided by research grant NB 06298 from the National Institute of Neurological Diseases and Blindness. We thank S. Turchin for technical assistance.

# 24

## *Lysergic Acid Diethylamide (LSD): No Teratogenicity in Rats*

J. WARKANY and E. TAKACS

The report of Cohen et al. (1) of chromosomal damage in human leucocytes, induced by lysergic acid diethylamide (LSD), prompted us to test this compound for teratogenicity in rats. A pilot experiment was planned to ascertain possible effects of the drug administered to pregnant Wistar rats during periods of embryonic organogenesis. Delysid (Sandoz; batch 65002), containing LSD at 0.1 mg/ml, obtained from the National Institute of Mental Health was administered intraperitoneally or orally in single doses on the 7th, 8th, or 9th day of gestation, or in multiple doses from the 7th to the 12th day. The total dosage to individual rats ranged from 1.5 to 300 μg.

Fifty-five pregnant rats were treated; four litters were completely resorbed; 47 rats were killed on the 21st day of pregnancy and their young were removed; four were allowed to deliver and raise their young. The mean litter size of the 21-day fetuses was 10.2 ± 1.8 (controls, 10.0 ± 2.8); their mean weight was 3.53 ± 0.44 g (controls, 4.14 ± 0.71 g). The differences between experimental and control animals are not significant.

Of the 508 21-day fetuses, 504 (409 dissected and 95 cleared for skeletal examination) were normal and only four were considered abnormal. One had hydrocephalus, but 12 of its littermates were normal; its mother had been injected once on the 7th day with 50 μg of LSD. Another fetus had short extremities and syndactylism; there were nine normal littermates; the mother had been injected daily from the 7th to the 11th day with 50 μg of LSD. Two fetuses were small, weighing 1.7 and 2.1 g; they were from a litter of six, the other four being normal; the mother had been injected on the 7th and 9th days with 50 μg of LSD. There was no common pattern in the abnormalities of the four young and there was no dose-dependence.

The four treated rats that delivered had 44 apparently normal young, some of which could be raised and bred. Since an incidence of about 1 percent of congenital malformations in the offspring of untreated Wistar rats is not unusual, our pilot experiments did not prove that LSD is teratogenic in rats. Even dosage as great as 300 μg to rats did not harm their embryos. Such dosage is comparable to human dosage; on a weight basis it is more than 200 times larger.

Later we learned of the results of Alexander et al. (2) who gave single injections of LSD to rats early in pregnancy (4th day of gestation) and observed resorption of one litter and some stillborn, stunted young in others. On the 4th or 5th day of pregnancy we gave 34 rats doses ranging from 1 to 100 μg of LSD (Delysid), and obtained from 32 females a total of 335 young. Of these, 296 were removed on the 21st day by cesarean section; with the exception of one fetus that was small, all were normal on external inspection, dissection, or clearing. Thirty-nine young were delivered and raised; they remain alive and healthy. Two of the 34 rats had no litters. A resorption rate of 5.9 percent is not different for that for pregnant Wistar rats injected with saline solution.

Although most of the doses administered in these experiments were very large (the highest single doses administered by us were about 80 times larger than those given by Alexander et al.), we found no abnormalities other than reduction in size of one of the young. Alexander et al. (2) used a dry LSD dissolved in saline, while we administered Delysid. The stocks of rats used in their and our experiments also must differ since they mention that their control offspring weighed an average of 46 g at 10 days; rats in our laboratory weigh about 19 g at 10 days. Donaldson (3) cites weights of 15 g for 10-day-old rats. If the LSD-treated rats weighed 44 to 46 g at 10 days, as Alexander et al. (2) state, it would appear that the drug did not reduce the weight of these animals but more than doubled it.

Thus we did not find LSD teratogenic during the organogenetic period and found no abnormalities in the offspring of rats injected on the 4th or 5th day of pregnancy, although the doses administered to some of the pregnant rats were as high as those used by human beings.

We draw no conclusions from the negative results with rats, concerning teratogenicity of LSD in man, since it is known that a drug teratogenic in one species may not be so in another; this general rule applies to results with mice (4) and hamsters (5) also.

## REFERENCES AND NOTES

1. M. M. Cohen, M. J. Marinello, N. Back, *Science* **155**, 1417, (1967).
2. G. J. Alexander, B. E. Miles, G. M. Gold, R. B. Alexander, *ibid.* **157**, 459 (1967).
3. H. H. Donaldson, *The Rat, Memoirs of the Wistar Institute of Anatomy and Biology* (Wistar Inst., Philadelphia, 1924).
4. R. Auerbach and J. A. Rugowski, *Science* **157**, 1325 (1967).
5. W. F. Geber, *ibid.* **158**, 265 (1967).
6. Aided by NIH grant ROI-HD-00502.

# 25

# *Congenital Malformations Induced by Mescaline, Lysergic Acid Diethylamide, and Bromolysergic Acid in the Hamster*

W. F. GEBER

As part of (1, 2) an investigation of the various possible etiological factors involved in the induction of congenital malformations, I have studied the psychotomimetic alkaloid mescaline (MES), the active principle of the peyote cactus used in the rituals of certain Indian tribes, and the synthetic alkaloid lysergic acid diethylamide (LSD) used on a limited basis in drug therapy of mental disease. In addition, the monobromide derivative of LSD, 2-bromo-D-lysergic acid diethylamide (BOL), was also evaluated.

Pregnant hamsters were obtained from randomly bred stock of Lakeview Hamster Colony. All females were caged in air-conditioned quarters main-

From *Science*, Vol. 158, October 13, 1967, pp. 265–267. 

tained at 75°F. Water, Purina laboratory chow, cabbage, and carrots were available ad libitum throughout the experimental period. The animal quarters were illuminated by natural light (roof skylight). Noise was kept to a minimum since this factor has been repeatedly demonstrated to produce deleterious effects in reproductive studies (2, 3).

The compounds were dissolved in sterile saline solution 30 minutes before use and injected (MES, 0.45 to 3.3 mg/kg; LSD, 0.0008 to 0.24 mg/kg; BOL, 0.002 to 0.41 mg/kg) subcutaneously at 1 p.m. on the 8th day of pregnancy. This phase of pregnancy in the hamster is an effective period for the evaluation of the ability of a variety of compounds to cause teratogenesis (4). All of the control animals were injected with sterile saline. After the single injection of a drug or saline, the animal was returned to its cage and left undisturbed until the 12th day of gestation, when it was killed by an overdose of ether. As soon as maternal respiration ceased, the uterus was exposed by midline incision, and the number and distribution of fetuses was noted. Each fetus was carefully exposed and examined to determine both its viability and developmental status. The fetus was then placed in 10 percent formaldehyde for 3 days to allow for hardening so that it could be more completely examined for abnormalities.

No major congenital abnormalities were found in the 300 control fetuses, although there was a limited number of runts, dead fetuses, and resorbed fetuses found in this group (Table 1). In the experimental fetuses abnormalities of this type were many times greater (by percentage). The types of gross congenital defects found in the experimental litters were exencephaly, spina bifida, interparietal meningocele, omphalocele, hydrocephalus, myelocele, edema along spinal axis, edema in various body regions other than spinal area, and hemorrhages of local brain areas (parietal and frontal) and neck (sublingual area). Approximately 10 percent of the abnormal fetuses contained more than one type of defect, and several had four or five defects.

There is no correlation between the dose (milligrams per kilograms of body weight) of the drug administered to the pregnant female and the percentage of congenital malformations found in the fetuses. The lowest concentration of MES actually produced the largest number of defects. However, a dose-response relationship does appear in most cases when the other parameters are considered. The number of fetuses per litter decreased, and the percentage of resorptions, dead fetuses, and runts increased as the concentration of a particular drug administered to the pregnant female was increased.

Recent studies have shown the chromosomal effects of LSD on cultured leukocytes (5) and leukocytes obtained from LSD users (6). In addition, injections of LSD into rats early in pregnancy has produced runts and increased fetal mortality (7).

My results indicate that both lysergic acid diethylamide and its 2-brom derivative can induce a wide variety of congenital malformations in the hamster embryo. Mescaline, although a less potent teratogen as judged by the dose needed to produce anomalies, is nevertheless equipotent in the type and number of abnormalities produced. This difference in potency between mescaline and lysergic acid corresponds qualitatively to the relative psychotomimetic potency of the respective drugs, lysergic acid being the more potent.

**TABLE 1. Number and Types of Fetal Abnormalities Produced by Mescaline, LSD, and BOL**

| *Drug Concentration (mg/kg body wt)* | *Females (No.)* | *Fetuses (No.)* | *Congenital Abnormalities (%)* | *Resorptions (%)* | *Dead Fetuses (%)* | *Runts (%)* |
|---|---|---|---|---|---|---|
| | | | *Mescaline* | | | |
| 0.45 | 8 | 86 (10.8) | 28 | 7 | 5 | 5 |
| 1.33 | 8 | 76 (9.5) | 9 | 13 | 5 | 0 |
| 3.25 | 8 | 64 (8.0) | 11 | 25 | 10 | 12 |
| | | | *LSD* | | | |
| 0.000084 | 9 | 105 (11.6) | 6 | 8 | 7 | 7 |
| 0.0029 | 8 | 86 (10.8) | 8 | 12 | 15 | 10 |
| 0.021 | 11 | 110 (10.0) | 5 | 12 | 10 | 9 |
| 0.24 | 9 | 77 (8.6) | 6 | 14 | 17 | 10 |
| | | | *BOL* | | | |
| 0.002 | 8 | 87 (11.0) | 6 | 8 | 3 | 3 |
| 0.025 | 8 | 83 (10.4) | 7 | 12 | 4 | 1 |
| 0.41 | 7 | 63 (9.0) | 13 | 22 | 8 | 8 |
| | | | *Controls* | | | |
| Saline (0.9 percent) | 25 | 300 (12.0) | 0 | 2 | 1 | 1 |

Note: The numbers in parentheses are the average number of fetuses.

## REFERENCES AND NOTES


1. W. F. GEBER, *Amer. J. Physiol.* **202,** 653 (1962).
2. W. F. GEBER, *J. Embryol. Exp. Morphol.* **16,** 1 (1966).
3. B. ZONDEK and I. TAMARI, *Amer. J. Obstet. Gynecol.* **80,** 1041 (1960).
4. V. FERM, *Lab. Invest.* **14,** 1500 (1965).
5. M. M. COHEN, M. J. MARINELLO, N. BACK, *Science* **155,** 1417 (1967).
6. S. IRWIN and J. EGOZCUE, *ibid.* **157,** 313 (1967).
7. G. J. ALEXANDER, B. E. MILES, G. M. GOLD, R. B. ALEXANDER, *ibid.*, p. 459.


8. Supported by NIH grant FR-05365.
9. I thank Karin Landeen for technical assistance.

# 26

# *Drug-Motivated Behavior: The Effect of Morning Glory Seeds on Motor Activity of Chicks*

DOUGLAS W. MATHESON and JULIE THOMAS

Lysergic acid diethylamide (LSD-25) does not occur in nature but is prepared by semi-synthesis. The drug affects behavior in two basic ways. First, it acts as a predominant sympathetic nervous system stimulant and secondly, to a lesser extent, there is a central and peripheral depression. Morning glory seeds (*Ipomoea*) are known to contain certain alkaloids which are chemically similar to LSD-25 (Claus & Tyler, 1965), the major one being d-lysergic acid amide (Rice & Genest, 1965). Another alkaloid found in morning glory seeds is ergometrine, a known central nervous system stimulant. The ingestion of morning glory seeds facilitates a behavioral reaction very similar to that caused by LSD-25, and they have been used by both teenagers and adults to create visual hallucinations. One young woman who had taken 250 seeds felt very hyperactive, anxious, experienced an increased awareness of colors, and had a profound fear of losing her "mind." While under the influence of the seeds the woman had a rapid pulse and an accelerated respiration rate (Ingram, 1964). Rice & Genest (1965) reported observing both motor dysfunction and death in mice given heavy doses of morning glory seed alkaloids.

The present experiment studied the effects of morning glory seed ingestion on general sympathetic activity in chicks by measuring motor activity under controlled conditions. It was predicted that motor activity of chicks would increase with the ingestion of morning glory seeds when activity was measured in an open-field situation.

## SUBJECTS

Ten 3-day-old Leghorn rooster chicks (English strain), weighing 38–40 g each, were used in the experiment. All chicks were housed in a 30.5 x 30.5 cm box which was kept in a warm, well-lighted room. They were fed All-Age-Mash and given ad lib water in their home box.

## APPARATUS

The activity testing apparatus was an open-field maze consisting of an enclosed rectangular cardboard box (34.7 x 44.5 x 30.5 cm) which was marked

From *Psychonomic Science*, Vol. 15, No. 1, 1969, pp. 39–40. Reprinted by permission of authors and publisher.

off into eight nearly square 13.8 x 14.8 cm rectangles. Motor activity was measured by counting the number of rectangles crossed in a 3-min period. The chicks had to completely cross a line in order to get one activity count.

## PROCEDURE

The ten chicks were randomly assigned to two groups of five each, Group 1 serving as a control for Group 2. The two groups were separated in their home box by a partition and were provided with the same quantity of feed each day. Each chick was handled for 30 min on Day 1 and 10 min per day on 5 subsequent days (Days 2–6). Activity testing began on the third day of handling (Day 3). Each group was food deprived for 5 h. At the end of the 5-h period both groups were given access to food for ½ h and then were deprived of food for 2 additional hours. At the end of the 2-h period, each chick was placed individually in the open field testing apparatus where its spontaneous activity was measured by counting the number of rectangles traversed for 3 min. The placement of the chick in the testing apparatus for 3 min was defined as a trial and all chicks received one trial. On Day 4, the chicks were placed on the same deprivation schedule as Day 3. The procedure was the same except that during the ½-h feeding period each chick in Group 2 received 0.123 g of mashed "Heavenly Blue" morning glory seed which was uniformly mixed with 2 g of their regular feed. All chicks consumed the mixture within the ½-h period. Group 2 was given the same amount (2.123 g) of their regular feed without the seeds. The procedure for Days 5 and 6 was the same as for Day 4. The deprivation schedule began at the same time of day for Days 3–6. At the end of a trial each chick was placed in a temporary box until all chicks in that group were tested. The chicks were then given food ad lib until the deprivation schedule started the next day.

## RESULTS AND DISCUSSION

An analysis of the variance showed that Group 2's activity was significantly different from Group 1's over days [$F(1,8) = 7.095$, $p < .01$]. The analysis revealed that the activity of both groups changed over days. In addition, the linear component of the Group by Day interaction was significant [$F(1,24) = 9.24$, $p < .01$], which suggested that Group 2's activity increased significantly faster than Group 1's. That is, the two linear components differ significantly. A $t$ test between activity measures of the two groups for Day 3 was not significant, indicating that both groups' activity levels were initially the same. The mean number of rectangles crossed by each group for Days 3, 4, 5, and 6 are shown in Table 1.

Although the control group (Group 1) did show a significant increase in activity over days, the rate of change was not as large as for Group 2. The increase in activity shown by Group 1 may be attributed to adaptation or to novel stimuli in the experimental apparatus (Montgomery, 1954). That is, as the ani-

**TABLE 1. Mean Number of Rectangles Crossed per Day (Each mean is for N = 5 chicks)**

| | | Day | | | |
|---|---|---|---|---|---|
| | | *3* | *4* | *5* | *6* |
| Group | 1 | 1.6 | 3.0 | 4.0 | 11.4 |
| | 2 | 1.8 | 9.4 | 11.4 | 34.0 |

mals moved about in the open field, they came into commerce with novel stimuli which elicited increased exploratory behavior.

The rate of activity of Group 2, being significantly greater than that of Group 1, is attributed to the presence of alkaloids found in the seeds of the Heavenly Blue morning glory. Some of the components apparently can cause an increase in motor activity at a rate significantly greater than activity attributed to adaptation and novel stimuli alone. The results indicate that the drugs may have a cumulative effect on behavior. The agent or agents which facilitate the activity might be stored in the organism and could have a residual effect on subsequent days. Although there is no data for additional days, one might predict that the animals would have continued to increase their activity until severe motor dysfunction or death occurred.

In summary, morning glory seeds were found to increase motor behavior of chicks in an open-field situation. The increase in activity is in addition to activity attributed to adaptation or to novel stimuli. It also appears that the drug components in the seeds might have a cumulative effect on activity which could have a deleterious effect.

## REFERENCES


Claus, E. P., & Tyler, V. E., Jr. *Pharmacognosy.* (5th ed.) Philadelphia: Lea & Febiger, 1965.

Ingram, A. L. Morning glory seed reaction. *Journal of the American Medical Association,* 1964, 190, 1133–1134.

Montgomery, K. C. The role of the exploratory drive in learning. *Journal of Comparative & Physiological Psychology,* 1954, 47, 60.

Rice, W. B., & Genest, K. Acute toxicity of extracts of morning-glory seeds in mice. *Nature,* 1965, 207, 302.

# 5
# *Narcotic Analgesics*

So much has been written about opiate addiction (especially diacetylmorphine [heroin] addiction) that it would be impossible to cover the area adequately in a book of readings. With this in mind, we will very briefly describe several methods of treatment, some designed primarily to treat heroin addicts and the others designed for drug abusers in general.

## NARCOTIC ANTAGONISTS

Several methods have been tried in the treatment of opiate addiction. The least successful seems to be "cold turkey," short-term withdrawal with the aid of central nervous system depressants or tranquilizers. The heroin addict "shoots up" to prevent physical withdrawal, but after he withdraws, the dependence factor is usually so strong that the user returns to heroin as soon as he has the opportunity.

Other methods of treatment may hold promise in the treatment of heroin addiction. One method is the use of narcotic antagonists. The most experimentally used narcotic antagonists are nalline (nalorphine), cyclazocine, and naloxone (Zaks et al., 1969; Fink et al., 1968; Freedman et al., 1967. Antagonists partially or totally block the euphoric effect of heroin. The idea behind the use of a narcotic antagonist is that heroin acts as a reinforcer in reducing the physical and psychological effects of withdrawal, and, as a result, taking heroin becomes a conditioned response. That is, addiction may be a conditioned response in which the addict has learned to respond to stressful stimuli by using heroin to obtain relief and euphoria (Zaks et al., 1969). The narcotic antagonist prevents heroin from acting as a reinforcer, and theoretically the conditioned response can be extinguished. The antagonists have been tested with heroin challenges (injecting heroin) and have had varying degrees of effectiveness. Nalline brings on immediate heroin withdrawal. Cyclazocine has many undesirable side effects such as dysphoria, increased sex drive, constipation, anxiety, vivid imagery, and hallucinations. In spite of these difficulties, cyclazocine is useful in the treatment of heroin addiction (Fink et al., 1968). Naloxone is a potent, short acting, narcotic antagonist that has few of the side effects of cyclazocine and some of its advantages, such as potency and rapid starting action. However, its short duration and high cost are disadvantages (although the advantages may outweigh them), which may diminish with increased demand for the drug. The antagonists could show great promise if research is pursued along the lines that addiction is a conditioned response.

## METHADONE

In recent months the narcotic methadone has become a household word with heroin addicts. Methadone is a synthetic analgesic developed by the Germans (during the second World War) when their morphine supply dwindled. Methadone acts as a blocking agent to the effects of heroin by preventing the euphoria associated with heroin sniffing or injection (Dole and Nyswander, 1965; Zaks et al., 1969; Freedman et al., 1967). Several methadone maintenance programs have been set up throughout the United States to aid in social rehabilitation. Methadone treatment is inexpensive and clearly seems to offer a positive alternative to heroin addiction. The articles that follow are concerned with treatment of drug users. The first is from *The Medical Letter* (1969). This very short note supports the implementation of methadone programs. Nyswander (1971) and Dole (1971) discuss methadone treatment programs now in existence and anticipate problems arising from the expansion of such programs. Brill (1971) presents editorial comment on Dole's article. Fink (1970) presents an interesting analysis of the possibility that narcotic addiction is a conditioned phenomenon and revives the literature of research on narcotic antagonists. Matheson et al. (1970) present an experiment done by the editors of this book of readings which suggests a behaviorally oriented treatment model to be used in conjunction with methadone treatment. The study provides a general model for the treatment of drug users regardless of the specific drug problem. Steinfeld (1970) concludes the book with an illustration of an adroit use of behavior modification with narcotic addicts.

## REFERENCES

DOLE, V. and NYSWANDER, M. A medical treatment for diacetylmorphine (heroin) addiction. *Journal of the American Medical Association*, 1965, 193, 646–650.

FINK, M., ZAKS, A., SHAROFF, R., MORA, A., BRUNER, A., LEVIT, S. and FREEDMAN, A. Naloxone in heroin dependence. *Clinical Pharmacology & Therapeutics*, 1968, 9, pp. 568–577.

FREEDMAN, A., FINK, M., SHAROFF, R., and ZAKS, A. Cyclazocine and methadone in narcotic addiction. *Journal of the American Medical Association*, 1967, 202, pp. 191–194.

ZAKS, A., BRUNER, A., FINK, M., and FREEDMAN, A. Intravenous diacetylmorphine (heroin) in studies of opiate dependence. *Diseases of the Nervous System*, 1969, 30, pp. 89–92.

# 27

# *Methadone in the Management of Opiate Addiction*

Methadone therapy now offers substantial hope of rehabilitation for heroin and other opiate addicts. Despite the fact that it substitutes one addiction for another, *Medical Letter* editors and consultants are convinced that no other presently available therapy offers comparable promise for the many thousands of heroin addicts who are seeking help. Legally, methadone therapy is still experimental in the United States; practically, its effectiveness has been adequately established, and its benefits clearly outweigh its hazards.

## EFFECTS OF METHADONE

Methadone hydrochloride (Dolophine—Lilly; and others) is an opiate-type narcotic drug with analgesic effects similar to those of morphine. Its effectiveness against heroin addiction results from its ability to block the euphoriant effects of heroin and the craving for the opiate without heroin's deleterious physical and mental effects. Because methadone is addicting (though less so than heroin or morphine), its use in the treatment of addicts must be carefully supervised.

Unlike most other narcotics, methadone is highly effective when taken orally and it is relatively long-acting (12 to 48 hours, depending on dose). Usually, a single daily oral dose is sufficient to prevent euphoria if the patient uses heroin. This effect is specific for opiate-type narcotic drugs; methadone offers no benefits to patients who are dependent on such drugs as barbiturates or amphetamines, or who are alcoholic.

When properly administered, methadone allows the patient to function without sedation or euphoria and with no impairment of vigilance, reaction time, affect, or intellectual function. The originators and chief investigators of methadone therapy, V. P. Dole and M. Nyswander, have treated more than 2000 heroin addicts since 1964. None of their patients became readdicted to heroin so long as they remained under methadone treatment, and most have been able to return to school or work. About 10 percent of patients abuse other agents such as amphetamines or barbiturates, and another 10 percent use alcohol excessively. Almost all of the patients who left the program, about 17 percent, have shown a return of craving for heroin when methadone was discontinued. Many treatment centers have been established in areas where heroin addiction is common, and their results have generally confirmed those reported by Dole and Nyswander. In all centers, the therapeutic program includes aid in social rehabilitation.

From *The Medical Letter*, Vol. 11, No. 24 (Issue 284), November 28, 1969, pp. 97–99.

## SELECTION OF PATIENTS

Methadone maintenance has proved effective in the management of chronic addicts (in some studies, with an average period of addiction of 10 years) who have failed with other treatments and who have volunteered for methadone therapy. It is not recommended for the occasional user of narcotics, or for those with a short history of dependence; with such persons the effort should be made to cure heroin addiction by more conventional means, such as individual or group psychotherapy.

## DOSAGE AND ADMINISTRATION

The dosage of methadone needed by the new patient to avoid abstinence symptoms during the first few days of treatment depends on how much heroin or other narcotic he has been taking. Most investigators start with a dose of 10 to 20 mg of methadone orally and repeat the dose in four to eight hours if necessary, with the patient under close observation. The primary objective at first is to make the patient comfortable without excessive drowsiness or clouding of sensory and intellectual faculties. During the subsequent four to six weeks, the dose is slowly increased as tolerance develops. Initially, the daily dose is divided into morning and evening portions, but after several days or weeks, when the final maintenance dose (usually 80 to 120 mg/day) is reached, the two portions are gradually consolidated so that the patient can be maintained on an ambulatory basis with a single morning dose (V. P. Dole et al., *JAMA*, 206:2708, 1968).

Some investigators start treatment of ambulatory patients with a single oral dose of 10 mg the first day, increasing the dose by about 50 percent on each successive day until a maintenance dose of about 100 mg/day is reached. No effort is made to restrict the use of heroin during this period. As tolerance to methadone and cross-tolerance to heroin develop, however, the patient gradually gives up the heroin. Several experimental programs using methadone in lower maintenance doses have been reported, but there is as yet insufficient information on which to evaluate their effectiveness. The drug must be taken daily for an indefinite period, possibly for the rest of the patient's life, though further investigation may show that methadone can eventually be withdrawn from some patients without relapse to heroin or other opiates.

## ADVERSE EFFECTS

If the dose of methadone is increased too rapidly, especially at the beginning, the patient may become over-sedated and confused. These symptoms usually disappear if a dose is omitted and therapy then resumed at a lower dosage level. Tolerance to the smooth-muscle and autonomic effects of methadone develops more slowly than to the sedative effects, and excessive sweating and constipation are frequent complaints. Studies of the central nervous and neuromuscular systems and of the respiratory tract, liver, kidney, and bone marrow have thus far shown no adverse effects due to the use of methadone in patients who have been on the drug for as long as five years or more.

## TREATMENT OF METHADONE OVERDOSAGE

The patient maintained on a supervised methadone program is highly tolerant and thus is protected against overdoses of methadone or other narcotics; the daily maintenance dose is, however, dangerous to a person who has not built up tolerance. Ingestion of 80 mg can be fatal to a child. The specific antidote for respiratory depression, the most serious toxic effect of large doses of methadone taken by a nontolerant person, is nalorphine (Nalline); the dose for adults is 2 to 10 mg intravenously, and for children under 12, 0.1 mg/kg repeated once or twice if necessary during the following hour. It is important to note that nalorphine is effective for only one to two hours, and that poisoning by methadone can depress respiration for as long as 48 hours. The patient must therefore be observed continuously, and nalorphine given repeatedly in doses sufficient to control respiratory depression. The use of nalorphine in the methadone-tolerant patient may precipitate a severe withdrawal syndrome.

## LEGAL STATUS OF MAINTENANCE TREATMENT

There are ambiguities in both federal and state laws governing the right of physicians to prescribe narcotic drugs for the maintenance of addicted patients. In any event, it is difficult for the physician in private practice to provide adequate medical supervision of the patient during therapy, or the social supervision and rehabilitation assistance most patients require. Nevertheless, where methadone therapy is unavailable for an addict who otherwise qualifies for therapy, there should be no legal barriers preventing the private physician from administering the drug with guidance from experts. In New York State, methadone treatment programs carried out by medical institutions are accredited by the State Narcotic Addiction Control Commission. Similar accreditation has been obtained in other states.

## CONCLUSION

Methadone has proved highly effective in the treatment of heroin addiction, but it is still unavailable to most addicts. Government and private agencies concerned with the problem should do everything possible to speed the extension of treatment facilities.

# 28

# *Methadone Therapy for Heroin Addiction: Where Are We? Where Are We Going?*

MARIE E. NYSWANDER

In the absence of a cure for a crippling medical condition, it is traditional medical practice to attempt to ameliorate the symptoms or effects of the disease and to rehabilitate the patient as far as possible to a plausible way of life. The hope may be to keep him alive, functioning, and comfortable until such time as a better treatment, or a cure, may be found. Methadone maintenance therapy offers an effective means of managing the illness of heroin addiction—not to cure it, but to counter its effects. Although the use of methadone for maintenance therapy represents the substitution of one addiction for another, by eliminating narcotic hunger and euphoria and by blocking heroin's kick, methadone maintenance therapy has permitted large numbers of patients to change some behavioral patterns and to restructure their lives.

Methadone maintenance programs have proliferated rapidly in the past year or two. This therapy is based on the dual rationale that (1) opiate addiction may indicate an acquired metabolic dysfunction or deficiency, for which the only present management is replacement by the opiate or medication, and (2) the supply of the replacement substance is a ticket to functional rehabilitation.

Our early work was predicated on this dual rationale. Years of work as a psychiatrist at the federal hospital at Lexington, Kentucky, and later in New York's Harlem, had persuaded me that existing approaches to addiction treatment were yielding virtually no gains: almost all addicts fell back into their habits shortly after leaving treatment. And the return to addiction was accompanied by a return to the usually desperate life patterns of the addict—disrupted social behavior and sporadic or constant criminal activity to support the costly demands of the heroin hunger. I wondered whether some of the traits charged to the addict's character might not derive from the drug hunger itself. Perhaps within a system of regular and certain supply of opiates some of this behavior might be controlled and the addict's life regularized. He might become more accessible to treatment or rehabilitation in a less stressful situation.

Dr. Vincent P. Dole, a metabolic researcher at Rockefeller Institute, had in the meantime become interested in the possibility that addiction represented a particular metabolic deficiency, either predisposed or induced by heroin use. Together we investigated the condition of two patients maintained on opiates. We tried morphine and heroin but were unable to eliminate their drug hunger or the extremes of euphoria and the withdrawal syndrome. At the beginning I thought that simply supplying the addict to the level of his narcotic hunger would make a great difference. But whatever we tried, the story was the same: euphoria, a short "straight" period, then sick. Within a few hours of medication

From *Drug Therapy*, January 1971. Reprinted by permission of the author and publisher.

the patient was sitting around anxiously watching the clock, apprehensive of withdrawal symptoms, waiting to be relieved. In Britain, heroin maintenance was an accepted therapy; a certain number of certified addicts were having their needs relieved, but they could not be described as functioning either. These narcotics were not the answer. Their effectiveness was too brief. We needed to find an agent with the longest possible action, to give the patient a proportionately longer "straight" time before the threat of withdrawal appeared. As a parallel, if insulin medication were only effective for 3 or 4 hours, the diabetic who depended on it could barely function—it is extremely difficult, physically and emotionally, to live and work properly when the equilibrium between well-being and sickness is so short-lived.

It was then that we tried methadone hydrochloride, a long-acting synthetic narcotic with analgesic effects similar to those of morphine.

## CHARACTERISTICS OF METHADONE

We found that, taken orally, methadone could assuage narcotic hunger without giving the disabling euphoria of heroin. Also, while dosage had to be increased regularly for a while to achieve this effect, it eventually could be leveled off to a stable requirement. And through a mechanism of cross-tolerance for other opiates, methadone blocked the effect of a heroin shot. Despite large challenge doses of morphine, heroin, dilaudid, or methadone, patients and physicians both reported that the euphoric effects of those narcotics were absent.

Most important, methadone is effective for as long as 36 to 48 hours. Thus the patient has a sustained period—usually at least 24 hours—of normal alertness and well-being, and the leisure to get his next dose without panic over approaching withdrawal. And throughout that time the patient is immune to the euphoria that heroin produces. This long action makes methadone particularly suitable for a large-scale outpatient maintenance program, as patients need come in only once a day for treatment.

### Safety

Properly administered—that is, in oral doses that do not exceed the patient's tolerance—methadone is safe. Patients studied after at least 5 years in treatment showed no adverse effects on the liver, kidney, bone marrow, or respiratory tract, or in the central nervous and neuromuscular systems.

Tests have been shown that methadone patients function without impairment of reaction time, intellectual capacity, affect, or vigilance.

There are virtually no contraindications: methadone is apparently compatible with all other medications and conditions, including surgery and anesthetics. When medical procedures require it, narcotics such as morphine and Demrol may be superimposed for their pain-killing effects, which are still retained (for reasons which are not yet clear).

Because of the blockading action of methadone, it is practically impossible for a maintained patient to overdose himself; he may take a 2- or 3-day supply at once with little harmful effect. *However, this is not true of nonaddicts:*

*any child or nonaddict who accidentally ingests methadone, or any narcotic, should be hospitalized immediately and treated with repeated doses of nalorphine (Nalline), a specific antidote for all narcotics.*

Side effects due to methadone are minimal and are usually dosage-related. In the early weeks of treatment, while tolerance is being built up to large maintenance doses, some oversedation or confusion may appear. This can be managed by a slight decrease in medication—about 10 mg—for a few days, and then resuming build-up at a somewhat slower rate thereafter. Autonomic or smooth-muscle tolerance apparently takes somewhat longer to build up, and constipation from this source may be treated symptomatically by hydrophilic colloids, laxatives, or enemas.

The course of pregnancy and delivery have been normal for women on the methadone maintenance program. Babies thus far born to mothers on high methadone dosage have shown normal alertness and no congenital abnormalities, although one third of the babies have been born premature by weight, perhaps unrelated to methadone therapy. And despite the similarity of methadone to heroin, withdrawal symptoms have been absent or relatively minor in newborns.

A few patients report low sexual appetite in the early months. Here too a slight reduction in dosage and the passage of time are helpful.

## LARGE-SCALE MAINTENANCE THERAPY

Methadone has rarely shown any toxic effects, and by its characteristics is highly suitable for large-scale maintenance therapy. Our program, at present the largest in New York, developed out of Beth Israel Medical Center's Bernstein Institute and has grown to include 13 other hospitals and 22 satellite clinics. Some 20 new units are planned under its umbrella. The central facility still shelters the joint administrative, data, and laboratory services, while local units treat 50 to 150 patients. This arrangement ensures continued high medical standards while allowing the staff in the outlying clinics to know their patients personally and to develop their own treatment styles to some degree.

While elements of the program are subject to constant evaluation and adaptation, certain general procedures can be described.

Criteria for admission to the program are minimal: age 18 or over, an addiction history of at least 2 years, with no severe psychiatric problem or severe multiple addiction. When he is inducted into the program, the patient's job, family, housing, and legal situations are reviewed and he is given a complete medical workup and psychiatric evaluation.

It might be noted here what a medical examination generally reveals, based on the patient population in such programs as that at Beth Israel. The general health of patients at induction is poor. Pulmonary disease is probably the most common condition—untended respiratory infections are aggravated, and some patients harbor tuberculosis. Liver disease and history of hepatitis are common, as are skin and gastrointestinal disorders. There is a high incidence of malnutrition, venereal disease, and dental, foot, and vision problems. As a group, addicts have poor relations with the medical community, both because of the problem of illegality and because they tend not to follow up on appointments for care. Once in a maintenance program which takes responsibility for their care—and works hard to keep them returning for it—they show marked improvement in general health. These patients often suffer from the many other difficulties associated with housing, jobs, and sustenance, but to the degree that the program can help them to regularize their lives and their health management, their general physical condition improves.

*Phase I* The patient is given an initial low dose of methadone, usually 30 to 40 mg, in a glass of fruit juice, and his response is monitored to determine his level of tolerance. Gradually, over the next 3 to 6 weeks, the dosage is escalated until it levels off and remains stable. Stabilization is determined by the patient's reports that he is comfortable, feels no further craving for narcotics, and experiences no euphoria if he tries a heroin shot. This dosage level is usually between 60 and 100 mg per day. Some persons are inducted as inpatients for this period, but most are ambulatory.

*Phase II* For about a year thereafter, the patient comes to the clinic daily to take his stabilized dose of methadone. He leaves a urine sample to be tested for a confirmation of a constant level of methadone and for the possible presence of abuse substances such as other narcotics, alcohol, amphetamines, or barbiturates.

He is also under continuing medical care for other conditions, and he makes lesser or greater use of the facilities for social rehabilitation—job consultation or training, educational guidance, and counselling—according to his needs. Counselling is provided by trained therapists when needed, but the patient is also guided by a "research assistant" who is usually an ex-addict or a long-time maintenance patient experienced in the difficulties the patient encounters.

For most patients, secondary drug use falls off sharply in the early months of treatment, mainly because narcotics cease to provide a kick in the presence of the methadone blockade. But some patients continue to experiment with them, or to seek gratification from substances—cocaine, methedrine, LSD, for example—which are not blocked by methadone. If such use continues at a regular and important rate, the patient's counsellors attempt to bring him to recognize and deal with it as a problem. Those patients who persist in this activity, and those who continue to engage in antisocial or criminal behavior, are potential failures. Concentrated efforts are made to support their rehabilitation and to understand what is needed to do so.

*Phase III* When a patient has shown consistent ability to sustain stable behavior for a year or so, he is considered to be largely rehabilitated. Then he may move into the third phase, that of taking home his medication for a day or two at a time, and eventually several days' supply. He continues to appear at the clinic each week to have his urine checked, to pick up his supply, and, importantly, to drink a full dose under staff supervision. This ensures that he is maintaining himself regularly at the full dose. Signs of narcotic effects may mean that some methadone is being diverted or that the patient is undermedicating himself to get an occasional heroin kick, and in such a case he will need more attention.

Otherwise, although he may still be using the center's social rehabilitation facilities, the patient is generally working or maintaining a home life. He has rejoined the community to some degree.

His maintenance may go on indefinitely. Some patients whose lives have grown more manageable may want to try detoxification and abstinence, and the program offers them help and support in this effort. Asymptomatic withdrawal may be accomplished by a decrease in dosage of 10 mg a week.

## EVALUATION OF THE PROGRAM

An independent evaluation unit at the Columbia University School of Public Health examines the records of the New York City programs to establish which are the crucial components of the programs and what degree of success is achieved in the rehabilitation of narcotics addicts in treatment. Its most recent report, presented at the Third National Conference on Methadone Treatment (November 1970), stated that "*the successes of the program far outweigh the failures*" despite rapid expansion in size and in criteria for patients and in ambulatory induction. The report goes on:

> A majority of the patients have completed their schooling or increased their skills and have become self-supporting. Their pattern of arrests has decreased substantially [from a rate of 120 per 100 patient-years to a rate of 4.5 per 100 patient-years]. This is in sharp contrast to their own previous experience as well as their current experience when compared with a matched group from the detoxification unit, or when compared with those patients who have left the program.

(Statistics show that 20 percent of our patients at intake time are engaged in productive activity—work, school, or homemaking. Productivity for patients in the program for 3 months to 2 years ranges between 70 and 85 percent.)

> Less than 1% of the patients who have remained in the program have reverted to regular heroin use. A small proportion of the patients (10%) present continued evidence of drug use—and another 8% demonstrate continued problems from chronic alcohol abuse. These two problems account for the majority of failures in rehabilitation after the first few months.

The report concludes:

> Many questions continue to remain unanswered with reference to the role of methadone maintenance in the attack on the total problem of heroin addiction; nevertheless the data presented on [this] group . . . continues to demonstrate that this program has been successful in the vast majority of its patients.

Although the 18 percent failure rate of the New York program is low compared to the apparent dropout from other kinds of programs, it is still a matter for concern. Considering that these patients are a fifth of a population that has been somewhat selected in the first place—in that they volunteered for treatment and met certain minimal criteria for admission—the number is significant.

What is to be done to help control the antisocial behavior of perhaps a quarter or more of the country's total heroin-addict population, even supposing that maintenance treatment should eventually become accessible everywhere? The question of how much of the full addict population can actually be aided with methadone will depend on finding out what will help this segment of the population to profit by medication as an aid to rehabilitation.

Both the successes and the failures of the New York program will be amplified and clarified by the many other projects across the nation. Flexibility of approach is the key to the development of a therapy as young as this one. Conceiving and trying new approaches should yield many useful ideas and adaptations.

The concern with patients who find it difficult to stay with the program has spurred efforts to combine methadone treatment with the therapeutic community residence, as, for example, in New York City, at Bronx State Hospital and the Addiction Research and Treatment Corporation of Brooklyn. Such protective settings can support the patient who is having trouble reintegrating himself into a world in which he has had limited success, by offering concentrated attention with such techniques as psychotherapy and group encounters. A study of the case histories of discharged patients shows that few, if any, were pharmacologic failures; rather, they were discharged for persistent and disruptive antisocial behavior or abuse of non-narcotic drugs for which methadone has no blockade effect.

Quick-induction techniques, with only holding doses of methadone, are being tested widely to absorb the large waiting lists in established centers until the patients can join full rehabilitation services.

In a program being developed in Chicago by Dr. Jerome Jaffe, a wide range of modalities is being offered. Besides methadone maintenance there are detoxification and withdrawal systems, residential settings, psychotherapy, and use of the drug cyclazocine, a short-duration antagonist to heroin.

Dr. Robert Dupont, a psychiatrist in Washington, D.C., has developed a crash program for that city. The program admitted 2,500 patients in its first year and aims at reaching the city's entire addict population, an estimated 10,000, within 3 years. For its rehabilitation and laboratory needs this program makes use of existing agencies and community groups. There are no criteria for admission except age. In fact, the program has a clinic open 24 hours a day which will relieve a panicky addict who is on a heroin hunt by giving him a holding dose of methadone, without promises or commitment on his part. (After several such spot visits, he may be asked to confront the fact that he is nibbling at real treatment.) Halfway houses in the program will care for patients who find it hard to make it on the maintenance program, and for parolee patients whose failure will mean a revocation of parole.

The idea of long-term maintenance for adolescents is especially sensitive. Several research projects are currently investigating the needs of young addicts. Since their addiction is often only 2 or 3 years old, it would seem possible to reverse it and try for eventual abstinence. But most workers feel that attempts at withdrawal should not be pressed at the cost of driving patients out of the program altogether.

## WHAT IS A GOOD PROGRAM?

What is a good program, and what a bad? Clearly, at this moment when new methods and approaches are being tried everywhere, any definition of a good program that is based solely on its components risks being outmoded in a year or two. We do know that careful medical procedures lie at the heart of successful maintenance. As to what other rehabilitative services may be essential, most present programs involve general medical care, counselling, and support in solving practical living problems. We believe all these elements, and more, are probably necessary. Of course, experience could show a high success rate from the new quick-induction and holding programs, which supply methadone medication without services while the patient waits to be included in the full program. That possibility would have to be examined. Meanwhile, a program must be judged in terms of how many patients it helps, not by the number of ancillary services it offers.

Where treatment is less effective, it is far from the point to accuse the patient's "low motivation" or "poor character." A bad program imposes rules which favor the staff's convenience but are not essential to the patient's treatment. A program may adhere rigidly to unrealistic standards, and seek to punish or exclude the patient when he does not conform. Such behavior is manipulative, and in the end destructive. That a methadone patient continues to use drugs occasionally, for instance, is not a matter for punitive reaction. He is living a life full of stress, trying to reintegrate himself into a fairly unfriendly world. He may need to test the protection he is receiving from methadone; he may want drug support in a crisis; he may still move in a society of users. What matters is whether the patient is moving toward what he came to the program to achieve—a more stable life, a plausible pattern of social behavior, hopefully a life without crime and the desperation that leads to it. Eventually, the abuse of other drugs could cease altogether.

Motivation is, of course, a major element in a voluntary program. At present there are great numbers of addicts who are waiting for treatment until the existing programs can take them in; their motivation is obvious. But if we hope to reach all those whom maintenance treatment could help, some investigation is needed to tell us what motivates some addicts to ask for treatment and not others. We need to develop methods to interest a still greater proportion of the addict population. Installing centers for voluntary treatment in high-addiction neighborhoods, and publicizing the experience of patients who benefit by them, will do much in this direction. It might be useful to offer detoxification programs in all hospitals. For many, the experience of the treatment for a few months—a few months free of narcotics craving—might be a new and exhilarating option. In all situations, of course, the line between persuasion and coercion is a delicate one, and care must be exercised to protect personal liberties.

## EXPANSION OF FACILITIES

According to present determinations, methadone maintenance therapy has shown itself largely effective, nontoxic, and inexpensive. It costs about 10 cents per daily dose for the medication, with an estimated full service and administrative expense of $1,200 per patient in the first year, and less thereafter. Presented as a major, though not exclusive, modality, it could achieve wide acceptance in target communities. There are about 9,000 patients presently receiving methadone care. But there are an estimated 1 million narcotics addicts in the United States, and most of these cannot get methadone. Expanding its availability is crucial. As formal treatment facilities proliferate in the next few years, the problem will be to develop administrative techniques flexible enough to expand while maintaining high medical and rehabilitation standards. A degree of decentralization must be effected in the presence of governmental fears of misuse and probable reluctance to relinquish controls.

We need a widely deployed system of facilities, but to meet the demand we will have to find ways of rationally including the private practitioner in that system. Decentralization has so far been successful in the New York program, with laboratory work and data collection shared at the main unit. Such centralized services could probably be expanded to allow private physicians to treat patients in their offices and refer them for counselling and laboratory work to the local unit. Many rehabilitated patients now being maintained on public funds could pay a small fee for their maintenance care privately; this would free such monies for more treatment services.

At present, official medical and government opinion stands against the enrollment of private physicians. But many more outlets will be needed than centers will provide; and many a doctor is confronted with a patient he has tended since childhood who now needs help with addiction. The demand is so great already that no program can meet its waiting list, and a surprising number of addicts find their way to doctors' offices to ask, not for heroin, but for methadone care.

We would like to pilot out procedures now to include the private doctor under the administrative umbrella. A clear and well-founded code should be developed immediately, for without it private treatment may be inadequate, or downright bad.

A private physician considering maintenance care for some of his patients may apply to the Food and Drug Administration for a license to use an Investigational New Drug for this purpose. He should not attempt treatment entirely on his own, but inform his back-up hospital and enlist the support of his department chief. Such support, together with evidence of strict medical safeguards and full treatment records, will usually get him through the licensing restrictions. Alternatively, he can find out what services or Investigational New Drug licenses are available in his area and link up with them if he can.

## OUTLOOK

The goals of methadone maintenance therapy are many, and emphasis varies among the different workers. One program may accent a local drop in addiction-related crimes: another may stress the maintained patients' achievement of more socially productive behavior, and a crime-free personal record; still another may have as its eventual goal abstinence from narcotics altogether. All of these purposes relate to the honorable medical ethic of the patient's well-being, and with it, society's.

The methadone program should not deteriorate into a methadone dispensary program. It is a multifaceted treatment and service program. Responsible medical determinations, full medical care on site or through attentive referrals, and, above all, resourceful encouragement are essential to the patient's proper treatment. If the staff is energetic and kindly in outlook, the patient will find the most favorable atmosphere for integrating his life with a maintenance program.

# 29

# *Methadone Maintenance Treatment for 25,000 Heroin Addicts**

VINCENT P. DOLE

Methadone[1] maintenance programs in the United States and Canada are now treating about 9,000 former heroin addicts. The data from these studies amply document the safety of this medication and its efficacy in stopping heroin addiction when it is given under good medical control.

Detailed statistics have been collected in New York City by our central data office and made available to the independent evaluation committee directed by Dr. Frances Gearing. This committee has recommended continued support and expansion of the maintenance programs. The New York State Narcotics Addiction Control Commission has allocated an increased proportion of its next year's budget to maintenance treatment, and political leaders have called for an immediate expansion of maintenance programs in New York to a caseload of 25,000.

It would seem from all this that the only remaining problems of the methadone programs are to live with prosperity, and forget old arguments, now obsolete. The future, however, will not be this easy. The projected expansion of methadone programs to 25,000 in the next three years or sooner will confront us

From the *Journal of the American Medical Association*, Vol. 215, No. 7, February 15, 1971, pp. 1131–1134. 

* This investigation was supported by grants from the Health Research Council (City of New York Department of Health) and the New York State Narcotics Addiction Control Commission. Conclusions stated herein are not necessarily those of the commission.

[1] Nonproprietary and trade names of methadone: *Adanon, Althose, Amidone, Dolophine.*

with difficulties of greater magnitude than any that we have met during the first six years of this work. The problems will be administrative, not medical. The larger that the programs become, the more they will interact with other social agencies and political interests.

For example, if the programs in New York City grow to 25,000, they will be responsible for twice as many individuals with antisocial problems as the total present caseload of the Department of Corrections. How are criminal addicts to be treated and under whose control? General rules for bringing 25,000 criminal addicts into methadone treatment certainly do not exist at present. Is it proper for a judge to force treatment on an addict by sentencing him to a maintenance program? Is it advisable for a physician to accept patients on these terms? I would say definitely no to both of these questions. The rights of addicts must be respected, and the importance of abstinence programs must be recognized. I would object to the imposition of methadone maintenance treatment just as strongly as I have objected in the past to its unavailability when the needs of motivated volunteers could not be met.

Our responsibilities will also have common ground with the duties of narcotics control bureaus. With a caseload of 25,000, methadone programs will be dispensing approximately 9 million doses per year of a potent narcotic. We know that this medication is therapeutic when taken by the right person in a good medical program, but we also must recognize the need for adequate control of its usage. Law enforcement agencies of federal, state, and city governments quite properly have been concerned with the dangers of diversion and misuse of this medication. We must work with them to reduce this danger to a minimum.

So far, we have done well in our programs to ensure good medical control, but I am not sure that we have solved the problem for 25,000 patients. We have efficient, computerized record systems with continuous accountability for all patients, and treatment units that are small enough for all patients to be known personally. We would welcome suggestions from concerned agencies as to how our system of follow-up and data control could be improved without diminishing the effectiveness of the rehabilitation program. As to the medication, we have always insisted that it be dispensed in a form suitable for oral use only, and in the past three years we have been testing various noninjectable tablets which, in addition to medical advantages, can be more accurately controlled by identifying code numbers.

We have given much thought to the quantity of medication that should be dispensed to patients to take at home. Unreliable patients obviously should be required to take all medication under direct observation, but to impose this rule on all patients would be counterproductive. Crime reduction is correlated with rehabilitation. Certainly it would be against the public interest to make the dispensing rules so restrictive that a responsible patient could not hold a full-time job. Here again is a need for communication between law enforcement agencies and medical treatment programs.

We have in common the goal of enabling previously criminal persons to lead socially acceptable, crime-free lives. This will not be done simply by dispensing methadone. If crime is to be reduced significantly, we need an effective rehabilitation program, and this includes specifically the authority to dispense a week's supply of medication to responsible working patients whose conduct in treatment has shown that they merit this trust. At the same time, we must use this authority with good judgment, and recognize the concern of law enforcement agencies that this medication be used only as prescribed.

Under the best circumstances it will be difficult to maintain effectiveness of the rehabilitation services with a rapid expansion to 25,000. How can we be sure that the programs will continue to be as effective as they are now when the number is five times as great? Methadone programs could grow into cumbersome bureaucracies treating more patients than are now being treated by all of the federal, state, municipal, and private programs combined, or, alternatively, methadone might be dispensed without any attempt at rehabilitation. Neither extreme would provide good treatment for addicts. How are quality standards to be maintained?

At the moment, methadone programs are subject to controls exercised jointly by the Bureau of Narcotics and Dangerous Drugs and by the Food and Drug Administration, their authority being based on the proposition that the treatment is still only experimental. Privately, officials of these bureaus concede that the inherent safety and efficacy of the medication are no longer in doubt, but hold that the fiction of experimental status is needed as a legal basis for preventing misuse.

There is some merit in their contention, but in any event, the IND permit which now serves as a license for methadone treatment cannot be retained indefinitely as a control device. Expansion to a caseload of 25,000 in New York, and an equal number elsewhere in the country, is inconsistent with the concept of experimental status. Either the treatment is experimental or it is ready for large-scale use, but not both.

Methadone programs have already brought out strong differences in opinion as to how the treatment should be regulated, and even as to the capacity of the medical profession to define its own standards. The pessimists see only disaster if private physicians are allowed to prescribe methadone, and therefore insist upon controls by governmental agencies with power to prosecute offending physicians. The optimists see addiction becoming part of the inventory of chronic diseases, like diabetes and arthritis, some cases needing institutional care, while other cases are treated by physicians in general practice. It is futile to argue the assumptions that underlie these positions, but this much is clearly before us: Either the leadership of the medical profession and administrators of methadone programs will work together to guide an orderly expansion of methadone services, or the pessimists that view the medical profession as incompetent will win by default.

Let us review the evolution of methadone treatment in New York to learn what we can about the administrative problems in expansion (Figure 1). During the first two years, a few of us working together informally provided good medical services for a small, research-sized group (10 to 50 patients). Like teachers in a one-room school, we knew each patient personally. The ones in trouble were seen more often, the successful ones, less often; all were followed closely enough for us to know what they were doing. With growth to the pilot-program stage (50 to 500), and even more so on becoming a large-service program (500 to

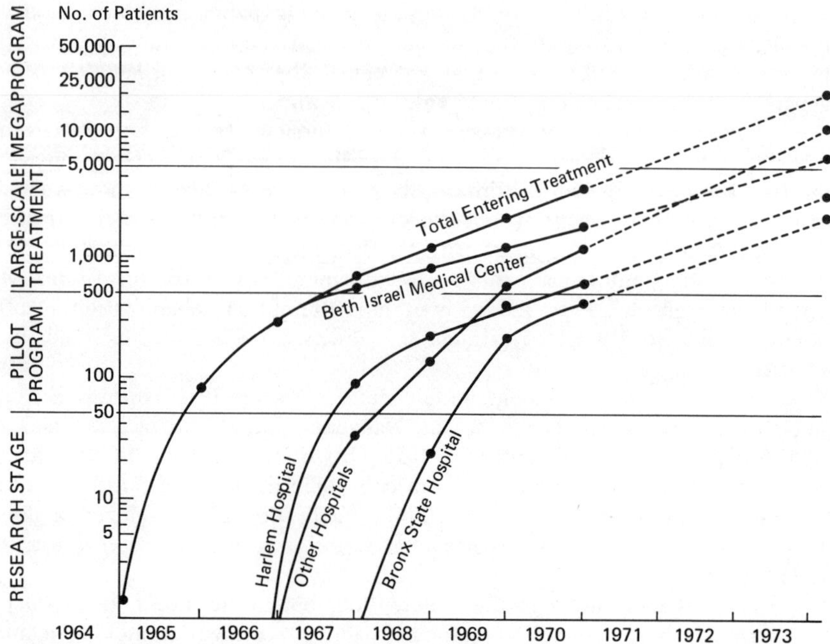


**Figure 1** Expansion of methadone maintenance programs in New York City.

5,000), our administrative structure changed. No longer could any single person know all of the patients or have time to hear their problems. Administrators by necessity delegated the actual treatment to other physicians, and gave their own time to budgets and the details of staff work, laboratory services, data control, and public relations.

The net effect has been a healthy decentralization of the program into small treatment units (50 to 150) which retain the personal qualities of the original research-sized group. The theater for the patient's rehabilitation is his own clinic. These are small enough for him to be known as an individual and independent enough for him to respect the authority of the physician in charge (Figure 2).

With decentralization, the rehabilitation techniques have also become diversified in details—another healthy trend. While general standards of medical practice have been maintained by the sharing of administrative services—data control, central laboratories, staff meetings, and consultations—local units have developed their own styles of counseling. The data and laboratory services could easily be extended to private practitioners affiliated with institutional programs if administrators of existing programs and officials of government wished to encourage this trend. Many rehabilitated patients now being carried on publicly funded programs could pay a reasonable fee for continued treatment by private practitioners.

The problem before us is that decentralization of methadone programs,

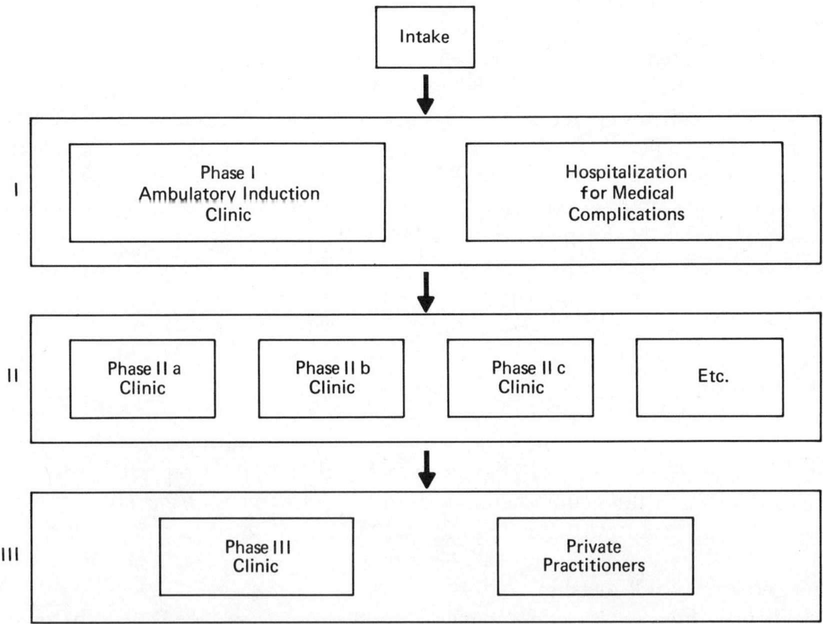


**Figure 2** Organization of methadone maintenance programs.

and specifically the inclusion of private practitioners in the system, would diminish the power of governmental agencies to regulate the treatment. At stake is control over a large program with a growing budget (for the country as a whole, perhaps $100 million per year by 1973) and with political significance at all levels of government. Decentralization of services might bring treatment to more addicts, but it would weaken the bureaus. History fails to disclose a precedent in which any bureau has cooperated in a reduction of its power.

Another concern for the future, this one internal to the medical profession, is the rivalry that has existed between different theories of addiction and different modalities of treatment. With growth to 25,000-patient size, methadone programs might be seen as a threat to the existence of programs using other techniques. This is wrong. We must find ways to work together in the public interest. Those of us who have been directly involved in methadone programs are well aware of the need for other programs, especially those that can prove effective in preventing heroin addiction.

We do not forget that 18% of the patients admitted to methadone programs in New York City during the past six years have been discharged as failures. Although this is a relatively low failure rate as compared to what appears to be the dropout from other programs, the problem becomes a major one for society as the methadone program grows. What is to be done to control the antisocial behavior of 5,000 addicts discharged as failures from a group of 25,000 admitted to methadone treatment?

Analysis of the case histories of patients discharged from methadone programs in New York City shows that few of them, if any, were pharmacological failures. These patients were discharged for persistent and disruptive antisocial behavior, or for persistent abuse of non-narcotic drugs (alcohol, barbiturates, amphetamines) for which methadone has no blockade effect, but even in the worst cases the regular use of heroin was stopped while the patients were taking their daily dose of methadone. This means that additional techniques for control of psychopathic behavior and for treatment of non-narcotic abuses must be developed if the overall program is to be made more effective. Combinations of methadone blockade with residential support and various psychotherapeutic techniques are now being studied by research groups in New York and other cities. We need this research, and a climate of scientific objectivity. We need reliable data on the effectiveness and the cost of non-methadone techniques alone and in combination with blockade treatment.

All of these problems have been with us in some degree since the beginning of the methadone research. Our relation to other social agencies, the maintenance of quality standards and reliable statistics, the effort to separate medicine from politics, the rivalries and jealousies among professionals, have always complicated the basic problem of treating addicts. With growth in size of methadone programs, these divisive problems will be intensified, but can be met with good will and good medical leadership.

There is however a serious danger that treatment programs will become subordinated to power struggles. So far the programs have been effective because their direction has been medical. The procedure has been developed by physicians with personal experience in treatment of addicts, not by governmental agencies or the medical administrators chosen by them. The success of this treatment in rehabilitation of addicts will decline significantly if methadone programs cease to be medical institutions, and instead become the instruments of another bureaucracy.

I call upon the leaders of our major medical institutions, the deans and professors of medical schools, the administrators of teaching hospitals, the officials of medical societies, to take an active interest in the treatment of heroin addicts. The medical profession cannot ignore the leading cause of death in urban adolescents and young adults. Enough research has been done to show how heroin addicts can be treated successfully in a medical setting. If we apply what we know now, effectively and on a large scale, we can begin to control heroin addiction and related crime in our large cities.

# 30

# *Methadone Maintenance: A Problem in Delivery of Service*

HENRY BRILL

Virtually every issue which relates to drug dependence is suffused with emotion that turns differences of opinion into controversy and leads to distortions, exaggerations, and misunderstandings. In methadone maintenance one can see an excellent example of the process. The drug has been known for years as a synthetic capable of producing addiction (full morphine-type drug dependence) (1) but very useful as a transitional drug in withdrawal from heroin. (2) It remained for Dole and Nyswander to show that methadone could be used in a radically different way and that addicts could be maintained on it in such a way as to promote their rehabilitation. The initial series of six cases was started in January 1964, and by December 1970 an estimated 10,000 US addicts in more than 60 programs across the country were receiving methadone maintenance.

The development of these programs has been accompanied by active controversy. The method, on the one hand, has been proclaimed by some to be a virtual panacea for all opiate addiction, and some writers even have mistakenly described the drug as a non-narcotic antiaddiction medication. On the other hand, opponents have declared it to be little better than an outright fraud which does nothing more than replace heroin addiction with methadone addiction, and they compare it to the earlier "heroin cure" of morphine addiction. Some black communities have branded methadone maintenance as a white racist plot to keep blacks down, although other black groups have promoted use of the drug in their own indigenously controlled clinics.

Even among those who apply the method, there are important differences of opinion as to certain details, such as the proper dose range, the exact criteria of case selection, the required type of case supervision and support, and the nature of the mechanism which accounts for the favorable results. Substantial agreement, however, does exist among authorities with respect to two crucial issues.

The first is that when methadone maintenance is correctly applied it produces striking effects in confirmed heroin addicts and leads to social, economic, and psychological rehabilitation in a high proportion of cases.

The second is that to produce such effects, methadone must be given in such a way as to produce physical dependence without the mental experiences of addiction. To achieve this essential condition the drug is given orally in gradually increasing doses over a period of weeks until full tolerance at the desired

From the *Journal of the American Medical Association*, Vol. 215, February 15, 1971, pp. 1148–1150. 

dose level is reached. This level is then maintained by oral medication from that time forward. Under these conditions the addict experiences no "rush," no "high," no "nodding," and no euphoria. The major demonstrable psychological effect is a return to capacity for normal adjustment.

Methadone maintenance is thought to act by saturating body receptors for opiate. Although it has been demonstrated that addicts receiving methadone maintenance are indeed nonresponsive to the usual street doses of heroin intravenously, (2) there has been no pharmacological explanation of why patients receiving methadone do not, for the most part, turn to other drugs or to alcohol for "kicks." The problem of interpretation is further complicated by reports that many addicts do well with relatively low doses which would saturate the receptors to a far lesser degree. (4) It does seem clear that the special value of methadone depends on its prolonged action and the stable state of tolerance and physical dependence it can produce when taken by mouth, and only when taken by mouth. This so-called narcotic blockade does not occur when the drug is taken by injection by addicts or when taken by injection or orally by nonaddicts. In the latter case, methadone is capable of producing the full syndrome associated with heroin or morphine addiction.

Thus methadone can be seen as a double-edged sword. Used in the right way, it can control and terminate an existing addiction syndrome. Used in the wrong way, it can initiate such a syndrome in persons not previously addicted or can maintain an ongoing addiction syndrome with all of its physical, psychological, and behavioral aspects.

This double potential has given rise to perhaps the sharpest and most important controversy which methadone has yet aroused. Methadone maintenance has been controlled as an experimental procedure and permission to apply it has been granted only to those who have been able to meet criteria set by federal agencies, including the capacity to provide necessary supervision and support services.

Now, however, in view of the uniformly favorable reports from various treatment groups, and because of the urgent nature of the problem, including the criminal behavior of heroin addicts, many persons are calling for an end to special controls on methadone maintenance, and asking that all physicians be permitted to prescribe maintenance for addicts with no restrictions beyond those which apply to any other medical use of narcotics. Opponents of such a move fear that it could create a serious hazard to public health through the diversion of a considerable amount of methadone into the street.

A solution to the controversy would seem to require the design and testing of a system of delivery which will provide this kind of medical care on the required scale without hazard to public health.

In this connection the comments by Dole [article 29, this text] are worthy of review. He points out that New York state political leaders now call for an expansion of the methadone case load from the current 5,000 to 25,000 within three years. This, he says, will be twice the case load of the Department of Corrections, and will require the dispensing of 9 million doses of a potent narcotic annually.

"So far," he writes, "we have done well in our programs to ensure good medical control, but I am not sure that we have solved the problem for 25,000 patients." He continues, "We have . . . the goal of enabling previously criminal persons to lead socially acceptable, crime-free lives. This will not be done simply by dispensing methadone."

The twin issues of drug control and adequate staffing, implicit in the Dole statement on 25,000 cases, would have to be faced on an even larger scale if the special controls were to be terminated abruptly. New York alone has an estimated total of 50,000 to 100,000 addicts, and the higher figure is thought closer to the truth. The potential number of cases for methadone could be far larger than the 25,000 that worry Dole, and the amount of drug prescribed would be correspondingly greater than 9 million doses.

Furthermore, without controls the case load might well reach its full potential in the first year, not the third year. This would give increased grounds for concern about large-scale failure of the method through perfunctory and mechanical procedures and the related hazard of correspondingly large diversion of methadone into the black market.

Concern about diversion finds some foundation in published papers (5–7) and in some informal reports which, though exaggerated, apparently are not totally without foundation. It should be noted that in each instance the problem even when quite extensive appears to stem from the poor judgment of a relatively few individual practitioners.

Such considerations must give one pause, and underline the need for careful evaluation of any new system for delivery of methadone maintenance. In seeking a solution to the problem, we should take into account the experience now available to us through programs operated by hospital groups and organized clinics. These agencies have already demonstrated their capacity to provide methadone maintenance adequately and safely. Although further experience may well identify types of cases which do not require such formal organization in treatment systems, for the present, and certainly for the management of the massive problem that lies immediately ahead, it would seem prudent to join Dole in his appeal to hospitals and medical schools to become involved with this work, rather than to take the risks of an untested system. Medical organizations should become involved not only to forestall a possible bureaucratic takeover of the service but because they have the special resources required to meet this urgent social need. The feasibility of such operations by hospital groups has been more than adequately demonstrated by Dole and Nyswander, and by those who have followed.

The urgent question of the moment is how methadone maintenance can be provided on the scale that is required without endangering others through diversion of the drug and without losing the therapeutic value through inadequate support services. At this stage of our experience it appears that the medical organizations have the potential to provide the answer safely and rapidly. It is to be hoped that they will be able to respond to this challenge and to meet the current need. An expanded methadone maintenance through this means is neither a panacea nor is it a final answer, but it is an obvious next move.

## REFERENCES

1. Sapira, J. M., Ball, J. C., Cottrell, E. S.: Addiction to methadone among patients at Lexington and Fort Worth. *Public Health Rep.* **83**: 691–696, 1968.
2. Isbell, H., Volgel, V. H.: The addiction liability of methadone (Amidone, Dolophine 10820) and its use in the treatment of the morphine abstinence syndrome. *Amer. J. Psychiat.* **105**: 909–914, 1949.
3. Freedman, A. M., Zaks, A., Resnick, O., et al: Blockade with methadone, cyclazocine, and naloxone. *Int. J. Addict.* **5**: 507–515, 1970.
4. Jaffe, J. H.: Further experience with methadone in the treatment of narcotic addicts. *Int. J. Addict.* **5**: 375–389, 1970.
5. Richman, A., Humphrey, B.: Epidemiology of criminal narcotic addiction in Canada. *Bull. Narcot.* **1**: 31–39, 1969.
6. Spear, H. B.: Growth of heroin addition in the United Kingdom. *Int. J. Addict.* **64**: 245–255, 1969.
7. Pierce, J.: Suicide and mortality amongst heroin addicts in Britain. *Brit. J. Addict.* **62**: 391–398, 1967.

# 31

# *Narcotic Antagonists in Opiate Dependence*

M. FINK

The use of narcotic antagonists in the treatment of heroin addiction was the subject of a symposium sponsored by the National Institute of Mental Health and the Department of Psychiatry, New York Medical College, on 4 June 1970, in New York.

Narcotic antagonists were introduced into the treatment of opiate dependence in 1965 after extensive studies of the conditioning aspects of addiction. Himmelsbach (1) showed that autonomic changes persist in opiate addicts for as long as 6 months after withdrawal. Environmental contingencies, frequently associated with the repetitive injection of opiates, were shown to possess qualities of a nonspecific conditioned stimulus to reactivate neural mechanisms that mediate abstinence from opiates (2). Wikler and Pescor (3) showed that the natural syndrome of morphine withdrawal could be conditioned. It was the interaction of physical dependence and conditioning to environmental factors that was the basis for relapse after withdrawal from opiates (4). The conditioning factors in relapse were also seen as the reason why psychotherapy had been unsuccessful in treating addicts, for the opiate-seeking behavior of the addict is determined largely by processes of which neither he nor the therapist is aware (5).

Within this framework and from the standpoint of behavior theory, Wikler (4) suggested that successful treatment would require extinction of both conditioned abstinence and opiate-seeking behavior for lack of reinforcement. N-allylnormorphine (nalorphine, Nalline) would not be suitable for carrying out such extinction because early studies showed that, for chronic spinal dogs, this narcotic antagonist had to be given every 3 hours to block the effects of morphine given every 6 hours and to prevent the development of tolerance and physical dependence to morphine.

The application of this concept was made possible by observations by Martin and his co-workers (6) that former addicts maintained on cyclazocine were protected against both the narcotic effects of opiates and those properties which produced dependence. Wikler predicted that such addicts who assay self-administration of opiates would soon extinguish the operant aspects of their drug-seeking behavior for lack of reinforcement and because of associated reduction of conditioned abstinence and anxiety.

After initial successful reports by Jaffe and Brill (7), Martin et al. (6), and Freedman et al. (8), more extensive clinical trials were undertaken. At this meeting, the ongoing clinical trials with former addicts on cyclazocine were reported by Laskowitz (Lincoln Hospital, Bronx, N.Y.); Petursson (Manhattan State Hospital, Ward's Island, N.Y.); Resnick, Fink, and Freedman (New York Medical College); Jacobsen (Lillian Wald Clinic); and Jaffe (University of Chicago). These trials, since 1968, showed an overall acceptance and continued treatment rate of 40 percent of more than 450 adult male addicts. Sixty patients have been maintained in treatment for more than 1 year, and 20 for more than 3 years. The initial trials in many units were marred by the experimentation necessary to establish an adequate daily dosage (now set at 4 to 8 mg) and duration of antagonism to heroin (22 to 28 hours for 4 mg given orally), as well as the need to develop rehabilitation facilities.

Almost all former addicts report continued experimentation with opiates, with decreasing frequency the longer they continue using cyclazocine, but without readdiction, provided they maintain a daily intake of cyclazocine. A rate of readdiction of 20 percent was associated with discontinued use of cyclazocine.

A daily intake of cyclazocine was accompanied by a variety of agonistic drug actions, chiefly irritability, insomnia, and illusions, which were reported early in treatment. Adaptation occurred rapidly. Resnick described a successful 4-day schedule for increasing the dosage of cyclazocine to 4 mg by the concurrent use of oral naloxone to antagonize the agonistic effects of cyclazocine. In some patients, rhinitis, muscle aches, and malaise persisting for 12 to 36 hours was described after withdrawal. Simeon (New York Medical College) reported antidepressant activity for cyclazocine in clinical trials in in-patient and out-patient depressives (9).

A second narcotic antagonist, *n*-allylnoroxymorphone (naloxone) was reported in clinical trial by Zaks and Fink (New York Medical College), Kleber (Yale University), and Kurland (Maryland Psychiatric Research Institute, Baltimore). Single intravenous doses of naloxone are effective in antagonizing opiates for 3 to 5 hours. Intravenous doses of 0.7 to 1.0 mg effectively antagonize 50 mg of heroin. When given orally the drug's potency is significantly less. Zaks reported that 3.0 g/day was required by addicts to achieve 24-hour antagonism to injected heroin (25 mg/2 ml per 2 minutes). Kleber and Kurland successfully treated 30 former addicts with dosages of up to 400 mg daily. The outstanding characteristics of naloxone were its specificity as an antagonist and the absence of any agonistic effects. Because of short supply and expense, however, these trials have been limited and have been performed with only a few subjects. The clinical use of parenteral naloxone in anesthesia, which provides extensive data on safety and efficacy, was reported by Foldes (Montefiore Hospital, New York) and Kallos (University of Pennsylvania).

Reviewing the clinical data, Freedman and Yolles (National Institute of Mental Health) concluded that these trials, particularly with cyclazocine, supported the clinical applicability of the conditioning hypothesis and suggested that an ideal antagonist would be one that exhibited antagonistic efficacy for weeks or months, without agonistic actions.

Harris (University of North Carolina), Blumberg (Endo Laboratories), Villareal (University of Michigan), Archer (Sterling-Winthrop), and Gray (Lederle Laboratories) reported that other *n*-allyl and cyclorphan derivatives of opiates were now in animal assay for their potency in antagonizing opiates. Jacobsen (Endo Laboratories) and Yolles (University of Delaware) described studies aimed at the development of long-acting formulations by delaying absorption from material implanted in body tissues; in successful trials in animals absorption has been extended over 2 to 3 weeks.

The application of implants of antagonists in the prophylaxis of opiate dependence in high-risk populations, particularly juveniles, the development of an "immunization" procedure, and the need for more extensive laboratory studies were discussed by Martin (Lexington), Fink, and Cochin (Boston University).

In the present chaos of treatment and prophylaxis of heroin addiction, therapeutic trials with narcotic antagonists represent a unique opportunity to test a rational theory of relapse in opiate dependence, a means for prophylaxis, and a way to reduce the incidence of juvenile dependence on opiates, and of opiate-related deaths.

## REFERENCES AND NOTES


1. C. K. Himmelsbach, *Arch. Int. Med.* **69**, 766 (1942).
2. A. Wikler, *Amer. J. Psychiat*, **105**, 329 (1948).
3. A. Wikler and F. T. Pescor, *Pharmacologist* 7, 171 (1965); A. Wikler, *Psycho-pharmacologia* **10**, 255 (1967).
4. A. Wikler, in *Narcotics*, D. M. Wilner and G. G. Kassebaum, Eds. (McGraw-Hill, New York, 1965), pp. 85–102.

5. A. Wikler, in *The Addictive States*, A. Wikler, Ed. (Williams & Wilkins, Baltimore, 1968), p. 280.
6. W. A. Martin, C. W. Gorodetsky, T. K. McLane, *Clin. Pharmacol. Therap.* 7, 455 (1966).
7. J. H. Jaffe and L. Brill, *Int. J. Addictions* 1, 99 (1966).
8. A. M. Freedman, M. Fink, R. Sharoff, A. Zaks, *J. Amer. Med. Ass.* **202**, 191 (1967); *Amer. J. Psychiat.* **124**, 1499 (1968).
9. M. Fink, J. Simeon, T. Itil, A. M. Freedman, *Clin. Pharmacol. Ther.* **11**, 41 (1970).
10. This meeting was conducted in the course of development of a long-acting narcotic antagonist—part of the addiction research program which is supported by contract with the New York State Narcotic Addiction Control Commission.

# 32

## *A Behavior Change Participation Model for Drug Users Undergoing Pharmacological Therapy**

DOUGLAS W. MATHESON, ROBERT W. EARL, STEPHEN J. LYNCH, MEREDITH DAVISON, ROBERT G. AUSTIN

This project investigated motivational factors affecting the voluntary participation of inpatient drug abusers and narcotic addicts in behavioral and pharmacological therapy at Stockton State Hospital. High drop-out rates and frequent readmissions characterize all voluntary treatment systems (Freedman, Fink, Sharoff, and Zaks, 1967). To engage the patients in therapy, this study utilized two methods of learning, participation versus passive, and three "therapeutic" drugs, methadone, apomorphine, and atropine sulfate. Presumably, the learning methods generated two degrees of intrinsic motivation while the drugs controlled in different degrees the aversive drives, pain and anxiety, associated with heroin withdrawal.

Grant and Grant (1967) presented a model for participation learning in their report on the New Careers Development Project. The "self-study" model states that an individual's motivation to learn (i.e., to exhibit systematic changes in performance) increases with amount of (a) his active participation as a teacher in the learning process (e.g., Efthin, 1968), (b) his effort to find answers to self-initiated questions, (c) self-study directed toward achievement rather than

Stockton State Hospital Research Report STO-50. Reprinted by permission of authors.
* The opinions or conclusions stated in this paper are those of the authors and are not to be construed as official or as necessarily reflecting the policy of the Department of Mental Hygiene.

self-cure, (d) group sharing of the individual's actual progress towards self-selected goals, and (e) real and simulated task performance (as opposed to abstract or theoretical instruction). Accordingly, the behavioral therapy sessions for the experimental group employed the participation model while the sessions for the control group did not. The control group received lectures on the identical subject matter under traditional schoolroom methods of "passive" learning.

The theoretical and practical considerations behind the selection of drugs and dosage levels for control of the pain and anxieties associated with heroin withdrawal may be summarized as follows: (a) Methadone hydrochloride has recently received qualified experimental support as a narcotic substitute and effective antagonist to narcotic withdrawal symptoms and the euphoric or systemic effects of opiates. Ausubel (1966) and Dole and Nyswander (1965) have recommended initial dosages of 10–20 mg, twice daily, to control abstinence symptoms and avoid euphoric and addicting effects. The smallest dosage, 10 mg/cap, 1 b.i.d., was used in the present study to reduce the aversive drives due to heroin abstinence. (b) Apomorphine is an emetic used to induce vomiting in case of poisoning. Burroughs (1959, p. XLII ff.) reported that apomorphine has also been used in combination with minute amounts of morphine as an effective agent in an eight-day cure for heroin addiction and antagonist to withdrawal cramps, fever, and idiosyncratic abstinence symptoms. The reported "cure," if valid, may represent successful avoidance conditioning mediated by the aversion to the apomorphine, the morphine serving as the conditioned stimulus. In order to investigate the possibility of other sub-emetic therapeutic effects of apomorphine in heroin withdrawal, this study used 6.5 mg/cap, 1 b.i.d. The expectation, however, was that even a sub-emetic dosage could increase the aversive drives due to heroin abstinence. (c) Atropine sulfate was used as the placebo for purposes of experimental control. Superficial similarities to the experimental drugs in appearance, taste, and certain peripheral physiological effects made atropine the logical choice for the placebo. Any motivational effects due to atropine, however, were expected to mediate between those due to methadone or apomorphine. The dosage was 0.4 mg/cap, 1 b.i.d.

The experimental hypotheses were that any real differences in class attendance or program drop-out rate due to the (a) learning methods would favor the participation model and (b) drug treatments would favor methadone over atropine and both of these over apomorphine.

## METHOD

### Subjects

Several male and six female voluntary inpatients at Stockton State Hospital served as subjects. The mean age of the subjects was 22.23 years, with a range from 16–41 years. The average subject had completed 10th grade education, with a range from 5th to 12th grade. Three males and one female were heroin addicts; the remainder were classified under drug abuse. Only the three male addicts received methadone, two out of the three being assigned at random to the participation learning condition. The female heroin addict and the nine drug abuse patients were assigned randomly to the four remaining conditions.

The patients were exhaustively interviewed and medically examined prior to acceptance in order to determine the extent of their drug involvement and their psychological and physical suitability as subjects. All available candidates qualified and subsequent analysis of psychological test scores showed that the randomization procedures satisfactorily equated subgroups on the variables measured, namely, (a) Peabody Picture Vocabulary Test, (b) Digit Span, WAIS, (c) Memory for Designs Test, (d) Shipley-Institute of Living Scale, and (e) Julian Rotter-Internal-External Locus of Control Scale.

## Procedure

The subjects were randomly assigned to the six conditions (two learning methods and three drug treatments) under restrictions that (a) only verified (by abstinence symptoms) heroin addicts could receive methadone, (b) subclass n's should be equal or proportional, and (c) prior to termination of the experiment, the pharmacist alone should know the exact assignments. Table 1 shows the actual subclass n's, the unverified female heroin user having fallen into the atropine group under participation learning. Since each behavioral measure summarized a subject's performance from Monday through Friday for each of the three weeks of behavioral therapy, the experimental plan conformed to a 2 x 3 x 3 factorial design with repeated measures on the third factor.

The drug therapy program commenced with all subjects receiving atropine sulfate, 0.4 mg/cap, 1 b.i.d., for seven days, followed by 24 days of differential drug therapy under the dosage described in the third paragraph of this paper. The behavioral therapy sessions began on day 13 and ended on day 31, terminating the experiment.

The three treatment drugs were dispensed in identical blue capsules. The contents were similar in taste and capable of inducing similar, although minor, physiological and psychological reactions that served to mask the identity of the drugs from the subjects and nursing staff alike.

The dependent variable was the percentage of the one-hour long therapy sessions a subject voluntarily attended on Mondays through Fridays in each of the three-week periods of the behavioral therapy program. Additional performance scores besides attendance included (a) before and after measures of the subjects' retention of the material covered in the therapy sessions and (b) ratings,

**TABLE 1. Mean Percentage Attendance at Daily Therapy Sessions**

| *Drug* | *Learning Method* | *N* | *Weeks* $C_1$ | $C_2$ | $C_3$ | $\bar{X}$ |
|---|---|---|---|---|---|---|
| $A_1$ (Methadone) | $B_1$ (Participation) | 2 | 100 | 90 | 100 | 97 |
| | $B_2$ (Passive) | 1 | 80 | 20 | 60 | 53 |
| $A_2$ (Apormorphine) | $B_1$ | 2 | 80 | 40 | 50 | 57 |
| | $B_2$ | 2 | 100 | 60 | 0 | 53 |
| $A_3$ (Atropine) | $B_1$ | 3 | 100 | 87 | 93 | 93 |
| | $B_2$ | 3 | 93 | 53 | 60 | 69 |

made by two research assistants, of various characteristics of the intrasession behaviors of each subject during 9 out of the 15 sessions. These characteristics included anxiety symptoms such as depression, apathy, hostility, negative contributions, and complaints, as well as intrinsic achievement-motivation indices such as goal setting, planning ahead, positive contributions, and sociability. The subjects also attended more traditional therapy sessions conducted by non-research personnel, all six groups being treated alike on these occasions.

### *Passive Learning Method*

Two research assistants alternated as lecturers during these sessions. The course content included instruction on (a) established research results on drug effects, therapy, and rehabilitation, (b) psychological research and theory on addiction and related personality disorders, and (c) New Careers goals, sub-goals, and ten skill areas requisite to goal attainment.

### *Participation Learning Method*

Two research assistants alternated as guides, catalysts, reinforcers, resource individuals, moderators, and change agents operating under quasi-socratic methods. The subjects, working in three teams of sizes 2, 2, and 3, were given initial library research assignments in the subject areas covered by the lecturers under the passive learning method. Emphasis was on team efforts towards development of (a) group skills, (b) research skills, (c) organizational dynamics, (d) strategies for planned change, (e) knowledge of social trends and issues, (e) interview skills, (f) self-awareness, (g) writing skills, (h) speaking skills, and (i) reading skills. This program was obviously overly ambitious for the 15 one-hour sessions; but the criticism is irrelevant. For the purpose of this research was to study the effectiveness of the participation process as a motivational technique, regardless of short-term improvement or differential group performance in the skill areas listed.

## RESULTS

Table 1 shows the mean weekly attendance of the six treatment groups over three weeks of behavioral therapy. ANOVA revealed no differences in performance between the methadone ($A_1$) and atropine ($A_3$) groups, but both of these groups performed differently from the apomorphine group ($A_2$) ($p < .05$); the mean attendance rates were 82%, 81%, and 55%, respectively. Furthermore, under the participation learning condition, the methadone ($A_1B_1$) and atropine ($A_3B_1$) groups attended the therapy sessions at least 87% of the time, while the apomorphine group's ($A_2B_1$) attendance dropped to 50% ($p < .05$) by the third week. Under the passive learning condition, all three groups show a sharp drop in attendance ($p < .001$), but the apomorphine group ($A_2B_2$) declined at a significantly faster overall rate (i.e., linear trends differed significantly, $p < .05$) than either the methadone ($A_1B_2$) or atropine ($A_3B_2$) group did during the three weeks of behavioral therapy. Finally, the apomorphine group showed even a sharper decline in attendance under passive learning

**TABLE 2. Mean Percentage Attendance at Daily Therapy Sessions (Drugs Ignored)**

| | | Weeks | | |
|---|---|---|---|---|
| *Learning Method* | *N* | $C_1$ | $C_2$ | $C_3$ |
| $B_1$ (Participation) | 7 | 94 | 74 | 83 |
| $B_2$ (Passive) | 6 | 93 | 50 | 40 |

($A_2B_2$) than they did under participation learning conditions ($A_0B_1$): that is, the linear trends differed significantly ($p < .05$).

The learning method by trials interaction (BXC), shown in Table 2, was significant ($p < .05$); but the superiority of the participation method over the passive method depended upon drugs (i.e., the A x B x C interaction was significant, ($p < .05$).

ANOVA of the anxiety symptoms data showed that variation among subjects exceeded the variation among group means, even though the negative correlation found between the means of the six groups and the attendance means listed in the right hand margin of Table 1 was large, Pearson's $r = -.933$, and significant ($p < .05$). Consistent with the ANOVA results, individual anxiety scores correlated poorly with individual attendance scores, $r = -.258$ (n.s.).

The subjects learned more under participation learning, 4.86 points increase, than they did under passive learning, 2.36 points increase in knowledge; but the difference was not statistically significant. Group differences in performance on the remaining measures of behavior were entirely attributable to chance.

## DISCUSSION

The results supported the experimental hypothesis that participation learning would motivate the higher rate of attendance between the two learning methods under study. Our interpretation of the results is that intrinsic motivation dominated anxiety under participation learning conditions, although far less effectively in the case of the apomorphine drug group, while anxiety dominated intrinsic motivation under the passive learning conditions, regardless of drug treatment. The large negative correlation found between the anxiety symptoms and attendance supported this interpretation and was furthermore consistent with the results of other research where anxiety was measured during task performance (Atkinson, 1964, pp. 241, 248–251), as in the case of the present study.

The results were also consistent with the second experimental hypothesis that any significant difference in attendance due to drugs would favor methadone over atropine and both of these over apomorphine. The effects due to apomorphine differed significantly from the effects due to either atropine or methadone, and both differences were in the direction predicted. Even the nonsignificant difference in effects due to atropine and methadone was in the predicted direction. Again we interpret drug effects in terms of the hypothetical construct "anxiety." The effect of methadone, as antagonist to the symptoms of withdrawal, was to reduce anxiety and the attendant task-avoidance responses; while apomorphine, by contrast, induced anxiety in the nonaddicted patients. Apparently, however, the amount of methadone used in this study was insufficient to induce the euphoria that would separate the performances of the methadone and atropine groups.

The present results bear upon "the applicability of the medical model of drug action as a rationale for the use of chemical agents to accomplish psychological (as opposed to physiological) alterations" (Lennard, Epstein, Bernstein, and Ransom, 1970, p. 439) of behavior. Our results suggest that drugs may serve to increase or reduce anxiety and thereby determine whether an individual will avoid a task situation or not under conditions of free choice. Anxiety may even motivate involuntary task-orientation if the individual is confined in an anxiety provoking situation and must perform the task in order to escape. Voluntary engagement in achievement oriented activity depends, however, upon the arousal of intrinsic motivation in sufficient strength to dominate anxiety (Atkinson, 1964, pp. 246–247). Arousal, in turn, depends upon complex, yet specifiable, relationships between cognitive states and environmental cues (Atkinson, 1964; Dember, 1960; Dember and Earl, 1957; Dember and Jenkins, 1970, pp. 631–640). The New Careers participation learning method proved to be a powerful realization of the intrinsic motivation model and a mandatory adjunct to the drug therapies used in the present study. Clearly, the specificity of actions that develops when anxiety is controlled or achievement-motivation aroused cannot be due to physiological or psychological effects of drugs alone; for the specificity, variability, and development of behavior sequences depend upon many other conditions of the laws of learning, the principle of reinforcement, in particular. The behavioral model also suggests the use of an euphoric agent such as methadone as a powerful reinforcing stimulus to shape "desirable" means-end behaviors in narcotic addicts.

## REFERENCES

Atkinson, J. W. *An introduction to motivation.* New York: Van Nostrand, 1964.

Ausubel, D. P. The Dole-Nyswander treatment of heroin addiction. *Journal of the American Medical Association*, 1966, **195**, 165–166.

Burroughs, W. S. *Naked lunch.* New York: Grove Press, 1959, Evergreen Black Cat Edition, 1966.

Dember, W. N. *The psychology of perception.* New York: Holt, Rinehart and Winston, 1960.

Dember, W. N. and Earl, R. W. Analysis of exploratory, manipulatory, and curiosity behaviors. *Psychological Review*, 1957, **64**, 91–96.

Dember, W. N. and Jenkins, J. J. *General psychology: modeling behavior and experience.* Englewood Cliffs, N.J.: Prentice-Hall, 1970.

Dole, V. P., and Nyswander, M. A medical treatment of diacetylmorphine (heroin) addiction. *Journal of the American Medical Association*, 1965, **195**, 646–650.

Efthin, A. *The homework helper program.* Mobilization for Youth, New York City, 1968.

Freedman, A. M., Fink, M., Sharoff, R., and Zaks, A. Cyclazocine and methadone in narcotic addiction. *Journal of the American Medical Association*, 1967, **202**, 191–194.

GRANT, J. D., and GRANT, J. *Report on the New Careers Development Project.* NIMH Research Grant OM-01616 (*Training Offenders for Crime and Delinquency Work*), 1967.

LENNARD, H. L., EPSTEIN, L. J., BERNSTEIN, A., and RANSOM, D. C. Hazards implicit in prescribing psychoactive drugs. *Science,* 1970, **169,** 438–441.

# 33

# *The Use of Covert Sensitization with Institutionalized Narcotic Addicts*

GEORGE J. STEINFELD

Maladaptive approach and avoidance responses have both been systematically treated with behavior modification techniques for more than a decade. Avoidance behaviors such as phobias and specific fears of particular realistic situations have been effectively dealt with by Wolpe's (1958) technique of reciprocal inhibition. The specific methods include systematic desensitization, assertive training, thought stopping, the use of sexual responses, and aversion-relief therapy.

Maladaptive approach responses such as cigarette smoking (Franks et al., 1966), homosexuality (Freund, 1960), alcoholism (Franks, 1966), transvestism (Blakemore et al., 1966) have been subjected to aversive stimulation in order to reduce and/or eliminate faulty approach behavior. With the usual technique of aversive conditioning the aversive stimulus is presented contiguously with the socially undesirable stimulus. Anant (1968) has recently summarized the work with chemical aversion therapy and faradic stimulation for the treatment of alcoholism, sexual deviancy, smoking, and self-injurious behavior. MacCulloch et al. (1965), treating cases of alcoholism with aversive electrical stimulation (shock), reported no success, even though shock was successfully used with homosexuals.

Recently, Cautela (1966) has developed a procedure called Covert Sensitization (C.S.) to treat maladaptive approach behavior. With this procedure, the undesirable stimuli are both presented covertly, i.e., in imagination only. The intent is to "sensitize" the person to the undesirable stimulus so he can build up an avoidance response to it where previously it was pleasurable. In other words, whereas the usual aversive conditioning technique utilizes external stimuli, in Covert Sensitization the pairing of the aversive and undesirable stimuli is internal.

From *The International Journal of the Addictions,* Vol. 5, No. 2, June 1970, pp. 225–232. By courtesy of Marcel Dekker, Inc., and author.

Cautela (1966) has employed Covert Sensitization in the treatment of alcoholism, obesity, and homosexuality, and reports success with all of these behaviors. Ashem and Donner (1968) replicated Cautela's experiment with alcoholics and found significant decreases in drinking behavior with this technique. Though Covert sensitization is a relatively new method of aversive conditioning, and the results have not always been consistent, it may warrant use with another group of people manifesting a maladaptive approach response, namely, narcotic addicts.

As we know, the habit of narcotic ingestion, once started, is extremely powerful. The "pleasure" experienced by the person is so intense that it serves as the reward that creates and maintains the addiction. Coupled with the positive reinforcement of getting high is the escape from painful experiences deriving from the psychophysiological discomfort of withdrawal, as well as escape from anxiety-provoking, stressful, interpersonal relationships and distressing environmental conditions.

In the treatment of heroin addiction, methadone has been used to rehabilitate addicts by satisfying the physiological need, the craving, without the high (Dole et al., 1966). Aversive conditioning, as already mentioned, has been employed in the treatment of alcoholism by the use of Antabuse and other chemicals such as emetine. Varying degrees of success have been reported, however. Raymond (cited by Liberman, 1968) used apomorphine and aversive conditioning to cure a woman addicted to methadone (report after a 2½ year follow-up). Wolpe (1965) used electric shock as the aversive stimulus and produced temporary abstinence (12 weeks) in an addicted physician. In this case, whenever the desire for narcotics arose, the subject shocked himself.

Liberman (1968) in a report on some pilot work with two patients attempted to make the narcotic fix unsatisfying and noxious instead of gratifying. The subjects were conditioned to associate the unpleasant effects of apomorphine (nausea, cold sweats, dizziness) with the drug-taking ritual. Liberman found that aversive conditioning did occur (subjects felt nausea when thinking about drugs) in both his patients, and the effects generalized outside the treatment setting (subjects had the ability to watch friends taking drugs without feeling the yen).

The question arises as to the effectiveness of aversive conditioning for a person who is not middle class in his background (as they were in the Liberman report), who may have come into conflict with the law, and who is incarcerated. Covert Sensitization may offer hope to the troubled narcotic addict in a relatively short period. Anant (1968) has described his work with this so-called "verbal aversion technique" and although he reports "encouraging" results, "out of 26 patients treated with this technique, only one was a drug addict." Undertaking a behavior modification program has the added feature, in theory at least, of permitting rather clear evaluation of treatment without having to wait for years to pass only to have the person be found lying dead with a syringe in his arm. It will become obvious that due to follow-up difficulties, we have not yet evaluated this treatment. The following is a description of the procedures used with two individuals and two groups. All subjects were addicted to heroin before coming into the institution. All (but case No. 2 who was a voluntary patient in a mental hospital) were residents at Mid-Hudson Rehabilitation Center, Beacon, New

York. They were incarcerated under law for approximately nine months, being treated as part of a program which also included aftercare.

## PROCEDURE—INDIVIDUAL

The description of the procedure used with L. R. is offered as the prototype of work with subsequent subjects. The patient, male, in his mid-twenties, had a history of addiction to a wide variety of drugs, and continued conflict with the law. He was asked to describe the typical setting in which he took heroin and to do so in detailed steps. From this description, the author constructed the to-be-imagined scene which, following Cautela (1967), integrated drug-taking stimuli with the aversive condition of nausea induction. With this as the model, another scene, described below, was created which took other subjects through the steps toward the drug-taking act, yet left enough gaps so that each person could add his own individualized features to the imagined scene.

L. R. was taught to relax in the manner prescribed by Wolpe and Lazarus (1960). In accord with previous work (Cautela, 1967) it was decided that four relaxation training sessions would be given. He was informed that the way to eliminate his problem would be to associate the pleasurable drug with an unpleasant experience. If he could do this, that is, build up a strong negative association, he would no longer want to take drugs.

Covert Sensitization was then begun with L. R. while in a state of deep relaxation. He was asked to visualize, as clearly as possible, a scene in which he was taking a sun bath on a beach. The image was presented to help induce relaxation. Once the subject was fully relaxed, the beach scene was erased and he was told to visualize the following scene as clearly as possible.

> You are walking toward the place where you are going to get off (get high). Your friend is with you. As you approach the place, you start getting a funny feeling in the pit of your stomach. You start taking out the works, the bags of dope (heroin, H, stuff, etc.), the cotton, the cooker, the dropper, and your stomach feels queasy and nauseous. You throw the bags into the cooker, add just enough water, and, as you start to cook up, some liquid comes up into your throat. It feels bitter and sour. You sit down and start rolling up one of your sleeves, and you try to swallow that sour liquid down. But as you do this, food particles start coming up into your throat and you feel them in your mouth. You continue feeling nauseous, feeling the bitterness in your mouth. You tie up your arm to get a good vein. Now, as you reach for the dropper, puke comes into your mouth. You try to keep your mouth closed and swallow it down, but there's nothing to wash it down with. As you're about to tap the spike into that vein, you can't hold it down any longer. You open your mouth and start to puke. It goes all over your hand, all over the dropper, and the rest of the works. You see the puke floating in the cooker, snot and mucus come out your nose. Your shirt and pants are full of vomit. Your friend has some on his clothes, and he's looking at you kind of funny. You're sick again, and you vomit some more. Now you have the dry heaves. The puke is running down all over. Your eyes are watery, your stomach hurts as you heave and heave, spit drools from your

> mouth, your hands feel sticky, the smell is awful. You finally turn away from the works and immediately start to feel better. As you rush out of the room, you start to feel better and better. When you get out into the clean fresh air you feel wonderful. You go to a comfortable place where you clean yourself up and you feel great.

The scene was rehearsed twice for each of two sessions. Although he was encouraged to practice the C. S. procedure, no data is available on this. L. R. left the rehabilitation center after the second week of training with this scene. He has not been heard from since, and whether he has returned to drugs is an open question.

D. R. was a 36-year-old male, divorced, bright, and articulate, with several years of college, though he had not received his degree. His life history questionnaire (Wolpe and Lazarus, 1966) reported a history of stomach trouble, insomnia, tension, inability to relax, bad home conditions, financial problems, and a history of the taking of a variety of drugs, from alcohol to mind expanders, to amphetamines, to barbiturates, and finally heroin. His life was "all messed up" and he signed himself into a hospital for treatment. When the program was outlined, he readily grasped its significance and volunteered as an experimental treatment subject.

The procedure with D. R. was the same as reported with the first case. The one outstanding difference was D. R.'s level of felt anxiety was below 10%. The above scene was introduced, with modifications specific for him (whom he saw to get drugs, where he shot drugs, etc.). At the 5th week, a modification in the scene included a respected friend coming thru the door and seeing him about to take the heroin and him vomiting all over the furniture, his friend, etc.

Although D. R. practiced, he felt he was not getting as "tight" as he thought he should. Nausea did not seem to be a situation which he felt would prevent him from using drugs if he wanted to. It was decided to use one of D. R.'s own fears, his fear of bees and wasps, as the aversive stimulus to be paired with the drug taking scene. The following scene was given to D. R.

> You wake up in the morning, and you feel as though you want to get off (get high, get a shot of heroin). As you're getting dressed, you sense something funny about the room, and you feel kind of edgy. Still, you get dressed, take the bus to the man's house, and make the score. All the time, though, you still feel kind of funny, as if something isn't right today. You get back on the bus, to return to the place where you're going to get off. You're walking toward the place and feel a strange apprehension.
>
> As you approach the door, you hear a faint buzzing from inside. You hesitate, feeling quite nervous, but you open the door and enter anyway. You start taking out the works, and the buzzing seems louder now. Still feeling uneasy, you throw the bags into the cooker, add just enough water, and start to cook up. But now you notice the buzzing has grown very loud, and is ringing in your ears. You're afraid to look up, because it sounds as tho some wasps may be around. You sit down, start rolling up one of your sleeves, and all of a sudden you see a large wasp. It's across the room, buzzing around, just flying and buzzing around, as if it is waiting for something. You continue to tie up your arm and as you reach for the dropper, more wasps enter thru a space near the window. It's as if they're coming thru the